NurseNotes

Maternal–Newborn

Core Content At-A-Glance

NurseNotes

Maternal–Newborn
Core Content At-A-Glance

Irene Bobak, RN, PhD, FAAN
Professor Emerita, Women's Health and Maternity Nursing
San Francisco State University
San Francisco, California

Edited by
Sally Lambert Lagerquist, RN, MS
Former Instructor of Undergraduate and Graduate Programs
    and Continuing Education in Nursing
University of California, San Francisco, School of Nursing
President, Review for Nurses, Inc., and RN Tapes Company
San Francisco, California

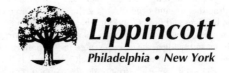
Lippincott
Philadelphia • New York

Acquisitions Editor: Susan Glover
Assistant Editor: Bridget Blatteau
Project Editor: Tom Gibbons
Production Manager: Helen Ewan
Production Coordinator: Nannette Winski
Design Coordinator: Doug Smock
Indexer: Nancy Newman

Library of Congress Cataloging in Publications Data
Bobak, Irene M.
    Nurse notes : maternal-newborn / Irene M. Bobak, Marianne K. Zalar ; edited by Sally L. Lagerquist.
        p.   cm.
    Includes bibliographical references and index.
    ISBN 0-7817-1128-2
    1. Maternity nursing—Outlines, syllabi, etc. 2. Maternity nursing—Examinations, questions, etc. I. Zalar, Marianne K. II. Lagerquist, Sally L. III. Title.
    [DNLM: 1. Maternal-Child Nursing—examination questions. 2. Maternal-Child Nursing—outlines. 3. Neonatal Nursing—examination questions. 4. Neonatal Nursing—outlines. WY 18.2 B663n 1997]
RG951.B666   1997
610.73'678'076—dc20
DNLM/DLC
for Library of Congress   96-9117
                                                                                                                 CIP

Care has been taken to confirm the accuracy of the information presented and to describe generally accepted practices. However, the authors, editors, and publisher are not responsible for errors or omissions or for any consequences from application of the information in this book and make no warranty, express or implied, with respect to the contents of the publication.

The authors, editors and publisher have exerted every effort to ensure that drug selection and dosage set forth in this text are in accordance with current recommendations and practice at the time of publication. However, in view of ongoing research, changes in government regulations, and the constant flow of information relating to drug therapy and drug reactions, the reader is urged to check the package insert for each drug for any change in indications and dosage and for added warnings and precautions. This is particularly important when the recommended agent is a new or infrequently employed drug.

Some drugs and medical devices presented in this publication have Food and Drug Administration (FDA) clearance for limited use in restricted research settings. It is the responsibility of the health care provider to ascertain the FDA status of each drug or device planned for use in their clinical practice.

9 8 7 6 5 4 3 2 1

This book is dedicated to . . .

the memory of my parents, Susan and Joseph Bobak, who
provided a good beginning;

to my family and friends:
Albert B. Bobak
Irene L. Bobak
Stephen J. Bobak
Veronica Bobak
Sister Mary Eleanor, VSC
Sally L. Lagerquist,
who encourage me and cheer me on;

to my colleagues who supply the professional inspiration;
to my students who motivated me.
I.M.B.

To my incredibly loving husband, Tom
L'Chaim and skòl!
We have so much to look forward to now that we can have time for "months of Saturdays." Thank you for your never-ending belief in me, for sharing a vision of what *is* and is *yet to be*, and for blending our lives all these 30-plus years!

To our daughter, Elana
Your love, caring, and complete emotional (as well as actual, task-related) support came through during unprecedented role reversal times—making it possible for me to put our priorities in order. I am so very grateful for having you as our daughter, and as *our* role model!
We are proud of your ever-unfolding abilities, interests, and ventures as a new teacher of children, as an artist, as a producer/director/actress, and your creative ideas for special books for children.
You've got the dreams, the creativity, and the follow-through to make it all come uniquely together for you.

To our son Kalen, our Woogie dragon
We are the grateful beneficiaries of your gifts of humor, sensitivity, and caring family ways when it counted the most! Your energy and enthusiasm have shown what you are capable of, as you convert your intellectual curiosity into scientific pursuit.
Congratulations upon joining the "club" of authors. We are both excited for you and proud of you as a newly published contributing author, in a significant resource book on environmental policy, about the long-term effects of global warming.

Sally

Reviewer

Deeann A. Gerken, MSN, RNCS
College of the Desert
Palm Springs, California

Preface

This book is written by Dr. Irene Bobak, a national nursing expert and author of best-selling maternity textbooks for over 20 years. It is intended for busy nursing students who need to cover the most important information in the shortest time.

Purpose

1. To help nursing students learn *faster, easier,* and retain vital information with this guided study written in an easy-to-read format. This will enable students to use their other large textbooks as reference sources.
2. To help graduate nurses update and build on their nursing knowledge as they prepare for certification exams.

Features

1. **Time-savers:** Numerous charts (25), illustrations (20), and extensive pharmacology boxes (4) outline a great deal of information in few pages. Save valuable study time with quick-access *index* to instantly locate pages that cover key content such as 36 *diets*, over 60 *diagnostic tests*, 30 maternal-newborn *emergencies*, 20 *positions*, and *hands-on care.*
2. **Visual:** Unique use of icons throughout the content review sections helps important content stand out.

●	Nutrition	*!*	Alert
	Home care	ꙮ	Diagnostic tests
⚡	Hazard		Warning
	Lab values	✉	Steps of nursing process
●	Drugs		Emergency
☞	Hands-on care		

There is also a purposeful use of **bold face** and *italics* within the text to identify content related to *diets, positions,* what to *avoid,* and *drugs.* These visual methods have proved to be particularly beneficial in boosting retention.

3. Most up-to-date, comprehensive coverage of a variety of topics, for *beginning* and *advanced* nurses already in practice as well as repeat test-takers.
4. **Self-assess:** Questions and answers at the end of every chapter include *fact-packed* rationale for *each* option. Learn more from the most complete explanations!
5. **Free disk:** An integrated exam covers all essential areas in maternity and newborn care.
6. One-of-a-kind sections in each chapter: *key points, summary, key words,* and *study and memory aids.*

7. An **extensive appendix** section includes a 26-page (over 1200 terms) *glossary*; 350 *acronyms* and *abbreviations*; *quick guide to common clinical signs* (e.g. Chadwick's); index to help locate *test questions* covering the nursing process, client needs, and categories of human functions; an index to 12 memory aids (mnemonics); list of *NANDA-approved diagnoses*; and a list of *health care agencies* and *resources*.

How to Benefit from this Book

1. Use the *key words* and *key points* section at the beginning of each chapter to *anticipate* the content that will be covered in the chapter.
2. Use the extensive *glossary* (over 1200 definitions of terms relevant for maternal–newborn care) in the appendix as an *end-of-course review* to ensure that you have retained what you need to know.
3. Use the various *indices* in the appendices to pull out for study and review *separate* key topics such as *diets, diagnostic tests and medical procedures, lab values,* and *nursing skills and procedures* (hands-on care) necessary for beginning nursing students to master.

I wish you much success as you prepare for nursing exams with the aid of *NurseNotes: Maternal–Newborn.*

Sally Lambert Lagerquist, RN, MS
Editor, *NurseNotes* series

Acknowledgments

This book was indeed a collaborative team effort.

It is especially important for me to acknowledge our gratitude to Bonnie Bergstrom, our special project coordinator, who "did it all" during the beginning phases of manuscript preparation and book production.

She worked intensively on a one-to-one basis with Dr. Bobak and with me as editor, to research and pull together "proven-to-be-the-best" parts of our Nursing Review Live-by-Satellite programs as well as what we created for our national nursing review courses. Bonnie researched reference sources, did fact-checking and line-by-line editing, and made many substantive suggestions. She presided over the word processor many a night and weekend and produced all the drafts and revisions leading to the final manuscript that was turned in for publication at deadline times!

A separate and special paragraph is dedicated to Sue Glover, Senior Nursing Editor, and Tom Gibbons, Associate Managing Editor, at Lippincott-Raven Publishers. Their noteworthy flexibility and patience with a complex project that came with "inheriting" this book in midstream (as well as their good humor and commitment to excellence!) sustained me through some otherwise difficult times. I am excited and proud to be on the same team with Sue and Tom—who made this book a reality to fill a needed niche as a nursing study guide for students who are in nursing school and graduate nurses who are studying for their certification exams.

Sally Lagerquist

Contents

List of Illustrations

List of Tables

Growth and Development

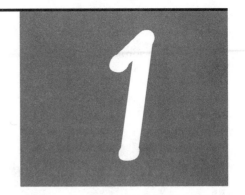

Chapter Outline

KEY POINTS

- Knowledge of female reproductive anatomy and physiology is essential to health promotion/maintenance.
- Factors such as immunizations, life-style, environment, and nutrition affect the functioning of the immune defense system.
- Common etiologic factors of impaired fertility include *male* factors (e.g., decreased sperm production, varicocele) and/or *female* factors (e.g., tubal occlusion, short luteal phase, endometriosis).
- Preconception counseling is designed to promote/maintain good health to afford the developing embryo/fetus the best environment for development/growth (one that allows the newborn to achieve his/her genetic potential).

Key Words

"ACHES"
BBT (basal body temperature)
Calendar method
Contraception
Dysmenorrhea
Fertile days (of menstrual cycle)
Fibrocystic breast disease
Hot flushes (flashes)
Impaired fertility
Interruption of pregnancy
Living ligature
Mammography
Menstrual cycle
 Menarche
 Menopause
 Menstruation
 Ovulation
Mittelschmerz
"PAINS"
PID (pelvic inflammatory disease)
Preconception care

1

Premenstrual syndrome (PMS)
Safer sex practices
Spinnbarkeit
STD (sexually transmitted disease)
Sterilization
TSS

Biologic Foundations of Reproduction

General overview: This review of the structures, functions, and important assessment characteristics of the reproductive system provides essential components of the database required for accurate nursing judgments. Comparing normal characteristics and established patterns with nursing assessment findings assist in identifying patient needs and in planning, implementing, and evaluating appropriate goal-directed nursing interventions.

Female Reproductive Anatomy

I. Structure of pelvis (Figure 1.1)
  A. Two hip bones (right and left innominate: sacrum, coccyx).
  B. *False pelvis*—upper portion above brim; supportive structure for uterus during last half of pregnancy.
  C. *True pelvis*—below brim; pelvic inlet, midcavity (curved passage having a short anterior wall and a much longer concave posterior wall), pelvic outlet

comprise this structure. Fetus passes through during birth.
II. Pelvic measurements
  A. Diagonal conjugate—12.5 cm or greater is adequate size; measured by examiner.
  B. Conjugate vera (true conjugate)—11 cm is adequate size; measured by X-ray.
  C. Obstetric conjugate—measured by X-ray.
  D. Tuber-ischial diameter—9–11 cm indicates adequate size; measured by examiner.
III. External genitalia (vulva, pudendum) (Figure 1.2)
  A. *Mons veneris* (mons pubis)—fatty subcutaneous tissue covered with pubic hair; protects symphysis.
  B. *Labia majora*—folds of adipose tissue; form internal borders of vulva; cover and protect labia minora.
  C. *Labia minora*—two located within labia majora; lubricate vulva and protect with bacteria-fighting secretion; sensitive to stimuli.
  D. *Clitoris*—small erectile tissue; sensitive to sexual stimulation; analogous to the male's glans penis.
  E. Vestibule—between labia minora; contains:
    1. *Urinary meatus*—opening of urethra.
    2. *Skene's glands*—paraurethral glands.
    3. Vaginal opening (*introitus*).
    4. *Hymen*—thin membrane at opening of vagina.
    5. *Bartholin's glands* (paravaginal)—produce alkaline secretions that enhance sperm viability, motility.
IV. Internal structures (Figure 1.3)
  A. *Vagina*—outlet for menstrual flow, depository for semen; lower birth canal.
  B. *Cervix*—uterine outlet.

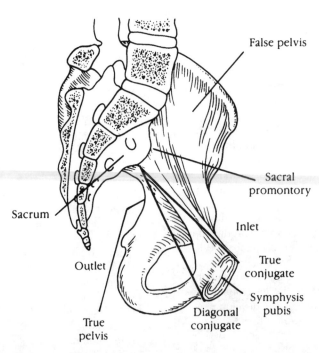

FIGURE 1.1   THE FEMALE PELVIS. (From SL Lagerquist [ed]. *Little, Brown's NCLEX-RN Examination Review*. Boston: Little, Brown, 1996. P 387.)

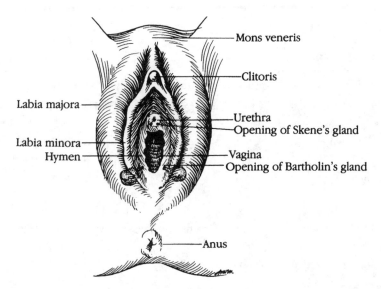

FIGURE 1.2   **EXTERNAL FEMALE GENITALIA.** (From R Judge, G. Zuidema, F Fitzgerald. *Clinical Diagnosis* (5th ed). Boston: Little, Brown, 1989. P 389.)

C. *Uterus*—muscular organ, composed of corpus (body), isthmus (lower uterine segment during pregnancy), and cervix; houses and nourishes embryo and fetus during gestation.
  1. The thick uterine myometrium consists of elastic and connective tissue, blood, and three smooth muscle layers (longitudinal, figure-eight [transverse], and circular [oblique] fibers).
  2. The primary function of the outer longitudinal fibers is to assist with effacement and dilatation of the cervix and to expel the fetus. These fibers are found mostly in the fundus.
  3. The figure-eight fibers of the middle layer (also known as the "living ligature") provide hemostatic action because the interlaced fibers encircle large blood vessels.
  4. The primary function of the circular muscle fibers of the inner layer is to retain uterine contents during pregnancy and prevent regurgitation of menstrual blood through the fallo-

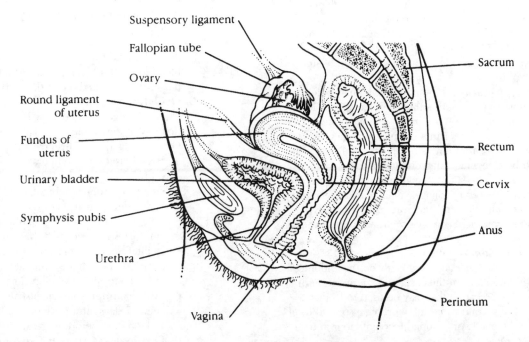

FIGURE 1.3   **FEMALE INTERNAL REPRODUCTIVE ORGANS.** (From SL Lagerquist [ed]. *Little, Brown's NCLEX-RN Examination Review.* Boston: Little, Brown, 1996. P 388.)

TABLE 1.1   MENSTRUAL CYCLE: A FEEDBACK MECHANISM

Phases/Events	First "Half" Cycle			Second "Half" Cycle	
Length	NOTE: 8 d to several weeks or months		O V U L A T I O N	NOTE: Constant: 14 d	
Anterior pituitary hormones	Follicle stimulating (FSH): follicular phase			Luteinizing hormone (LH): luteal phase	
Ovarian hormones	Estrogen			Progesterone and estrogen until start of ischemic phase 3 d before menstruation	
Endometrial response	Bleeding → 5 days (range: 3–6 d)	Proliferative phase →		Secretory phase →	Ischemic 3 d
Cervical mucus response	Dry (no mucus)	Increasingly viscous, opaque; no ferning		Cloudy, sticky; impenetrable to sperm; no ferning	
BBT	Individualized; often below 98.6°F (37°C)			After slight drop, rises about 0.4° to 0.8°F (0.2–0.4°C)	

pian tubes into the abdomen during menstruation.

   D. *Fallopian tubes*—two tubes stretching from cornua of uterus to ovaries; transport ovum; site of fertilization is in the outer two-thirds (in the ampulla of the tubes).

Female Reproductive Physiology

I. Reproductive hormones
   A. *FSH* (follicle stimulating hormone)—secreted during the first half of cycle; stimulates development of graafian follicle; secreted by anterior pituitary.
   B. *ICSH or LH* (interstitial cell stimulating hormone, luteinizing hormone)—stimulates ovulation and development of corpus luteum; secreted by anterior pituitary.
   C. *Estrogen*—assists in ovarian follicle maturation; stimulates endometrial thickening; responsible for development of secondary sex characteristics; maintains endometrium during pregnancy. Secreted by ovaries and adrenal cortex during cycle and by placenta during pregnancy.
   D. *Progesterone*—aids in endometrial thickening; facilitates secretory changes; maintains uterine lining for implantation and early pregnancy; relaxes smooth muscle. Secreted by corpus luteum and placenta.
   E. *Prostaglandins*—substances produced by various body organs that act hormonally on the endometrium to influence the onset and continuation of labor. A medication that may be used to facilitate onset of second trimester abortion; also used to efface the cervix prior to induction of labor in term pregnancies.

II. Menstrual cycle
   A. The **menstrual cycle** is a complex interplay of events that occur simultaneously in the hypothalamus and pituitary glands, the uterine endometrium and cervix, and the ovaries. The menstrual cycle—a feedback mechanism—is presented in Table 1.1.
   B. Important terms
     1. Menarche—onset of menses; occurs at about age 13. Initial cycles are irregular, unpredictable, painless, and anovulatory in the majority of girls. Ovulatory periods tend to be regular, monitored by progesterone; may be associated with *dysmenorrhea* (painful uterine cramping).
     2. Menstruation—vaginal discharge of blood and fragments of the two upper layers (the functional layer) of the endometrium; cyclic; occurs in response to dropping levels of estrogen and progesterone. *Menses* refers to the normal flow during menstruation. Average blood loss: 50 mL (range: 20–80 mL). First day of bleeding is the first day of the cycle.
     3. Ovulation—maturation and release of egg from ovary; generally occurs 14 days *before* first day of next cycle (first day of bleeding).
     4. Ovulation-associated events:
       a. BBT (basal body temperature)—slight drop.
       b. Cervical mucus—abundant, thin, clear (egg-white) mucus with **spinnbarkeit** (mucus stretchable from 4 cm, often up to 10 cm); dries in a fern pattern (arborization); facilitates sperm transport; pH rises (becomes more alkaline) from about 7.0 to 7.5 to facilitate sperm viability and mobility.
       c. Mittelschmerz (intermenstrual pain) occurs 1.7 days after peak of cervical mucus and 2.5 days before increase in BBT.
       d. Fertile days: 3 days before through 1 day (24 hr) after ovulation.
     5. Fertilization—impregnation of ovum by sperm.

    6. Implantation—fertilized ovum attaches to uterine wall for growth.

III. Menopause—normally occurring cessation of menses with gradual decrease in amount of flow and increase in the time between periods at end of fertility cycle; average age, 53. Early menopause rare but may be influenced by hypothyroidism, surgical ovarian removal, overexposure to radiation.

    A. Women say that the most distressing symptoms are hot flushes ("flashes") and night sweats. These are due to hormonal stimulation of the sympathetic system resulting in vasomotor instability with changeable vasodilation and vasoconstriction.

    B. Treatments during menopause for symptom relief: hormonal replacement therapy, *vitamins B* and *E* for hot flushes, vaginal creams for dyspareunia (painful intercourse), and exercise and calcium for osteoporosis.

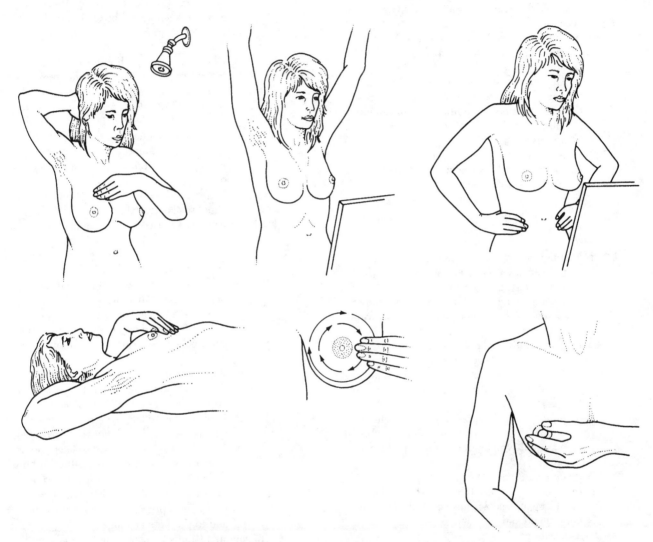

FIGURE 1.4   **BREAST SELF-EXAMINATION. (A)** Examine breasts during bath or shower since flat fingers glide easily over wet skin. Use right hand to examine left breast and vice versa. **(B)** Sit or stand before a mirror. Inspect breasts with hands at sides, then raised overhead. Look for changes in contour or dimpling of skin. **(C)** Place hands on hips and press down firmly to flex chest muscles. **(D)** Lie down with one hand under head and pillow or folded towel under that scapula. **(E)** Palpate that breast with the other hand using concentric circle method. It usually takes three circles to cover all breast tissue. Include the tail of the breast and the axilla. Repeat with other breast. **(F)** End in a sitting position. Palpate the areola areas of both breasts, and inspect and squeeze nipples to check for discharge. (From SL Lagerquist [ed]. *Little, Brown's NCLEX-RN Examination Review.* Boston: Little, Brown, 1996. P 203.)

Neoplasms

See also Cancer and Pregnancy (Chapter 3).

　See medical-surgical texts for in-depth discussions of these conditions.

I. Breast

　A. *Fibrocystic breast disease* (mammary dysplagia, chronic cystic mastitis)

　　1. *Incidence:* most common of the benign breast lesions. Affects 1 : 3 premenopausal women. Peak incidence between 30 and 50 yr.

　⋈ **2. Assessment**

　　a. *Symptoms:* dull heavy pain, a sense of fullness, tenderness that increases premenstrually.

　　b. *Palpation:* cysts are soft, well differentiated, movable. Deeper cysts are harder to palpate; must be differentiated from carcinomas.

　〰 **3.** *Diagnosis*

　　a. Surgical biopsy.

　　b. Mammography: visualization of breast tissue by X-ray examination.

　　c. Ultrasonography: can differentiate cysts from solid tumors.

　　d. History.

　　e. Physical examination.

　⋈ **4. Management/Intervention**

　　a. Conservative: *diet*—eliminate dimethylxanthines (e.g., caffeine and theophylline) and nicotine; eliminate foods containing these: coffee, cola, tea, chocolate (still controversial).

　　▱ **b.** Conservative: *vitamin E*—increase to between 400 and 600 units qd.

　　▱ **c.** *Medications:* danazol (Danocrine), tamoxifen, oral contraceptives (Pharmacology Box 1.1).

　　d. *Education:* emphasize breast self-examination (BSE) and report any changes in breast mass and symptoms; comfort—padded bras.

　B. *Malignant conditions*

　　1. *Incidence:* will affect 1 : 8–1 : 9 women during the life span; leading cause of death in women between 35 and 54 years.

　⋈ **2. Assessment**

　　a. *Symptoms:* pain, nipple discharge—bloody or clear.

　　b. *Palpation:* lump or thickening, hard and fixed or soft and spongy, well-defined or irregular borders, usually in the upper outer quadrant. If fixed to skin, dimpling, "orange peel"–appearing skin, retraction.

　〰 **3.** *Diagnosis:*

　　a. BSE (Figure 1.4): only approved screening method to date; should be performed once each month throughout the life span.

　　b. Mammography (see schedule under **C**).

　　c. Needle aspiration, needle localization, followed by open breast biopsy, the most definitive test.

⋈ **4. Management/Intervention**

　▱ **a.** *Medications: estrogens* or *progestins* (if neoplasm has estrogen or progesterone receptor sites); an *anti-estrogen* such as tamoxifen. See Pharmacology Box 1.1, pp. 7–8.

　b. *Surgery:* lumpectomy (tylectomy), quadrectomy (segmental resection), total (simple) mastectomy, and radical mastectomy. Five-year survival rates for women following lumpectomies are statistically similar to those following total breast removal.

　c. Hormone/surgical procedures in combination.

　d. Chemotherapy and hormonal therapy may improve cytotoxicity of chemotherapy.

　▱ **e.** Chemotherapy: *cyclophosphamide, methotrexate, doxorubicin* (Adriamycin), *5-fluorouracil,* and *vinblastine*. In addition to their antineoplastic qualities, these cytotoxins have some immunosuppressive side effects. Episodes of thrombosis can be expected to occur.

　f. *Radiation:* 2–3 wk following lumpectomy.

　g. Emotional support!

⋈ **5. Postoperative care,** including discharge planning

　a. Safety: protect arm during hospital stay and at home—due to lack of feeling.

　☞ **b.** Exercise: to maintain full range of motion; inactivity (secondary to pain, initially) could affect joint action, and alteration in lymphatic drainage leads to edema formation and further impairment of joint/arm movement.

　c. Woman needs to expect that she will have discomfort and a feeling of tightness in the arm and chest on the affected side.

　d. Explain that axillary node resection leads to edema because lymph flow is interrupted.

　e. Closed self-suction is used to keep the operative site free of fluid so that wound healing with approximation of tissue can occur.

　☞ **f.** Suture line is cleansed daily with hydrogen peroxide to prevent scar tissue formation and to promote healing.

C. Recommendations for screening for breast neoplasms, in addition to monthly BSE

　〰 **1.** Women at **average** risk:

Age	Mammography	Clinical Examination
29–39	Not recommended	Included with routine gynecologic examination
40–49	Joint decision by patient and her physician or nurse practitioner	Every 1–2 yr
50–74	Every 1–2 yr	Every 1–2 yr

Pharmacology Box 1.1   NEOPLASMS OF BREAST AND ENDOMETRIUM

Drug/Dosage	Indication/Action	⋈ Assessment: Side Effects	Nursing Management
Progestins *Hydroxyprogesterone caproate* (Delalutin) Injection—125 mg/ mL, 250 mg/mL IM—1–7 g/wk	Advanced endome- trial carcinoma (Stage III or IV) (DOC)	Stop therapy when relapse oc- curs or after 12 wk with no objective response Weight gain Mild depression	Be alert for signs and symptoms of hypercalcemia (polyuria, polydipsia, weakness, constipa- tion, mental sluggishness or disorientation) in patients with metastatic breast cancer being treated with tamoxifen or pro- gestins; perform periodic *se- rum calcium* determinations Monitor fluid intake and output
Medroxyprogesterone acetate (Provera, Depo-Provera) Tablets—2.5 mg, 10 mg Oral, IM—400–1000 mg/wk Injection—100 mg/ mL, 400 mg/mL Maintenance—400 mg/mo or adjusted to patient's needs	Endometrial carci- noma	Recommended only as adjunc- tive and palliative therapy in advanced inoperable cases; usually well tolerated even in large doses; gluteal abscesses have occurred Weight gain Mild depression	⬭ Recommend contraceptive measures for patients receiv- ing *estrogens, progestins, ta- moxifen,* and *mitotane* Diabetic patients receiving *pro- gestins* may have a *decreased glucose tolerance*; monitor urine sugar closely and notify physician immediately of any abnormalities
Megestrol acetate (Megace, Pallace) Breast cancer: 40 mg qid Endometrial cancer: 40–320 mg/d in 4 divided doses	Breast and endo- metrial carci- noma (DOC)	Continue treatment for at least 2 mo to determine efficacy Weight gain Mild depression	

(continued)

(continued)

		Clinical
75 +	Joint decision by patient and her physician or nurse practitioner	Joint decision by patient and her physician or nurse practitioner

⩗ **2.** Women at **high** risk:

Age	Mammography	Clinical Examination
29–39	Annually starting at age 35; earlier if breast cancer has occurred	Annually starting at age 35
40–49	Annually	Annually
50–74	Annually	Annually
75 +	Joint decision by patient and her physician or nurse practitioner	Joint decision by patient and her physician or nurse practitioner

II. Uterus
  A. *Endometrial carcinoma*
    1. Women at greatest risk: those who are obese and/or have hypertension.
    2. The *most* important sign of endometrial carci- noma is abnormal bleeding, e.g., reappearance of "menstrual-like bleeding" after 6 mo of menopause.
    ⬭ **3.** Oral contraceptive use may protect against such disorders as endometrial and ovarian can- cer and other conditions.
  B. *Cervix*
    Early treatment of cervical erosion is thought to prevent neoplastic changes. Treatment consists of cryosurgery, cauterization, and douches.

Nursing Process

⋈ **I.** Assessment
  A. Health history

Pharmacology Box 1.1   Neoplasms of Breast and Endometrium (*Continued*)

Drug/Dosage	Indication/Action	✉ Assessment: Side Effects	✉ Nursing Management
Tamoxifen (Nolvadex)—anti-estrogen Tablets—10 mg 10–20 mg bid	Advanced breast carcinoma (DOC) Postmenopausal women respond better than pre-menopausal women (who get better response from DES)	May *increase serum calcium* levels; transient "flaring" of disease may occur during initial therapy, usually subsides rapidly; ocular toxicity is associated with long-term, high-dose therapy Vaginitis, decreased libido, nausea, or anorexia	○ Be aware that *tamoxifen* may cause a *transient* flare of the disease with increased tumor and bone pain; advise the patient that this is not uncommon, and provide additional analgesics if needed
Danazol (Danocrine) Capsules—50 mg, 100 mg, 200 mg Endometriosis—400 mg bid for 6–9 mo Fibrocystic breast disease—100–400 mg/d in 2 divided doses for 3–6 mo	Suppresses release of FSH and LH, inhibiting ovarian function. Complete resolution of endometrial lesions in the majority of cases Symptomatic treatment of severe fibrocystic breast disease Treatment of infertility secondary to endometriosis	Anovulation and associated amenorrhea Flushing, sweating Virilization (acne, oily skin, hirsutism, deepening of the voice, decrease in breast size, clitoral hypertrophy), vaginitis, vaginal bleeding, edema, weight gain, nervousness Other effects for which a direct causal relationship has not been established are: loss of hair; changes in libido; pelvic pain; muscle cramps; back, neck, or leg pain; skin rash; nasal congestion; nausea; vomiting; gastroenteritis; dizziness; headache; tremor; paresthesias; and visual disturbances	**Contraindications:** carcinoma of the breast, pregnancy, lactation, undiagnosed vaginal bleeding, and markedly impaired cardiac, hepatic, or renal function Reassure that drug-induced anovulation and amenorrhea are reversible within 60–90 d after termination of therapy Observe for development of signs of virilization and advise physician; some of these symptoms may be irreversible

DOC = drug of choice; DES = diethylstilbestrol.

1. Menarche: onset and duration.
2. Menstrual problems.
3. Contraceptive use.
4. Pregnancy history.
5. Fertility problems.
〰 **B.** Physical examination and laboratory tests
  1. External, internal reproductive organs.
  2. Breast examination.
  3. Mammography: if at risk yearly ≥35 yr of age.
  4. Periodic Papanicolaou (Pap) smears.
  5. Tests for STD (sexually transmitted diseases).
✉ **II.** Analysis/nursing diagnosis
  A. *Health-seeking behaviors* related to health promotion.
  B. *Health-seeking behaviors* related to menopause.
✉**III.** Nursing care plan/implementation
  A. Discuss anatomy and physiology of reproductive tract.
  B. Review menstruation, ovulation, fertilization, "fertile" and "safe" days of cycle.

  C. Explain need for periodic Pap smears, annual gynecologic examinations, including mammography.
✉ **IV.** Evaluation/outcome criteria
  A. Woman displays basic understanding of anatomy and physiology.
  B. Woman understands menstrual cycle and its "fertile" and "safe" days.
  C. Woman understands her chosen method of contraception.
  D. Woman regularly seeks preventive care and performs monthly breast self-examinations.

Decision Making Regarding Reproduction

General overview: During the reproductive years, the sexually active woman often faces the decision to postpone, prevent, or terminate a pregnancy. The nursing role focuses on assisting her in making an informed decision consistent with individual needs.

Contraception

✉ **I.** Assessment
   A. Determine interest in and present knowledge of methods of family planning, e.g., planning for pregnancy, contraception.
   B. Identify factors affecting choice of contraceptive method: cultural and religious objections, contraindications for individual methods, motivation/ability to follow chosen method successfully, financial considerations.

✉ **II.** Analysis/nursing diagnosis: *knowledge deficit* regarding family planning methods/options.

✉ **III** Nursing care plan/implementation—goal: *health teaching*—to facilitate informed decision making, selection of option appropriate to individual needs, desires.
   A. Describe, explain, discuss options available and appropriate to the woman. Include information on advantages and disadvantages of each option (Table 1.2)
   B. Demonstrate, as necessary, method selected.
   ⬮ **C.** Quick health teaching reminders for missed oral hormone preparations°
      1. One pill should be taken at the same time every day for 21 (or 28) days.
      2. If woman misses one pill, she should take it as soon as she remembers it, and then take the next one at the usual time.
      3. If woman misses two or more pills in a row in the first 2 wk of her cycle, she should take two pills for 2 days, and use a backup method of contraception for the next 7 days.
      4. If woman misses two pills in the third wk, or three or more pills anytime
         a. *A Sunday starter* should keep taking pills until the next Sunday, then start a new pack that Sunday. She should use a backup method of contraception for the next 7 days.
         b. *A day 1 starter* should throw out the rest of the pack, and start a new pack that day. She should use a backup method of contraception for the next 7 days.
      5. *28-day pill pack:* If woman misses any of the seven pills that do not have any hormones, she should throw out the pills missed and keep taking one pill a day until the pack is empty. She does not need a backup method of contraception.
   D. Alert woman to discontinue use of *oral hormone contraceptive* preparations if any of the following symptoms occur and to report the symptoms to the physician STAT. Signs of potential problems: **"ACHES"**

   A—**A**bdominal pain: possible problem with the liver or gallbladder
   C—**C**hest pain or shortness of breath: possible clot problem within lungs or heart
   H—**H**eadaches (sudden or persistent): possibly caused by cardiovascular accident or hypertension
   E—**E**ye problems: possible vascular accident or hypertension
   S—**S**evere leg pain: possible thromboembolic process

   E. Alert woman to signs of potential problems related to *IUD* use: **"PAINS"**†
   P—**P**eriod (menstrual) late, abnormal spotting or bleeding
   A—**A**bdominal pain, pain with coitus (dyspareunia)
   I—**I**nfection, abnormal vaginal discharge
   N—**N**ot feeling well, fever or chills
   S—**S**tring missing (nonpalpable on vaginal self-examination, or not seen on speculum examination)

   F. Toxic shock syndrome (TSS)
   ✉ **1.** Alert woman to signs/symptoms
      a. Fever of sudden onset—over 102°F (38.9°C).
      b. Hypotension—systolic pressure <90 mm Hg; orthostatic dizziness; disorientation.
      c. Rash—diffuse, macular erythroderma (resembling sunburn).
      d. Sore throat; severe nausea, vomiting.
      e. Copious vaginal discharge.
   ✉ **2.** Instructions for prevention
      a. General
         (1) *Avoid* use of tampons, cervical caps, and diaphragms during the postpartum period (6 wk).
         (2) Do *not* use any of the above if you have a history of TSS.
         (3) Call physician if you experience sudden onset of a high fever, vomiting, diarrhea, or skin rash.
         (4) Insert clean tampons and contraceptive devices with clean hands.
         (5) Remove within prescribed time limits.
      b. Tampons
         (1) Change tampons every 3–6 hr.
         (2) Do *not* use superabsorbent tampons.
         (3) For overnight protection, substitute other products such as sanitary napkins or minipads.
      c. Diaphragm or cervical cap
         (1) *Avoid* use during your menstrual period.
         (2) Remove within 8 hr after intercourse (diaphragm must be removed no later than 24 hr; the cap, no later than 48 hr).

✉ **IV.** Evaluation/outcome criteria
   A. Woman avoids or achieves a pregnancy as desired.

° Modified from Family Health International. An Example of *OC Use Instructions for PPIs.* Research Triangle Park, NC: Family Health International, 1990.

† Modified from RA Hatcher et al. *Contraceptive Technology: 1994–1995* (16th ed). New York: Irving Publishers, 1994.

TABLE 1.2   CONTRACEPTION

Method	Action/Effectiveness	Advantages	Disadvantages and Side Effects
Hormonal Contraceptives Combination of *estrogen* and *progesterone*.	• Suppresses ovulation by suppressing production of FSH and LH • *Most efficient* form of contraception (99.7%) if used consistently	• Convenient • Easy to take • Withdrawal bleeding cycles are predictable • Not related to sex act • Safe for older non-smoking women until menopause • Many noncontraceptive health benefits	• **Absolute contraindications,** e.g., thromboembolic or coronary artery disease, some cancers or liver disease • **Relative contraindications,** e.g., migraines, hypertension, immobility of 4 wk or more, abnormal genital bleeding • Some decrease in glucose tolerance • Effectiveness decreased if taken during use of barbiturates, phenytoin, antibiotics • **No protection against STDs**
Estrogen only "Morning-after" pill: *estrogen* (diethylstilbestrol [DES]) in very high doses (25 mg)	• Antifertility; taken within 72 hr of unprotected coitus during fertile period	Available, prn	• Because of *DES* effect on fetus, elective abortion advised if method fails
Progestin only Minipill (O) qd Depo-Provera (IM) q3–6 mo Norplant (subdermal) up to 5 yr	• Impairs fertility • Thickens cervical mucus; decreases sperm penetration • Alters endometrial maturation • *Effectiveness:* undetermined; can reach 100% reliability if used exactly as prescribed	• (O): convenient, easy to take • (IM): 2–4 times/yr; lactation OK during this time • Subdermal: long-term • Not related to sex	• Ovulation may occur • Irregular bleeding • May change glucose and insulin values • **No protection against STDs**

(continued)

B. Woman expresses comfort and satisfaction with method selected.

Infertility

I. Definition: inability to conceive after 1 yr of unprotected intercourse.
II. Pathophysiology: contributing factors—hormonal deficiencies, reproductive system disorders, congenital anomalies, male impotence, sexual knowledge deficit, debilitating disease.
III. Assessment
   A. History—general health, reproduction, social history.
      1. Age at menarche

2. Common menstrual disorders
   a. Hypogonadotropic *amenorrhea* (absence of menstruation)—problem in central hypothalamic-pituitary axis (most often due to stress or deficit in critical body fat-to-lean ratio).
   b. *Dysmenorrhea* (painful menstruation): primary—occurs in absence of organic disease.
   c. *Dysmenorrhea*: secondary—associated with organic pelvic disease, e.g., endometriosis, pelvic inflammatory disease, cervical stenosis, uterine or ovarian neoplasms, and uterine polyps.
   d. *Premenstrual syndrome (PMS)*—begins

TABLE 1.2   CONTRACEPTION (*Continued*)

Method	*Action/Effectiveness*	*Advantages*	*Disadvantages and Side Effects*

Intrauterine Devices (IUDs)
Small T-shaped device inserted into uterine cavity.
Medicated with
  Copper
  Progesterone
	• Prevents fertility: damages sperm in transit to fallopian tube (*progesterone* alters cervical mucus and endometrial maturation)
	• *Effectiveness:* 90–99%
		• Can be used by women who cannot use hormonal contraception
		• Recommended for women who have had at least one child
		• No disruption of ovulation pattern
		• Less blood loss during menses and decreased primary dysmenorrhea
		• *Copper* can be used effectively for 10 yr; *progesterone* must be changed yearly
			• *Contraindications:* history of PID, pregnancy, undiagnosed genital bleeding, genital malignancy, abnormal uterine cavity
			• *Risks:* uterine perforation, infection (may be followed by PID) in the first 3 mo of insertion; unnoticed expulsion
			• *Side effects* (especially with *copper T*): heavy flow, spotting between periods, and cramping within first few months of insertion
			• Must check for string after each menses and before intercourse
			• **No protection against STDs**

Mechanical Barriers *Diaphragm*—shallow rubber device that fits over cervix	• Barrier preventing sperm from entering cervix (if it is correct size, undamaged, correctly placed, and is used with spermicide) • *Effectiveness:* 83–90%; 99% in highly motivated women	• Does not interrupt sex act, except to add spermicide just before act • Insert up to 6 hr before intercourse and leave in place for 6 hr after last intercourse, but do *not* leave in place longer than 24 hr[a] • Safe: no side effects from well-fitted device, if woman is not allergic to diaphragm or spermicide • Decreased incidence of vaginitis, cervicitis, PID	• Requires careful cleansing with warm water and mild soap; powder with cornstarch and store away from heat • Size/fit needs to be checked after: term birth, 2nd or 3rd trimester abortion, weight gain or loss of 20 pounds or more, and/or 2 yr • Spermicide must be reinserted for additional acts that may follow initial intercourse • **No protection against STDs**

(continued)

during luteal phase and ends with menses; gives rise to positive symptoms (e.g., heightened sense of creativity), or negative symptoms (e.g., symptoms related to edema or emotional instability).

  e. *Endometriosis*—presence and growth of endometrial tissue outside of the uterus; characterized by secondary amenorrhea, dysmenorrhea, dyspareunia, chronic pelvic pain, abnormal uterine bleeding, and infertility.

  3. *Sexually transmitted disease (STD) or pelvic inflammatory disease (PID)*

  4. Contraceptive methods used

  5. Obstetric history

B. *Maternal diagnosis*

  1. *Basal body temperature (BBT):* monitored throughout the cycle.

TABLE 1.2   CONTRACEPTION (*Continued*)

Method	Action/Effectiveness	Advantages	Disadvantages and Side Effects
Cervical cap—1¼–1½ in. soft, natural rubber dome with a firm but pliable rim	• Physical barrier to sperm • Spermicide inside cap adds a chemical barrier • *Effectiveness:* similar to that of diaphragm	• Worn for 8 hr, but *not* longer than 48 hr[a] • *No* need to add spermicide for repeated acts of intercourse	• Need a yearly Pap smear: higher rate of conversion from class I to class III[b] • If in place over 48 hr, it produces an odor, and might be associated with TSS[a] • *Cannot* be worn during menstrual flow (menses), or up to 6 wk postpartum • *Contraindications:* abnormal Pap smear, hard to fit, history of TSS or genital infection, allergy • Change after: genital surgery, birth, or major change in weight • Must be checked *yearly* • **No protection against STDs**
Female condom—vaginal sheath of natural latex rubber with flexible rings at both the closed and the open ends	• Barrier preventing sperm from entering vagina • *Effectiveness:* similar to other mechanical methods used with spermicide[c] • NOTE: Male and female condoms should *not* be used at the same time	• Apply well in advance of intercourse; spermicide added just before intercourse • Heightens sensation for man • About as satisfying for both woman and man as intercourse without it • **Provides protection from STDs**	• Cost is high • A new one *must* be used for every act of intercourse

(continued)

2. Endocrine studies: *FSH, LH;* performed before and following ovulation.

3. *Huhner's* (postcoital) test used to determine the adequacy of coital technique, cervical mucus, sperm, and degree of sperm penetration through cervical mucus; it is performed within 2 hr after ejaculation of semen into the vagina; it is synchronized with the expected time of ovulation.

4. *Rubin* test: a transuterine insufflation of the fallopian tubes with carbon dioxide to test their patency; it is performed before ovulation.

5. *Hysterosalpingogram:* a test to determine patency of fallopian tubes; scheduled before ovulation because there is no chance of an early pregnancy being disrupted by the test.

6. *Laparoscopic* examination: to visualize internal structures; can be used in conjunction with tests for tubal patency. Since air is insufflated into the abdominal cavity during this procedure, women can expect some shoulder (referred) pain or subcostal pain following the procedure. This discomfort usually lasts 24 hr and generally can be relieved with mild analgesics.

C. *Male diagnosis*
  1. History
    a. Parotitis (mumps): acute, communicable viral disease involving chiefly the parotid gland, but frequently affecting tissues such as the gonads, thus impairing male fertility.
    b. Tight clothing, sitting for prolonged periods

TABLE 1.2   CONTRACEPTION (*Continued*)

Method	Action/Effectiveness	Advantages	Disadvantages and Side Effects
Condom—thin, stretchable latex sheath to cover penis	• Barrier preventing sperm from entering vagina; is applied over erect penis before loss of preejaculatory drops and is held in place as penis is withdrawn • Spermicidal foam, jelly, or cream is also used[c] • *Effectiveness:* 64–98% when used with spermicide	• Safety—no side effects • **Provides protection from STDs;** with spermicide (0.5 g nonoxynol-9) added to interior or exterior surface, provides protection from STDs including human immunodeficiency virus (HIV)	• Check expiration date • Requires high motivation to use correctly and consistently • Must be properly applied and removed • Sheath may tear during intercourse
Chemical Barriers *Spermicide*—aerosol foams, foaming tablets, suppositories, creams, and films (C-Film)	• Physical barrier to sperm penetration • Chemical action to sperm (kills sperm) • Nonoxynol-9 has a bacteriostatic action • *Effectiveness:* 70–98% when used with diaphragm or condoms	• Increases effectiveness of mechanical barriers • Ease of application • Aids lubrication of vagina • Requires no medical examination or prescription • May be used during lactation • Backup for missed oral contraceptive pills • **May provide some protection from STDs**	• Messy • Some people are allergic to preparations • Tablets or suppositories take 10–15 min to dissolve • If it is the only method being used, each intercourse should be preceded (by 30 min) by a fresh application

Other Methods
Natural family planning methods
  Basal body temperature (BBT) each morning before any physical activity
 	
  Symptothermal variation —BBT plus cervical mucus changes
 	
  Calendar method[d]
 	
  Predictor test for ovulation
	• Require sexual abstinence during woman's fertile period (4 d before ovulation and for 3 or 4 d after ovulation)
	• *Effectiveness:* about 80%
		• Physically safe to use
		• No drugs or appliances are used
		• Meet requirements of most religions
			• *Effectiveness:* depends on high level of motivation and diligence
			• Requires a fairly predictable menstrual cycle
			• Calendar method also requires knowledge of cycle lengths and formula; formula must be worked for each cycle
			• **No protection from STDs**

[a] Although there is no direct link between *TSS (toxic shock syndrome)* and use of the diaphragm or cervical cap, a possible association remains (see p. 9).

[b] **Class I** Pap smear: no abnormal cells; **class III** Pap smear: suspicious abnormal cells present.

[c] Spermicide provides lubrication, but if additional lubrication is needed, use only water-based products, e.g., K-Y Jelly.

[d] **Calendar method:** Sperm remain viable in the woman's reproductive tract for approximately **3** days; they are most capable of fertilizing an egg during the first **24** hr, however. The egg is viable for about **24** hr; it is most likely to be fertilized during the first **12** hr. The calendar method considers the life spans of the egg and sperm and that the time of ovulation is unpredictable; the formula that recognizes these variations follows: Subtract 18 from the shortest cycle the woman experienced within the last year and subtract 11 from the longest cycle she had during the last year. The difference gives the "*fertile* days." NOTE: *Ovulation takes place 14 days before the next menstrual cycle.*

(cross-country truck drivers), or use of a hot tub may affect sperm count until the man changes these behaviors.

c. A large amount of alcohol may affect fertility in that it may affect the libido or erection potential.

2. Physical examination: secondary sex characteristics; anatomy.

3. *Laboratory tests:* especially semen analysis. Semen is assessed for sperm: number, morphology, motility; pH; volume. Specimen should be collected in the container provided by the clinic and brought to the clinic within 2 hr after ejaculation to support a more accurate semen analysis. If collected in a condom, it must *not* be coated with nonoxynol-9, which is spermicidal, and it must be delivered to the clinic within 1 hr.

IV. Analysis/nursing diagnosis: *altered sexuality* related to infertility.

V. Nursing care plan/implementation:

A. Provide emotional support.

B. Explain testing procedures for diagnosis.

C. Explain ordered drug therapy (Pharmacology Box 1.2).

D. Advise woman on use of medication to increase vaginal pH to a neutral or to slightly alkaline pH. Sodium bicarbonate douches help to optimize vaginal pH for sperm motility.

E. Assist with referral process, e.g., adoption agencies.

VI. Evaluation/outcome criteria

A. The couple conceives, or,

B. If the couple does not conceive, they accept referral for help with adoption, other reproductive alternatives, or childlessness.

Sterilization

I. Definition: process or act that renders a person unable to produce children (e.g., tubal ligation, hysterectomy, vasectomy).

II. Sterilization procedures, their effectiveness, advantages and disadvantages, and side effects, are presented in Table 1.3.

Interruption of Pregnancy

Also known as elective, voluntary, or therapeutic abortion. Once the diagnosis of pregnancy and the length of gestation are established, the woman faces the decision to interrupt or to maintain the pregnancy (Table 1.4).

I. Decision-making stage

A. Assessment

1. Health history

a. Determine woman's feelings about the pregnancy, reasons for considering abortion, level of maturity; if decision was already made before she came to clinic, how was decision made?; does she have a support system?

b. Identify factors influencing/complicating

her decisions (religious beliefs, cultural mores, peer and family pressures).

c. Information needs.

2. Physical examination.

3. Laboratory tests: blood type, Rh, hemoglobin, hematocrit, urinalysis, pregnancy test, antibody titer, other tests dependent on her health status.

B. Analysis: *Some examples of nursing diagnoses:*

1. *Ineffective coping* related to emotional conflicts associated with need for decision to continue/terminate pregnancy.

2. *Altered family process* related to intrafamily conflict associated with need for/decision to continue/terminate pregnancy.

3. *Anticipatory grieving* related to loss of pregnancy/child.

4. *Altered self-concept, self-esteem disturbance* related to possible guilt feelings, related to pregnancy/termination.

5. Knowledge deficit related to available options.

C. Nursing care plan/implementation

1. Goal: *emotional support to minimize impact on self-image and self-esteem.*

a. Maintain accepting, nonjudgmental attitude.

b. Encourage verbalization of feelings, perceptions, and values.

c. Support woman's decision.

2. Goal: *health teaching* to facilitate informed decision-making.

a. Explain and discuss available options as applicable (see Table 1.4).

b. Describe procedure selected and what to expect after procedure.

3. Goal: *minimize impact on intrafamily relations, family process.* Where applicable, encourage open communication between deciding partners.

D. Evaluation/outcome criteria

1. Woman states she understands all information necessary to give consent.

2. Woman expresses comfort and satisfaction with the decision.

II. Preoperative period

A. Assessment

1. Reassess emotional and physical status and current feelings regarding decision.

2. Determine current knowledge/understanding of authorization form, anticipated procedure, and consequences (informed consent).

3. Monitor physiologic and (if awake) psychological response to procedure.

B. Analysis: *examples of nursing diagnoses:*

1. *Anxiety/fear* related to procedure, potential complications.

2. *Knowledge deficit* related to ongoing procedure, sights, sounds, and sensations experienced.

C. Nursing care plan/implementation

1. Goal: *provide opportunity to reconsider decision regarding termination of pregnancy.*

Pharmacology Box 1.2   THERAPY FOR IMPAIRED FERTILITY

Drug/Dosage°	*Indication/Action*	*Assessment: Side Effects*	*Nursing Management*
Clomiphene Clomid Serophene *Adults:* 50 mg/24 hr PO for 5 d (if necessary may repeat with 100 mg/24 hr PO for 5 d, *after* at least 30-d rest period) Maximum: 100 mg/24 hr	Induction of ovulation	**Contraindicated** in abnormal uterine bleeding, severe liver dysfunction, patients with ovarian cysts, and pregnancy May cause multiple pregnancy in approximately 11% of patients; however, over 90% of these are twins Commonly causes abdominal discomfort, visual disturbances, and hot flashes	**Educate:** Monitor for abdominal discomfort Observe for hot flashes Observe for visual disturbances
Menotropins Pergonal IM 1 amp (FSH + LH)/day for 9–12 days (followed by 5000–10,000 U HCG; if ovulation does not occur, repeat with 2 ampules)	Human gonadotropic responses; treatment of secondary anovulation (induces ovulation); stimulation of spermatogenesis	Abortions occur in 25%; failure rate 55–80% of patients; possible multiple births; ovarian enlargement; gynecomastia in men.	☞ Assist in collection of urine to assess estrogen levels **Educate:** couple's need to have daily intercourse from day of HCG injection until ovulation
Bromocriptine Parlodel Initial dose: 1.25–2.5 mg/d; 2.5 mg as tolerated may be added q3–7d; usual dose: 5–7.5 mg/d, with a daily range of 2.5–15 mg	Short-term treatment of amenorrhea/galactorrhea associated with hyperprolactinemia	**Contraindicated** in presence of hypersensitivity to drug/ergot alkaloids, uncontrolled hypertension CNS: *dizziness, headache,* fatigue, lethargy, **epileptiform seizures,** nightmares, confusion; CV: hypotension, edema, palpitations. EENT: nasal congestion, visual disturbances; GI: *N/V/D,* cramps, anorexia, constipation, dyspepsia, dry mouth, metallic taste; GU: urinary frequency; other: symptoms of ergotism	Assess for hx of ergot alkaloid hypersensitivity *Avoid* exposure to heat, moisture, light in storage Administer with *meals/milk* Assess BP for stability before administration **Educate:** take with meals; *avoid* alcohol—may cause dizziness —use caution in potentially hazardous activities; *avoid* changing positions (lying/sitting/standing) rapidly

HCG = human chorionic gonadotropin.

°See Pharmacology Box 1.1 for danazol.

    a. Check to ensure all required permission (informed consent) forms have been signed/filed.

    b. Refer to physician if ambivalent or insecure in decision.

  2. Goal: *reduce anxiety/fear related to procedure.*

    a. Explain all anticipated preoperative, operative, and postoperative care.

    b. Assist with procedure; if awake, explain what is happening, and what she may be experiencing.

  3. Goal: *emotional support to facilitate effective coping.*

    a. Encourage verbalization of feelings, fears, concerns.

    b. Support woman's decision.

  ▷ **D.** Evaluation/outcome criterion

    1. Woman experiences no physiologic or psychological problems during procedure.

III. Postoperative period

  ▷ **A.** Assessment

TABLE 1.3   STERILIZATION

Procedure/Effectiveness	*Advantages*	*Disadvantages and Side Effects*
Male Vasectomy: vas deferens is occluded (ligated and severed; bands; clips) to prevent passage of sperm	• Relatively simple surgical procedure • Does *not* affect endocrine function, production of testosterone • Does *not* alter volume of ejaculate • Tubal reconstruction possible (90%)	• Sterility is *not* immediate; sperm are cleared from vas after several ejaculations • Some men become impotent due to psychological response to procedure • Fertility after tubal reconstruction (40–60%)
Female Tubal ligation: Both fallopian tubes are ligated and severed, or occluded with bands or clips to prevent passage of eggs; fulguration of the tubes at the cornu is most effective	• Abdominal surgery utilizing 1-in. incision and laparoscopy • Greater than 99.5% effective	• Major surgery (if done by laparotomy) with possible complications of anesthesia, infection, hemorrhage, and trauma to other organs; psychological trauma in some
Hysterectomy and/or oophorectomy	• Abdominal or vaginal surgery • Absolute sterility	• Success rate for pregnancy after tubal reanastomosis is about 15%

1. Monitor *physiologic* response to procedure (vital signs, blood loss, uterine cramping).
2. Determine *psychological* response (happy, relieved; guilt feelings, lowered self-esteem).
3. Determine desire for family planning information.
4. Determine need for Rho (D^u) immune globulin, *rubella* vaccination.

◄ **B.** Analysis: *examples of nursing diagnoses:*
  1. *Pain* related to procedure.
  2. *High risk for infection* related to lack of knowledge of postabortal self-care.

◄ **C.** Nursing care plan/implementation
  1. Goal: *provide and explain postoperative care.*
    ☞ **a.** Administer IV fluids.
    ◖ **b.** Administer medications prn for discomfort.
    ◖ **c.** Administer *oxytocic* for uterine atony, prn.
    d. If *Rh-negative mother*, 8 or more wk gestation, and laboratory tests indicate no current sensitization (i.e., she is Coombs negative):
      (1) Explain rationale for post abortion administration of *Rho* (*D* antigen) immune globulin (*RhoGAM*).
    ☞◖ (2) Administer *RhoGam*, as ordered.
    e. Provide and explain perineal care.
  2. Goal: *health teaching* to facilitate active participation in own health maintenance and informed decision making; provide predischarge anticipatory guidance (also provide in written form°)

    a. Immediately report any cramping, excessive bleeding, signs of infection.
    b. Provide name and phone number of person to call if she has questions.
    c. Schedule a postabortal checkup.
    d. Discuss contraception, if woman indicates interest, or give her place and name to call for information later.
    e. Discuss resumption of tampon use (3 d–3 wk as ordered) and sexual intercourse (1–3 wk as ordered).
    f. Discuss need to avoid douching.

◄ **D.** Evaluation/outcome criteria
  1. Woman returns for postabortal appointment.
  2. Woman suffers no adverse physical sequelæ to the procedure.
  3. Woman suffers no adverse psychological sequelae to the procedure.
  4. Woman is successful in achieving her goal of either contraception or conception at the time she desires.
  5. Postabortion psychological impact
    a. Majority—relieved and happy.
    b. Small number (5–10%)—negative feelings, such as guilt or low self-esteem.

Preconception Care

Preconception care is care designed for health maintenance for everyone, but especially for women and their potential fetuses. Healthy life-styles support immune system function and normal cell differentiation in the developing embryo/fetus.

° With attention to woman's level of reading skill and understanding, and in her language, whenever possible.

TABLE 1.4   INTERRUPTION OF PREGNANCY (ELECTIVE/VOLUNTARY ABORTION)

Method	Advantages	Disadvantages and Side Effects
First-Trimester Procedures *Menstrual extraction*—aspiration of endometrium through undilated cervix	• Performed for women who have not yet missed a menstrual period • 100% effective if implantation site is not missed	• Cervical trauma may occur and may lead to incompetent cervix • Hemorrhage
RU 486 (Mifepristone)[a]—a progesterone antagonist Taken up to 5 wk after conception	• Prevents implantation of fertilized egg • Most effective in early gestation, during luteal phase, within 10 d of first missed period • Softens cervix	• Slight nausea and fatigue during period of bleeding • Uterine aspiration may be needed if RU 486 does not work • Controversy over use continues
Uterine aspiration (vacuum or suction curettage)—cannula suction under local anesthesia, following cervical dilatation, usually with laminaria tent	• Relatively few complications—minimal bleeding, minimal discomfort • Done on outpatient basis	• Performed after 1 or 2 missed menstrual periods • Cervical and/or endometrial trauma possible
Surgical D & C—cervix dilated with laminaria tents; endometrium scraped with metal curette or flexible aspiration tip, under local anesthesia (paracervical block)	• After cervix is dilated, procedure time is about 15 min • Outpatient basis • Relatively few complications ($\leq$1%)—bleeding like a heavy period, some cramping	• Performed after 1 or 2 missed periods • Possible, but rare: cervical trauma, uterine perforation, infection, hemorrhage
Second-Trimester Procedures *Intraamniotic infusion* between weeks 14 and 16 Transabdominal extraction of 200 mL amniotic fluid and replacement with equal amount of *hypertonic NaCl* (20%; or 30% urea in 5% D/W)	• Does not require laparotomy • Women may ambulate until labor starts and during early labor • Abortion completed within 36–40 hr; two-thirds of fetuses are aborted in 24 hr • With *urea*: abortion usually occurs within 12 hr • Complications less common or serious than with NaCl	• Complications increase proportionately with weeks of gestation • **Risks** *Hypernatremia:* tinnitus, tachycardia, and headache *Water intoxication:* edema, oliguria ($\leq$200 mL/8 hr), dyspnea, thirst, and restlessness • Hemorrhage and possible disseminated intravascular coagulation (DIC) • Fever with sepsis • Experiences labor • May require D & C
Instillation of 40–45 mg *prostaglandin* F_2, E_2	• Labor is usually shorter than with hypertonic *NaCl* • Avoids complications of water intoxication and hypernatremia	• May cause vomiting, diarrhea, nausea • Fetus may be born alive

(continued)

TABLE 1.4   INTERRUPTION OF PREGNANCY (*Continued*)

Method	Advantages	Disadvantages and Side Effects
D & E (dilation and evacuation)—extends D & C and vacuum curettage up to 20 wk gestation[b]	• Does not experience labor • Hospitalization is shortened • With a skilled operator, complication rate is lower than with intraamniotic injection methods	• Requires 3 d to dilate cervix; • Procedure done on 3rd day
Second- and Third-Trimester Procedures *Hysterotomy*—cesarean delivery	• Available for gestations more than 14–16 wk • Preferred method if woman wishes a tubal ligation or hysterectomy to follow	• *Post:* major surgery complications —hemorrhage and infection possible • Fetus may be born alive, opening ethical, moral, religious, and legal problems

[a] *New:* Watch literature for use of a combination of two drugs—methotrexate, a folic acid antagonist used to treat cancer, and misoprostol, which is used to treat ulcers—to induce abortions.

[b] The House of Representatives passed a bill to ban this procedure late in pregnancy (October 1995).

Components of Preconception Care: Nursing Process

I. Assessment for risk factors
A. *Medical history*—immune status (e.g., vaccinations, *rubella* titer), infectious illnesses, genetic disorders, current use of medications (including over-the-counter drugs), medical/surgical conditions.
B. *Reproductive history*—contraceptive methods used; obstetric.
C. *Psychosocial history*—family or other support system; spouse/partner situation; assess for domestic violence, use of recreational (mind altering) drugs.
D. *Reproductive choice*—plans for having children or for childlessness, readiness for pregnancy (e.g., age, life goals, financial resources, stress).
E. *Environmental* (home/workplace)—safety hazards, toxic chemicals, radiation, noise.

II. Health promotion: general teaching
A. *Nutrition*—healthy diet; optimum weight.
  1. Important to the maximum functioning of the immune system; phagocytosis and humoral and cellular immunity depend on diet.
  2. Deficient or excessive intake of some dietary components, such as vitamins and minerals, can exert negative effects on the immune response.
  3. Protein deficiency alters immune defenses, such as reducing levels of immunoglobulin A (IgA) in secretions and abnormal ratios of lymphocytic white cells.
  4. Breast milk encourages growth of *Lactobacillus bifidus,* which converts lactose into lactic acid.

B. Exercise and rest.
C. Avoidance of substance abuse.
D. Practice of "safer sex" (Table 1.5).
E. Family and social needs.
F. Referrals: genetic counseling, family planning, family and social needs.
G. Immunizations (e.g., *rubella,* tuberculosis, hepatitis).
H. Medical/surgical therapy for existing conditions.

Summary

The nurse needs a basic knowledge of *anatomy and physiology* in order to understand *conception, contraception, impaired fertility, sterilization, interruption of pregnancy,* and life-styles that support the immune system. *Preconception care* plays an important role in helping people establish a healthy environment for reproduction. Selected conditions that affect the reproductive system are also reviewed: *breast conditions* and *uterine neoplasias.*

⚲ Study and Memory Aids

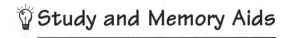

Menopause — from Greek:

men = month
pausis = to stop

TABLE 1.5   SAFER SEX GUIDELINES

If you are going to have sex, following these guidelines can reduce the risk of HIV transmission.

Always use a latex condom (rubber) for vaginal, oral or anal sex.

Do not get semen or vaginal fluids in your mouth.

Nonoxynol-9 is a spermicide that kills the virus. Always use spermicide with a condom; never use it alone.

Do not use Vaseline or vegetable or mineral oil with condoms. They make condoms break more easily. Use water-based lubricants such as K-Y Jelly.

Always leave some room at the tip of the condom to catch the sperm. This will decrease the possibility of the condom tearing.

Throw the condom away after using it. *Never* use the same condom twice.

Use a latex square (dental dam) or plastic wrap for oral sex with a woman. Vaginal fluid and menstrual blood can carry the virus.

From *Straight Talk about Sex and HIV.* San Francisco AIDS Foundation, 1995.

Decision Making Regarding Reproduction

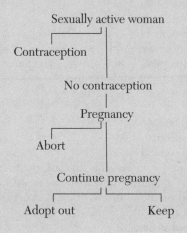

Oral Contraceptives: Signs of potential problems — "ACHES"

Abdominal pain
Chest pain
Headaches
Eye problems
Severe leg pain

IUDs: Signs of potential problems — "PAINS"*

Period late/abnormal
Abdominal pain
Infection
Not feeling well
String missing

Key Warning Signs of TSS

Sudden fever
Hypotension
Rash

Legal Aspects

"Conscience" clauses allow nurses to refuse to assist with procedures that go against their moral, religious, or medical judgment.

Questions

1. A woman asks why she needs to do arm exercises following axillary node dissection. The nurse tells her that the *most important* reason is to:
   1. Strengthen the muscles.
   2. Restore energy levels.

* Modified from RA Hatcher et al. *Contraceptive Technology: 1994–1995* (16th ed). New York: Irving Publishers, 1994.

3. Retain full range of motion.
4. Provide a diversional activity.

2. Nursing care of the woman with fibrocystic breast disease involves evaluation of a patient's response to the nurse's teaching. The patient has understood teaching when she eliminates which of the following from her diet?
1. Caffeine (methylxanthine): coffee, colas.
2. Whole grains and legumes.
3. Cigarettes (nicotine).
4. Milk and cheese (lactose).

3. The nurse is developing a teaching plan for a woman's health class. The health teaching plan should include explaining that an approved screening procedure for breast cancer is:
1. Ultrasound imaging.
2. Monthly breast self-examination (BSE).
3. Transillumination.
4. Thermography.

4. The nurse should teach women and their partners that breast self-examination (BSE) is best performed:
1. On the first day of menstruation.
2. At the time of ovulation.
3. About the 10th day after menstruation begins.
4. Just before menstruation begins.

5. The plan of care for a patient undergoing therapy for impaired fertility includes a prescription for Clomid (clomiphene citrate). The nurse knows that this patient's problem is:
1. Endometriosis.
2. Endometritis.
3. Short luteal phase of the menstrual cycle.
4. Anovulation.

6. The fertility clinic nurse reads the following assessment findings in the chart. Which finding should the nurse recognize as being linked to infertility in men?
1. Does not take multivitamins or vitamin E supplementation.
2. Had parotitis (mumps) at the age of 5 yr.
3. Prefers jockey-type shorts over boxer shorts.
4. Drinks one to three 12-ounce cans of beer per day.

7. To prepare a woman for tubal ligation, the nurse should include the following information:
1. The production of estrogen/progesterone will decrease.
2. Menstrual flow will be much lighter.
3. Ovulation will continue.
4. Menopause can be expected soon after the procedure is performed.

8. Predischarge teaching for the man who has just had a vasectomy includes:
1. Instructing him to avoid sexual intercourse for 4 weeks.
2. A reminder that he may have hematuria for 12–24 hr.
3. Explaining that fertility always returns after tubal reanastomosis.
4. Cautioning him that he is still fertile for several weeks, or until his semen is clear of sperm.

9. If a nurse's religious beliefs do not permit artificial means of family planning, which of the following would be the nurse's most appropriate response to a woman's

question about contraceptive methods?
1. "Personally, I don't believe in contraceptives. Please ask someone else."
2. "All artificial contraceptives have bad side effects. I recommend 'natural' family planning."
3. "There are several methods available. I'll tell you about them. Then you and your doctor can decide which is best for you."
4. "Norplant is the most convenient and effective. You can ask for it right away so that you will be protected the next time you have sex."

10. A woman is discussing feminine hygiene with the clinic nurse. Which statement by the woman indicates to the nurse that she correctly understands a concept?
1. "I should not take a bath and shampoo my hair during my menstrual period."
2. "I should use a feminine deodorant spray every day to make it effective."
3. "I need not use a vaginal douche in normal circumstances."
4. "Superabsorbent tampons need to be changed at least every 24 hr."

11. A woman is admitted to an acute care unit with a diagnosis of toxic shock syndrome (TSS). The nurse knows that the *first* priority of therapy for TSS is:
1. Fluid resuscitation.
2. Fever reduction.
3. Antimicrobial therapy.
4. Antihypertensive therapy.

12. A nurse is conducting a preconception class on sexuality. A woman states, "Men have it easy to get excited. The tip of the penis is so sensitive." The nurse's response is based on knowledge that the male's glans penis is analogous to the female's:
1. Clitoris.
2. Clitoral hood.
3. Vaginal meatus.
4. External cervical os.

13. While teaching a woman's health class, the nurse describes cervical mucus throughout the menstrual cycle, describing the cervical mucus at onset of ovulation as:
1. Thin, clear, and stretchable.
2. Decreased in amount.
3. Pinkish or yellowish in color.
4. Thickened, cloudy, and viscous.

14. A patient in the fertility clinic needs to know when her next fertile period will be. Her menstrual cycles are 30–32 days in length. Her last normal period (LMP) began on August 5. The nurse determines that her next fertile period will be:
1. August 14–16.
2. August 19–21.
3. August 21–23.
4. August 24–26.

15. A woman is interviewed by the nurse at her 6-wk postpartum check. She expresses a desire to have another child in the future and asks the nurse about birth control methods. Which response by the nurse is true?
1. "An intrauterine device (IUD) is a safe, reversible form of contraception."
2. "Birth control pills are completely safe for all women

under 40."

3. "The diaphragm should be removed just after intercourse."

4. "The basal body temperature (BBT) can help to determine when you ovulate."

16. A woman is admitted for an elective abortion after her second missed menstrual period. The nurse assists in preparing her for which type of procedure?
1. Hypertonic salt solution instillation.
2. Menstrual extraction.
3. Dilatation and extraction (D & E).
4. Dilatation and suction (vacuum) currettage (D & C).

17. The nurse knows that intervention with a battered woman has been successful when the woman:
1. Follows the advice of counselors.
2. Accepts her marriage vow to be with her husband "in sickness and in health. . . ."
3. Recognizes which of her behaviors deserve punishment.
4. Refers to herself specifically using phrases such as "I am. . . ."

18. In preconception counseling of sexually active adolescents, when discussing the Papanicolaou (Pap) smear, the nurse should advise them that Pap smears are:
1. Associated with a low false-negative rate.
2. Abnormal in 40% of adolescents.
3. Normal in 10% of women with human papillomavirus (HPV).
4. Best done annually.

19. After reviewing a woman's chart, the nurse's plan of care would include referral for investigation for endometrial carcinoma if her history shows:
1. Postmenopausal bleeding.
2. Use of combined oral hormonal contraceptives between ages of 16 and 30.
3. Use of an intrauterine device (IUD) for 8 yr.
4. Menopause that occurred at age 45.

20. The nurse should be alert to the fact that axillary node resection for breast cancer leads to edema because:
1. The arm is positioned over head during surgery.
2. Circulation to the arm is interrupted during surgery.
3. The arm is traumatized during surgery.
4. Lymph flow is interrupted.

21. A woman who has had breast surgery for cancer is taught to care for the suture line. The nurse knows that she has learned appropriate self-care when the woman:
1. Covers it with lanolin cream three times per day.
2. Cleans it every day with hydrogen peroxide (H_2O_2) diluted with water or normal saline (NS).
3. Reapplies a pressure dressing over it once a day for 7 days.
4. Ignores it.

22. When danazol (Danocrine) is prescribed for the management of endometriosis and fibrocystic breast disease, the woman is informed of the side effects. The nurse knows that her chief complaint is *not* related to danazol therapy when the patient describes the following:
1. Fluid retention.
2. Hypoestrogenic manifestations.
3. Dysmenorrhea.
4. Virilization.

23. After reviewing a woman's diagnostic test results, the nurse explains to her that the pH of the vaginal canal can be a factor in impaired fertility, and that to alter the vaginal pH the physician may order:
1. Vaginal instillation of clotrimazole (Gyne-Lotrimin).
2. Sodium bicarbonate douches.
3. Lactic acid douches.
4. Oral estrogen therapy.

24. The nurse should know that a woman is not a good candidate for using a diaphragm for contraception if she:
1. Gave birth 6 wk ago.
2. Did not like using the cervical cap.
3. Has frequent urinary tract infections (UTIs).
4. Is planning to go on a diet to lose 10 pounds.

25. The nurse tells the woman that a symptom to watch for that is indicative of a chlamydial infection is:
1. +1 protein in urine.
2. Burning on urination.
3. Purulent vaginal discharge.
4. Dependent edema.

26. A young woman has just been diagnosed as having diabetes mellitus. The nurse's teaching plan includes discussion of childbearing and contraception. The contraceptive choice for a diabetic woman is/are:
1. Combined hormonal oral contraceptive pills.
2. Sterilization.
3. Intrauterine device (IUD).
4. Spermicide and diaphragm or condoms.

27. A nurse is conducting an in-service class about contraceptives. One of the group asks how birth control pills affect mucus patterns. The nurse's response is based on knowledge that, under the influence of combination oral hormonal contraception, the dried cervical mucus pattern is:
1. Dependent on the phase of the menstrual cycle.
2. Markedly fernlike.
3. Minimally fernlike.
4. Amorphous.

Answers/Rationale

1. **(3)** Inactivity secondary to pain could affect joint action, and alteration in lymphatic drainage leads to edema formation and further impairment of joint/arm movement. Options **1, 2,** and **4** are also important, but the *most* important reason for arm exercises at this time is to retain full range of motion of the joint. **IMP, 3, SECE**

Key to Codes

Nursing process: AS, assessment; **AN,** analysis; **PL,** planning; **IMP,** implementation; **EV,** evaluation. (See Appendix E for explanation of nursing process steps.)

Category of human function: 1, protective; **2,** sensory-perceptual; **3,** comfort, rest, activity, and mobility; **4,** nutrition; **5,** growth and development; **6,** fluid-gas transport; **7,** psychosocial-cultural; **8,** elimination.

Client need: SECE, safe, effective care environment; **PhI,** physiologic integrity; **PsI,** psychosocial integrity; **HPM,** health promotion/maintenance.

2. **(1)** Women are advised to reduce their intake of caffeine when they are diagnosed with fibrocystic breast disease. Options **2, 3,** and **4** are not items specifically eliminated from the diet of a woman with this disease. **EV, 4, HPM**

3. **(2)** BSE is the only approved screening method of the procedures listed. Palpation of the breast has an estimated accuracy of 65–75%; it is considered to be the first step in the diagnostic survey. Options **1, 3,** and **4** are not approved screening methods. **IMP, 1, SECE**

4. **(3)** The best time to perform BSE is about the 10th day after the 1st day of the last menstrual period (LMP), when the hormonal effects on the breast are at the lowest; otherwise stated: about 5 days after menses stop. Options **1, 2,** and **4** are all incorrect: Hormonal effect on the breasts is lowest at about the 10th day after the LMP. **IMP, 1, HPM**

5. **(4)** Clomid, a nonsteroid estrogen analogue, is used to induce ovulation. Endometriosis **(1)** requires medications such as danazol or nafarelin that suppress the production of ovarian hormones, estrogen and progesterone. Endometritis **(2)** requires *antibiotic* therapy. Clomid has no effect on the luteal phase of the menstrual cycle **(3). AN, 5, HPM**

6. **(2)** Parotitis (mumps) is an acute, communicable viral infection involving chiefly the parotid gland, but frequently affects tissues such as the gonads. Vitamins, including E **(1),** are *not* linked to male fertility/infertility. Jockey-type shorts **(3)** are not specifically linked to infertility. (Tight clothing, sitting for prolonged periods, or use of a hot tub frequently may affect sperm count but this is reversed soon after the behavior is changed.) This amount of alcohol **(4)** may affect the libido or erection potential, but does not affect fertility itself. **AN, 5, HPM**

7. **(3)** Ovulation will continue, but the ovum will disintegrate within the abdominal cavity. Ovarian hormone production **(1)** is unaffected. Menses **(2)** should not be affected. The woman will experience menopause at the usual time; since ovarian function continues, tubal ligation does not induce menopause **(4). IMP, 5, HPM**

8. **(4)** He is still fertile until all the sperm in his vas deferens above the vasectomy and in the seminal vesicles are emptied. Option **1** is incorrect because he may wish to have sexual intercourse much earlier, after discomfort is past. They should continue to use contraception until his semen contains no sperm. Hematuria **(2)** is not associated with vasectomy. Option **3** is incorrect because he may develop autoantibodies against his own sperm (as he continues to produce sperm and his body must resorb them), so that he may still be infertile or sterile following the expensive operation for reanastomosis. **IMP, 5, HPM**

9. **(3)** The nurse needs to provide the information about all choices; then the woman (couple) makes the decision along with the physician. In option **1,** the nurse gives a personal judgment in what is the patient's right to choose; depending on the way it is said, the statement can sound very rude. In option **2,** the nurse is giving a personal opinion; the patient has the right to choose for herself. In option **4,** the nurse is giving a

personal opinion without giving the patient a chance to review all the options; in addition, the nurse is making an assumption that the woman will have intercourse soon and without protection. **IMP, 5, HPM**

10. **(3)** Under normal circumstances, vaginal douching is not necessary. (It should *not* be used during pregnancy.) Bathing and shampooing **(1)** are *not* contraindicated during the menstrual period. Feminine deodorants **(2)** are *not* necessary; they can cause an allergic reaction. Superabsorbent tampons **(4)** should *not* be used; tampons should be changed frequently, and perineal pads are recommended during the night so as to minimize the possibility of developing toxic shock syndrome (TSS). **EV, 5, HPM**

11. **(1)** The first priority of therapy for TSS is fluid resuscitation to combat hypotension. Reduction of fever **(2)** is the *second* concern, *then* antistaphylococcal infection therapy **(3).** *Hypo*tension, not hypertension **(4),** is characteristic of TSS. **PL, 6, PhI**

12. **(1)** The male's glans penis is analogous to the female's clitoris; each contains the same number of nerve endings, giving these structures an important role in sexual arousal. Options **2, 3,** and **4** are all incorrect: The glans penis and *clitoris* are analogous. **IMP, 5, HPM**

13. **(1)** Under estrogen influence, the cervical mucus at about the time of ovulation is thin, clear, and stretchable, like egg white. This mucus promotes sperm viability. The amount of mucus increases, *not* decreases **(2),** just before ovulation. The mucus is *clear* at this time, not pinkish or yellowish **(3).** Thick, cloudy, viscous mucus **(4)** is characteristic of progesterone influence *after* ovulation. **IMP, 5, HPM**

14. **(3)** Ovulation occurs 14 days *before* the next menstrual period (30 − 14 = 16; 32 − 14 = 18). Adding day 16 to Aug. 5 = Aug. 21; adding day 18 to Aug. 5 = Aug. 23. The patient will ovulate between August 21 and 23, depending on whether the next period was to be 30 or 32 days in length. Options **1, 2,** and **4** are incorrect: These dates do not take into account the expected date of ovulation based on her LMP. **AS, 5, HPM**

15. **(4)** A slight drop in the BBT, then a sustained rise (for 3 d or more) follows ovulation. The IUD **(1)** may predispose the patient to endometritis and pelvic inflammatory disease (PID), which may impair fertility. Birth control pills **(2)** have possible side effects for some women (e.g., smokers). A diaphragm **(3)** should be left in place for 6–8 hr after intercourse. **IMP, 5, HPM**

16. **(4)** The woman is in her first trimester; the procedure of choice is dilatation and suction (vacuum) curettage (D & C). Hypertonic salt solution via amniocentesis **(1)** is not possible during the first trimester, when the uterus is a pelvic structure; it is done during the second trimester when the uterus becomes an abdominal structure. Menstrual extraction **(2)** is best done around the time of the first missed period. D & E **(3)** is done during the second trimester. **IMP, 1, SECE**

17. **(4)** Goals have been met when the woman can use phrases such as "*I* am. . . ," which indicate a developing self-esteem, feelings of worth and personal adequacy,

and independence. Options **1**, **2**, and **3** reflect a continuation of learned helplessness, submissiveness, passivity, and dependence. **EV, 1, PsI**

18. **(4)** Because HPV-related lesions will not otherwise be detected at a manageable stage, the Pap smear must be done annually. Option **1** is incorrect because Pap results have a recognized false-negative rate of 8–50%. Option **2** is incorrect because between 3 and 20% of adolescents will have an abnormal Pap smear. Option **3** is incorrect because the Pap smear will be normal in *30%* of women with HPV. **IMP, 1, HPM**

19. **(1)** The most important sign of endometrial carcinoma is abnormal bleeding, e.g., reappearance of "menstrual bleeding" after 6 mo of menopause. Oral contraceptives **(2)** may protect against such disorders as endometrial and ovarian cancer and other conditions. Neither use of the IUD **(3)** nor menopause at age 45 **(4)** is associated with endometrial carcinoma. **AS, 1, HPM**

20. **(4)** Axillary lymph node resection for breast cancer often leads to edema because lymph flow is interrupted. None of the conditions in options **1**, **2**, and **3** should occur and interrupt lymph flow. **AN, 6, PhI**

21. **(2)** Cleaning it every day with H_2O_2 diluted with water or NS prevents scar tissue formation and promotes healing. (Some physicians order Betadine or nothing at all.) None of the actions in options **1**, **3**, and **4** are appropriate for the care of the incision site. **EV, 1, HPM**

22. **(3)** When the woman describes dysmenorrhea, the nurse knows that this is *not* a side effect of danazol. Fluid retention **(1)**, hypoestrogenic manifestations **(2)**, and virilization **(4)** *are* all side effects of danazol therapy. **EV, 3, HPM**

23. **(2)** Sperm motility is increased as vaginal pH approaches neutral or is slightly alkaline; sodium bicarbonate douches help to optimize vaginal pH for sperm motility. Vaginal instillation of clotrimazole **(1)** does *not* raise the pH to support sperm motility; this is an excellent treatment of infection with *Candida albicans.* Lactic acid douches **(3)** make the vaginal fluids more acid, a condition that does *not* optimize vaginal pH for sperm motility. Estrogen therapy **(4)** does *not* alter the vaginal pH. **IMP, 5, HPM**

24. **(3)** The diaphragm may place pressure on the urethra, preventing complete emptying and leading to UTI recurrence. She *can* be fitted for a diaphragm 6 wk after giving birth **(1)**. Her experience with the cervical cap **(2)** is not a contraindication (unless she did not like touching herself). A 10-pound loss **(4)** is not likely to cause a problem; she needs to have the diaphragm refitted after the gain or loss of *20* pounds. **AN, 5, HPM**

25. **(3)** The most obvious sign of an active chlamydial infection is a cervical vaginal discharge; the woman may be otherwise asymptomatic. Generally, there is no renal involvement **(1)**. Burning **(2)** is indicative of a urinary tract infection. Edema **(4)** is not related to vaginal infections. **IMP, 1, SECE**

26. **(4)** Spermicide and a diaphragm or condoms do not affect metabolism and are not associated with infection. Combined hormonal contraceptive pills **(1)** may affect metabolism. Diabetes mellitus usually can be controlled by patient compliance to her planned care; therefore, this condition should not keep a woman from having children if she so chooses **(2)**. Infection is possible during the first 3 mo after insertion of an IUD **(3)**, and this can compromise the diabetic condition. **IMP, 5, HPM**

27. **(4)** The combination of estrogen and progesterone gives an amorphous appearance in dried cervical mucus, a condition that prevents sperm penetration and mobility. There is no "phase of the menstrual cycle" **(1)**; the bleeding that occurs is known as withdrawal bleeding—it is *not* menstrual flow. Fernlike patterns **(2 and 3)** occur in response to estrogen alone; combination hormone contraception includes progesterone, which inhibits formation of this pattern. **AN, 5, HPM**

Normal Pregnancy

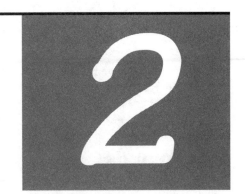

Chapter Outline

⚷ KEY POINTS

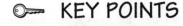

- The prenatal period is a preparatory one; both physically, in terms of fetal growth and maternal adaptations, and psychologically, in terms of anticipation of parenthood.

- Nutritional risk factors that compromise the well-being of the mother and her fetus include adolescent pregnancy; bizarre or faddist food habits; other risk factors include: abuse of nicotine, alcohol, or drugs; a low weight for height; and frequent pregnancies.
- The expected outcome of preparation for childbirth and parenting is "education for choice" and enhanced coping skills.

- Every woman/couple needs to know the warning signs of potential problems (e.g., preterm labor) and how and to whom to report these signs.

Key Words

Amniotic fluid
Birth plan
Conception
Expected date of birth
Fertilization
Fetal membranes
   Amnion
   Chorion
Gate control theory
Implantation
Kegel's exercises
Physiologic anemia
Placenta
Signs of pregnancy
   Presumptive
   Probable
   Positive
Supine hypotension

General overview: This review of the normal physiologic and psychosocial changes occurring during each trimester of pregnancy provides essential components of the database for accurate nursing judgments and anticipatory guidance during the prenatal period.

General Aspects of Nursing Care

I. Assessment—based on nursing knowledge of
  A. Biophysical and psychosocial aspects of conception and gestation.
  B. Parameters of normal pregnancy.
  C. Risk factors, signs, symptoms, and implications of deviations from normal patterns of maternal and fetal health.

II. Analysis/nursing diagnosis
  A. *Knowledge deficit* related to normal pregnancy-related alterations (physiologic and emotional alterations/trimester).
  B. *Pain* related to normal physiologic alterations in pregnancy.
  C. *Altered elimination* related to normal physiologic changes during pregnancy (polyuria, constipation).
  D. *Altered nutrition* related to increased metabolic needs due to pregnancy.
  E. *Impaired adjustment* related to altered self-image; anticipated role change; resurgence of old, unresolved conflicts.

III. **Nursing care plan/implementation**
  A. Goal: *emotional support.*

    1. Encourage verbalization of feelings, fears, concerns.
    2. Validate normalcy of behavioral response to pregnancy.
  B. Goal: *anticipatory guidance.*
    1. Facilitate achievement of developmental tasks.
    2. Strengthen coping techniques for pregnancy, labor, birth. Suggest appropriate resources (preparation for childbirth classes).
  C. Goal: *health teaching.* Describe, explain, discuss:
    1. Normal physiologic alterations during pregnancy.
    2. Common discomforts of pregnancy, management.

IV. Evaluation/outcome criteria
  A. Woman takes an active, informed part in her pregnancy-related care.
  B. Woman copes effectively with common alterations associated with pregnancy (physiologic, psychological, role change).
  C. Woman successfully carries an uneventful pregnancy to term.

Genetics, Conception, and Embryonic and Fetal Development

I. Basic genetic components
  A. *Chromosomes*—elements within the cell nucleus carrying genes and composed of DNA and proteins. The diploid number of 46 (23 pairs) in each cell: 22 pairs of autosomes (somatic cells) and 1 pair of sex chromosomes.
  B. *Genes*—factors on a chromosome responsible for hereditary characteristics of offspring.

II. Sex determination
  A. Established at time of fertilization by the male sex chromosome.
  B. Mature ovum: contains haploid number of 23 chromosomes, one of which is always an X.
  C. Mature spermatozoon: contains haploid number of 23 chromosomes, one of which is either an X or a Y type
    1. If spermatozoon contains an X, a female results (XX).
    2. If spermatozoon contains a Y, a male results (XY).

III. Fertilization and implantation
  A. *Before fertilization*
    1. *Ovum* (egg) life span: approximately 24 hr after ovulation.
    2. *Spermatozoon* life span: approximately 72 hr after ejaculation into female reproductive tract.
     a. *Acrosome reaction*—release of proteolytic enzymes that enable the sperm to digest the cumulus cells and penetrate the zona

pellucida (a thin layer of proteins and polysaccharides that surrounds the ovum and provides protection during transport in fallopian tubes).

    b. *Capacitation*—process that enables sperm to bind to the ovum.

    c. After one sperm has entered, changes occur within the zona pellucida that prevent other sperm from entering.

B. *Conception* (fertilization) usually occurs within 12–24 hr after ovulation, in the outer third (ampulla) of fallopian tube. With fertilization, the diploid number of chromosomes is reestablished; egg and sperm unite to form the single cell known as the *zygote.*

C. *Implantation* (nidation) usually occurs within 7 days after conception, or about day 21 of a 28-day menstrual cycle.

D. *Placenta*

  1. Functions:

    a. Endocrine gland: human chorionic gonadotropin (HCG), human placental lactogen (HPL), progesterone, estrogens.

    b. Metabolism: respiration, nutrition, excretion, and storage.

  2. Methods of exchanging nutrients, etc.:

    a. *Diffusion:* Oxygen diffuses from the maternal blood across the placental membrane into the fetal blood; carbon dioxide diffuses in the opposite direction.

    b. *Facilitated* and *active transport:* assist in the transfer of glucose, amino acids, calcium, iron, and substances with higher molecular weight.

    c. *Pinocytosis:* mechanism used for transferring large molecules, such as albumin and gamma globulins, across the placental membrane.

  3. A thin membrane, only one cell thick, separates maternal and fetal circulation; occasionally breaks occur, allowing fetal red blood cells to leak into the maternal circulation.

  4. Placental function depends on the maternal blood pressure.

  5. Placental "barrier" resembles other membranes. Small molecules, and lipid-soluble substances diffuse readily but water-soluble substances either do not diffuse or diffuse poorly. Examples:

    a. Heparin replaces use of warfarin (Coumadin) in treatment of coagulation problems during pregnancy.

    b. Anesthetics and analgesics readily cross both the blood-brain and placental barriers; e.g., morphine-induced respiratory depression and miosis (constriction of pupils) may occur in both the mother and her newborn.

    c. Newborns of narcotic-addicted mothers will be born with dependence on narcotics.

E. *Fetal membranes*

  1. *Chorion:* develops from the trophoblast and contains the chorionic villi on its surface.

  2. *Amnion:* develops from interior cells of blastocyst; forms a fluid-filled sac; covers umbilical cord and covers the chorion on fetal surface of the placenta.

F. *Amniotic fluid*

  1. *Composition:* albumin, urea, uric acid, creatinine, lecithin, sphingomyelin, bilirubin, fructose, fat, leukocytes, epithelial cells, enzymes, and lanugo hair.

  2. Forms initially by diffusion from maternal blood; fetus urinates into fluid, greatly enhancing its volume.

  3. *Volume:* normally between 800 and 1200 mL; slightly transparent, yellow liquid.

  4. *Functions:* cushions fetus, allows freedom of movement, keeps embryo from tangling with the membranes, helps maintain constant body temperature, acts as source of oral fluid as well as a waste repository.

IV. Stages of prenatal development

A. *Ovum* (preembryonic)—period until primary villi have appeared, usually about 12–14 d; embryonic membranes (chorion and amnion) and germ layers (ectoderm, mesoderm, and endoderm) form.

B. *Embryo*—period from end of ovum stage until measurement reaches approximately 3 cm: 54–56 d (8 wk).

C. *Fetus:* week 9 to birth.

D. Summary of development

  1. First trimester

    a. Susceptible to teratogens; malformation possible.

    b. Heart functions at 3–4 wk.

    c. Eye formation at 4–5 wk.

    d. Arm and leg buds at 4–5 wk.

    e. Recognizable face at 8 wk.

    f. Brain: rapid growth.

    g. External genitalia at 8 wk.

    h. Placenta formed at 12 wk.

    i. Bone ossification at 12 wk.

  2. Second trimester

    a. Less danger from teratogens after 12 wk; dysfunction possible, however.

    b. Facial features formed at 16 wk.

    c. Fetal heartbeat heard by 18–20 wk with a stethoscope.

    d. Quickening at 18–20 wk.

    e. Length: 10 in., weight: 8–10 ounces.

    f. Vernix: present.

  3. Third trimester

    a. Iron stored.

    b. Surfactant production begins in increasing amounts.

    c. Size: 15 in., 2–3 pounds.

    d. Calcium stored at 28–32 wk.

    e. Reflexes present at 28–32 wk.

    f. Subcutaneous fat deposits at 36 wk.

g. Lanugo shedding at 38–40 wk.

h. Average size: 18–22 in., 7.5–8.5 pounds at 38–40 wk.

Biophysical Foundations of Pregnancy

I. Anatomic and physiologic modifications

  A. *Bases of functional alterations*

    1. *Hormonal:* Table 2.1 explains the effects of estrogen and progesterone during pregnancy. Nursing implications provide the knowledge base for

      a. Anticipatory guidance regarding normal maternal adaptations.

      b. Early identification of deviations from normal patterns.

    2. *Mechanical:* enlarging uterus → displacement and pressure; increased weight of uterus and breasts → changes in center of gravity, posture and pressure.

  B. *Breasts:* enlarged darkened areola; secrete colostrum.

  C. *Reproductive organs*

    1. *Uterus*

      a. Amenorrhea. Occasional spotting common, especially at time of first missed menstrual period.

      b. Increased vascularity adds to increase in size and softening of the lower uterine segment (*Hegar's sign*).

      c. Growth is due to hypertrophy and hyperplasia of existing muscle cells and connective tissue.

      d. Fundal height measurement landmarks:

Uterus	Nonpregnant	Pregnant (at term)
Length	6.5 cm	32 cm
Width	4 cm	24 cm
Depth	2.5 cm	22 cm
Weight	50 g	1000 g

    2. *Cervix*

      a. Increased vascularity → softening (*Goodell's sign*) and deepened blue-purple coloration (*Chadwick's sign*).

      b. Edema, hyperplasia, thickening of mucous lining, and increased mucus production; formation of mucous plug by end of second month.

      c. Becomes shorter, thicker, and more elastic.

    3. *Vagina*

      a. Hyperemia deepens color (*Chadwick's sign*).

      b. Hypertrophy and hyperplasia thicken vaginal mucosa.

      c. Relaxation of connective tissue.

      d. pH acidic (4.0–6.0).

      e. Leukorrhea—nonirritating.

    4. *Perineum*

      a. Increases in size—hypertrophy of muscle cells, edema, and relaxation of elastic tissue.

      b. Deepened color—increased vascularization/hyperemia.

    5. *Ovaries*

      a. Ovum production ceases.

      b. Corpus luteum persists; produces hormones to week 10–12 until placenta "takes over."

II. Alterations affecting fluid-gas transport

  A. *Cardiovascular system* (Table 2.2)

    1. **Physiologic changes**

      a. Heart displaced upward and to the left.

      b. Circulation

        (1) Cardiac volume increases by 20–30%.

        (2) Labor—cardiac output increases by 20–30%.

      c. Hemoglobin and hematocrit values remain between 10–14 g and 35–42%; normal drop is 10% during second trimester.

      d. Hypercoagulability—increased levels of blood factors VII, IX, and X.

      e. Nonpathologic increased sedimentation rate—due to 50% increase in fibrinogen level.

      f. Blood pressure should remain stable with drop in second trimester.

      g. Heart rate often increases 10–15 beats/min at term.

      h. Compression of pelvic veins → stasis of blood in lower extremities.

      i. Compression of inferior vena cava when supine → bradycardia → reduced cardiac output, faintness, sweating, nausea (*supine hypotension*). *Fetal response:* marked bradycardia due to hypoxia secondary to decreased placental perfusion.

    2. **Assessment**

      a. Apical systolic murmur.

      b. Exaggerated splitting of first heart sound.

      c. Physiologic anemia.

      d. Dependent edema in third trimester (Table 2.3).

      e. *Vena cava syndrome* (supine hypotension)—drop in systolic blood pressure may occur due to compression of descending aorta and inferior vena cava when supine.

      f. Varicosities (vulvar, anal, leg).

    3. **Nursing care plan/implementation:** goal: *health teaching*

      a. *Elevate* lower extremities frequently.

      b. Apply support hose.

      c. *Avoid* excess intake of *sodium*.

      d. Assume *side lying position* at rest.

      e. Learn signs and symptoms of preeclampsia—eclampsia.

TABLE 2.1   HORMONES OF PREGNANCY

Primary Effects	*Clinical Implications for Nursing Actions*
Estrogen	
Level rises in serum and urine	Basis of test for maternal/placental/fetal well-being
Uterine development	Probable sign of pregnancy
Breast development	Probable sign of pregnancy; increased tingling, tenderness
Genital enlargement: increased vascularization, hyperplasia	Vaginal growth facilitates vaginal birth
Softens connective tissue	Results in back and leg ache; relaxes joints to increase size of birth canal and rib cage
Alters nutrient metabolism	*GI and metabolic changes*
Decreases HCl and pepsin	Digestive upsets
Antagonist to insulin—makes glucose available to fetus	Anti-insulin effect challenges maternal pancreas to produce more insulin; failure of beta cells to respond leads to "gestational" diabetes
	For the insulin-dependent woman, insulin requirements increase by an average of 67% during the second half of pregnancy
Supports fat deposition	Protect source of energy for fetus
Sodium and water retention; edema of lower extremities (nonpitting)	Meet increased plasma volume needs and maintain fluid reserve
Hematologic changes	
Increased coagulability	Increased tendency to thrombosis
Increased sedimentation rate (SR)	SR loses diagnostic value for heart disease
Vasodilation: spider nevi; palmar erythema	Resolves spontaneously after birth
Increased production of melanin-stimulating hormone	Resolves spontaneously after birth
Progesterone	
Development of decidua	High levels result in tiredness, listlessness, and sleepiness
Reduces uterine excitability	Protection against abortion/early birth
Development of mammary glands	Prepares breasts for lactation
Alters nutrient metabolism	*Nutritional significance*
Antagonist to insulin	Diabetogenic
Favors fat deposition	Energy reserve
Decreases gastric motility and relaxes sphincters	Favors heartburn and constipation
Increased sensitivity of respiratory center to CO_2	Increased depth, some dyspnea, increased sighing
Decreased smooth muscle tone	*Decreased tone can lead to*
Colon	Constipation
Bladder, ureters	Stasis of urine with infection
Veins	Dependent edema; varicosities
Gallbladder	Gallbladder disease
Increased basal body temperature (BBT) by 0.5°C	Discomfort from hot flashes and perspiration

(continued)

B. *Respiratory system*
   1. **Physiologic changes**
      a. Increased tidal volume, vital capacity, respiratory reserve, oxygen consumption, production of CO_2.
      b. Diaphragm elevated by ~3 cm, increased substernal angle → flaring of rib cage allowing for increase in tidal volume.
      c. Uterine enlargement prevents maximum lung expansion in third trimester.

✉ 2. **Assessment**
      a. Shortness of breath or dyspnea on exertion and when lying flat in third trimester.
      b. Nasal stuffiness due to estrogen-induced edema (Table 2.3).
      c. Deeper respiratory excursion.
✉ 3. **Nursing care plan/implementation:** goal: *health teaching*
      a. Sit and stand with good posture.
      b. When resting assume *semi-Fowler's position.*

TABLE 2.1   HORMONES OF PREGNANCY (*Continued*)

Primary Effects	*Clinical Implications for Nursing Actions*
Human Chorionic Gonadotropin	
Maintains corpus luteum during early pregnancy	Placenta must "take over" after a few weeks
Stimulates male testes	Increased testosterone in male fetuses
May suppress immune response	May inhibit response to foreign protein, for example, fetal portion of placenta
	Diagnostic value
	Biologic marker for pregnancy test
	Hydatidiform mole
	Decreased level with threatened abortion
	Increased level with multifetal pregnancy
Human Placental Lactogen	
Antagonizes insulin	Diabetogenic; may → gestational diabetes or complicate management of existing diabetes
Mobilizes maternal free fatty acids	Increased tendency to ketoacidosis in pregnant diabetic
Prolactin	
Suppressed by estrogen and progesterone	No milk produced before birth
Increased level after placenta is delivered	Milk production 2–3 d after birth
Follicle Stimulating Hormone	
Production suppressed during pregnancy; level returns to prepregnant levels within 3 wk after birth	No ovulation during pregnancy; ovulation usually returns: within 6 wk for 15%, within 12 wk for 30%
Oxytocin	
Causes uterus to contract when the oxytocin levels exceed those of estrogen and progesterone	Labor induction or augmentation; treatment for postpartum uterine atony
Melanotropin	
Increases after 8 wk gestation; activity increased by increase in adrenocorticotropic hormone (ACTH) during pregnancy	Responsible for chloasma ("mask of pregnancy"), linea nigra, deeper color of areola (around nipple) and genitalia
Deepens pigmentation	Women with histories of melanoma should delay pregnancy for about 3 yr following surgical excision

TABLE 2.2   BLOOD VALUES

Component	*Prepregnant*	*Pregnant*	*Postpartum*°
WBC	4–11,000	9–16,000 (25,000–labor)	20,000–25,000 within 10–12 d of birth, then returns to normal
RBC volume	1600 mL	1900 mL	Prepregnant level of 1600 mL
Plasma volume	2400 mL	3700 mL	Prepregnant level of 2400 mL
Hct (PCV)	37–47%	32–42%	At 72°, returns to prepregnant level of 37–42%
Hgb (at sea level)	12–16 g/dL	10–14 g/dL	At 72°, returns to prepregnant level of 12–16 g/dL
Fibrinogen	250 mg/dL	400 mg/dL	At 72°, returns to prepregnant level of 250 mg/dL

°Postpartum values depend on factors of amount of blood loss, mobilization, and physiologic edema (excretion of extravascular water). Normal blood loss for vaginal birth of one fetus is 300–400 mL.

TABLE 2.3   COMMON DISCOMFORTS DURING PREGNANCY

Discomfort and Cause	◁ *Health Teaching*
Morning sickness—first 3 mo; nausea and vomiting; may occur anytime, day or night; *cause:* hormonal, psychological, and empty stomach	Alternate dry carbohydrate and fluids hourly; take dry carbohydrate before rising, stay in bed 15 more minutes; *avoid* empty stomach, offending odors, and food difficult to digest (food high in fat, for example)
Fatigue (sleep hunger)—first 3 mo; *cause:* possibly hormones; often returns in late pregnancy when physical load is great	Iron supplement if anemic—foods high in iron, folic acid, and *protein;* adequate rest
Fainting (syncope)—early pregnancy; due to slightly decreased arterial blood pressure; late pregnancy, due to venous stasis in lower extremities	*Elevate* feet; sit down when necessary; when standing, do *not* lock knees; *avoid* prolonged standing, fasting
Urinary frequency—enlarging uterus presses on bladder, turgescence of structures from hormone stimulation; relieved somewhat as uterus rises from pelvis; recurs with lightening	*Kegel's exercises; limit fluids* just before bedtime to ensure rest; rule out urinary tract infection
Vaginal discharge—months 2–9, mucus, acid, and increases in amount (leukorrhea)	Cleanliness important; treat only if infection sets in; douche *contraindicated* in pregnancy
Hot flashes—heat intolerance, due to increased metabolism → diaphoresis	Alter clothing, bathing, and environmental temperature prn
Headache—cause unknown; possibly blood pressure change, nutritional, tension (unless associated with preeclampsia)	If pain relief needed, consult physician (avoid over-the-counter drugs without prescription); reduce tension
Nasal stuffiness—due to increased vascularization; allergic rhinitis of pregnancy	Antihistamines and nasal sprays by *prescription only*
Heartburn—enlarging uterus and hormones slow digestion; progesterone → reverse peristaltic waves → reflux of stomach contents into esophagus	Physician may prescribe an antacid; *"flying exercise"; avoid* use of antacids containing sodium; instead of leaning over, bend at the knees, keeping torso straight; sit on firm chairs; *limit fatty and fried* foods in diet; small, frequent meals
Flatulence—altered digestion from enlarging uterus and hormones	Maintain regular bowel habits, *avoid* gas-forming foods; antiflatulent may be prescribed
Insomnia—fetal movements, fears or concerns, and general body discomfort from heavy uterus	Medication by prescription only; exercise; side-lying *positions* with pillow supports; change position often; back rubs, ventilate feelings
Shortness of breath—enlarging uterus limits expansion of diaphragm	Good posture; cut down/stop smoking; *position*—supine and upright
Backache—increased elasticity of connective tissue, increased weight of uterus, and increased lumbar curvature	Correct posture, low-heeled, wide-base shoes, and diet; do pelvic rock often; *avoid* fatigue
Pelvic joint pain—hormones relax connective tissue and joints and allow movement within joints	Rest; good posture; will go away after giving birth, in 6–8 wk

(continued)

       c. *Avoid* overdistention of stomach.

III. Alterations affecting elimination

     A. *Urinary system*

       1. Physiologic changes

         a. Relaxation of smooth muscle results in conditions that can persist 4–6 wk after birth:

           (1) Dilatation of ureters.

           (2) *Decreased* bladder tone.

           (3) Increased potential for urinary stasis and *infection* (urinary tract infection [UTI]).

         b. *Increased* glomerular filtration rate (50%) during last two trimesters.

         c. *Increased* renal plasma flow (25–50%)

TABLE 2.3   COMMON DISCOMFORTS DURING PREGNANCY (*Continued*)

Discomfort and Cause	⋈ *Health Teaching*
Leg cramps—pressure of enlarging uterus on nerve supplying legs; possible causes: lack of calcium, fatigue, chilling, and tension	Stretch affected muscle and hold until it subsides; *do not rub* (may release a blood clot, if present)
Constipation—decreased motility (hormones, enlarging uterus) and increased reabsorption of water; iron therapy (oral)	*Diet*—prunes, fruits, vegetables, roughage, and fluids; regular habits; exercise; sit on toilet with knees up; *avoid* enemas, mineral oil, laxatives.
Hemorrhoids—varicosities around anus; aggravated by pushing with stool and by uterus pressing on blood vessels supplying lower body	As above, *avoid* constipation; pure Vaseline or Desitin, applied externally, is mild and sometimes soothing; use any other preparation with prescription only
Ankle edema—normal and nonpitting; gravity	Rest legs often during day with legs and hips raised
Varicose veins—lower legs, vulva, pelvis; pressure of heavy uterus; relaxation of connective tissue in vein walls; hereditary	Progressively worse with subsequent pregnancies and obesity; elevate legs above level of heart; support hose may help
Cramp in side or groin—round ligament pain; stretching of round ligament with cramping	To get out of bed, turn to side, use arm and upper body and push up to sitting position

during first two trimesters; returns to near normal levels by end of last trimester.
  d. *Increased* renal-tubular reabsorption rate —compensates for increased glomerular activity.
  e. Glycosuria common—reflects kidney's inability to reabsorb all glucose filtered by glomeruli (urine glucose *not* reliable index of diabetic status during pregnancy).
  f. *Increased* renal clearance of urea and creatinine (creatinine clearance used as test of renal function during pregnancy).
  g. Hormone-induced turgescence of bladder and pressure on bladder from gravid uterus (Table 2.3).
  ⋈ **2. Assessment**
  a. Urinary frequency, first and third trimesters (Table 2.3).
  b. Nocturia.
  c. Stress incontinence in third trimester.
  ⋈ **3. Nursing care plan/implementation:** goal: *health teaching*
  a. Void with urge to prevent bladder distention.
  b. Learn signs and symptoms of UTI.
  c. *Decrease fluid intake* in late evening.
  ☞ d. Perform Kegel's exercises to reduce incontinence (p. 42).
  B. *Gastrointestinal system* (Table 2.3)
    1. Physiologic changes
    a. General decrease in smooth muscle tone and motility due to actions of progesterone.
    b. *Intestines:* slowed peristalsis, increased water reabsorption in bowel.
    c. *Stomach*

      (1) Gastric emptying time is delayed (e.g., 3 hr vs. 1½ hr).
      (2) Gastric secretion of HCl and pepsin decreases.
      (3) Decreased motility delays emptying; increased acidity.
    d. *Cardiac sphincter* relaxes.
    e. Increasing size of *uterus* and displacement of *intraabdominal organs*.
    f. *Gallbladder:* decreased emptying.
  ⋈ **2. Assessment**
    a. Nausea and vomiting in first trimester.
    b. Constipation and flatulence.
    c. Hemorrhoids.
    d. Heartburn, reflux esophagitis, indigestion.
    e. Hiatal hernia.
    f. Epulis—edema and bleeding of gums.
    g. Ptyalism—excessive salivation.
    h. Jaundice.
    i. Gallstones.
    j. Pruritus due to increased retention of bile salts.
  ⋈ **3. Nursing care plan/implementation:** goal: *health teaching*
    a. Nausea and vomiting
      (1) *Avoid* fatty food; *increase* carbohydrates.
      (2) Eat small, frequent meals.
      (3) Eat dry unsalted crackers in A.M.
      (4) *Decrease* liquids with meals.
      (5) *Avoid* odors that predispose to nausea.
    b. Constipation and flatulence
      (1) *Increase* fluids (6–8 8 oz. glasses/d).
      (2) Maintain exercise regimen.
      (3) *Add fiber* to diet.
      (4) *Avoid* mineral oil laxatives.

(5) *Avoid* gas-producing foods (i.e., beans, cabbage).
  c. Heartburn and indigestion
  (1) *Eliminate* fatty or spicy foods.
  (2) Eat small, frequent meals (6/d).
  (3) Eat slowly.
  (4) *Avoid* gastric irritants (i.e., alcohol, coffee).
  (5) Perform "flying exercises."
  (6) *Avoid* lying flat.
  (7) Take antacids without sodium or phosphorus.
  (8) Sip milk or eat yogurt with heartburn.
  (9) *Avoid* sodium bicarbonate.
  d. Hemorrhoids
  (1) Increase *fluid and fiber* intake.
  (2) Maintain exercise regimen.
  (3) *Avoid* constipation and straining to defecate.
  (4) Take warm sitz baths.
  (5) Apply witch hazel pads.
  (6) *Elevate* hips and legs frequently.
  (7) Use hemorrhoidal ointments only with advice of health care provider.
IV. Alterations affecting nutrition (see also discussion, pp. 36; 37–42)
  A. Physiologic changes
  1. *Gastrointestinal system*
  a. Gingivae soften and enlarge due to increased vascularity.
  b. Increased saliva production.
  2. *Endocrine system*
  a. *Increased* size and activity of pituitary, parathyroids, adrenals.
  b. *Increased* vascularity and hyperplasia of thyroid.
  c. Pancreas: *increased* insulin production during second half of pregnancy, needed to meet rising maternal needs; placental HPL and insulinase deactivate maternal insulin; may precipitate *gestational diabetes* in susceptible women.
  3. *Metabolism*
  a. *Basal metabolic rate (BMR): increases* 25% as pregnancy progresses, due to increasing oxygen consumption; protein-bound iodine (PBI) *increases* to 7–10 µg/dL; metabolism returns to normal by sixth postpartal week.
  b. *Protein:* need *increased* for fetal and uterine growth, maternal blood formation.
  c. *Water retention: increased.*
  d. *Carbohydrates:* need *increases* in order to spare protein stores.
  (1) *First half of pregnancy*—glucose rapidly and continuously siphoned across placenta to meet fetal growth needs; may lead to hypoglycemia and faintness.
  (2) *Second half of pregnancy*—placental production of anti-insulin hormones;

normal maternal hyperglycemia; affects coexisting diabetes.
  e. *Fat: increased* plasma-lipid levels.
  f. *Iron:* supplements recommended to meet *increased* need for red blood cells by maternal/placental/fetal unit.
B. Assessment
  1. Weight gain: 20–30 pounds (average gain, 24 pounds).
  2. Normal pattern: first trimester, 1 pound/mo; remainder of gestation, 0.9–1 pound/wk.
C. Nursing care plan/implementation: goal: *health teaching*
  1. Evaluate diet for adequacy of nutrient and caloric intake.
  2. Evaluate cultural, religious, and economic influences on diet.
  3. Review dietary recommendation for pregnancy with woman.
  4. *Avoid* dieting in pregnancy (even if obese).
  5. Supplement diet with *vitamins, iron,* or *folic acid* on advice of health care provider.
  6. Ptyalism
  a. Suck hard candies.
  b. Perform frequent oral hygiene.
  c. Maintain adequate oral intake (6–8 8 oz. glasses/d).
  d. Use lip balm to prevent chapping.
  7. Epulis
  a. Frequent oral hygiene.
  b. Use soft toothbrush.
  c. Floss gently.
  d. See dentist regularly.
V. Alterations affecting protective functions—*integumentary system*
  A. Physiologic changes—estrogen-induced vascular and pigment changes.
  B. Assessment
  1. Increased pigmentation (see Table 2.1).
  2. Striae gravidarum (stretch marks).
  3. Increased sebaceous and sweat gland activity.
  4. Palmar erythema.
  5. Angiomas—vascular "spiders."
  C. Nursing care plan/implementation: goal: *health teaching*
  1. Bathe or shower daily.
  2. Reassure woman that skin changes decrease after pregnancy.
VI. Alterations affecting comfort, rest, mobility—*musculoskeletal system*
  A. Physiologic changes
  1. Progesterone, estrogen, and relaxin-induced relaxation of joints, cartilage, and ligaments.
  2. Function in childbearing: increases anteroposterior diameter of rib cage and enlarges birth canal.
B. Assessment
  1. Complaint of pelvic "looseness."
  2. Duck-waddle walk.
  3. Tenderness of symphysis pubis.

4. Lordosis (exaggerated lumbar curve)—*increased* weight of pelvis tilts pelvis forward; to compensate, woman throws head and shoulders backward; complaint of leg and back strain and fatigue (see Table 2.3).

▶ **C.** Nursing care plan/implementation: goal: *health teaching*

1. Good body alignment—tuck pelvis under; tighten abdominal muscles.
2. Pelvic-rock exercises.
3. Squat; bend at knees, *not* at waist.
4. Wear low-heeled, sturdy shoes.
5. Advise against tight-fitting clothing interfering with circulatory return in legs.
6. *Modify exercise programs* during pregnancy. Calisthenic exercise in water is encouraged; however, swimming in water that is too cold or too hot (above 85–90°F) is to be avoided. The serious jogger may jog with her physician's permission, but she must restrict herself to no more than 2 miles/d. The pregnant woman should *not* exercise if the temperature and/or humidity is *high*. Women should *avoid* exercising on hard surfaces and should limit repetitive movements to 10. Maternal exercise during pregnancy has been associated with fetal bradycardia. Maternal arrhythmia is not associated with maximal exercise; exercise is safe up to 148 beats/min (approximately 70% of maximal aerobic power).
7. Travel during pregnancy is safest during the second trimester.
   a. During the first trimester: Susceptible women may suffer *spontaneous abortion* if traveling to high altitudes or flying in unpressurized aircraft (some private planes).
   b. During the third trimester: Susceptible women may experience *preterm labor* if traveling to high altitudes or flying in unpressurized aircraft (some private planes).

Psychosocial-Cultural Alterations

I. Emotional changes—affected by age, maturity, support system, amount of current stresses, coping abilities, physical and mental health status. *Developmental tasks of pregnancy:*

A. Accept the pregnancy as real: "I am pregnant"; progress from symbiotic relationship with the fetus to perception of the child as an individual.

B. Seek and ensure acceptance of child by others.

C. Seek protection for self and fetus through pregnancy and labor ("safe passage").

D. Prepare realistically for the coming child and for necessary role change: "I am going to be a parent."

II. *Physical bases of changes*

A. *Increased* metabolic demands may result in anemia and fatigue.

B. *Increased* hormone levels (steroids, estrogen, progesterone) affect mood as well as physiology.

III. *Characteristic behaviors:* Table 2.4 describes behaviors commonly exhibited in each trimester.

IV. *Sexuality and sexual expression:* Feelings and expressions of sexuality may vary during pregnancy as a result of maternal adaptations.

V. *Intrafamily relationships*

A. Pregnancy a maturational crisis for the family.

B. Requires changes in life-style and interactions

1. Increased financial demands.
2. Changing family and social relationships.
3. Adapting communication patterns.
4. Adapting sexual patterns.
5. Anticipating new responsibilities and needs.
6. Responding to reactions of others.

Prenatal Management

I. Initial assessment goal: establish baseline for health supervision, teaching, emotional support, and/or referral.

II. Objectives

A. Determine woman's present health status and validate pregnancy.

B. Identify factors affecting and/or affected by pregnancy.

C. Describe current gravidity and parity.

D. Identify present length of gestation.

E. Establish an estimated date of birth (EDB); **Nagele's** determination of EDB—subtract 3 mo, add 7 days to date of last menstrual period (LMP).

F. Determine relevant knowledge deficit.

▶ **III.** Assessment: *history*

A. *Family:* inheritable diseases, reproductive problems.

B. *Personal:* medical, surgical, gynecologic, past obstetric, average nonpregnant weight.

1. *Gravida*—a pregnant woman.
   a. *Nulligravida*—woman who has *never* been pregnant.
   b. *Primigravida*—woman with a *first* pregnancy.
   c. *Multigravida*—woman with a *second or later* pregnancy.
2. *Para*—refers to *past pregnancies* (not number of babies) that reached viability (20–22 wk; whether or not born alive).
   a. *Nullipara*—woman who has *not* carried a pregnancy to viability; e.g., may have had one or more abortions.
   b. *Primipara*—woman who has carried *one* pregnancy to viability.
   c. *Multipara*—woman who has had *two or more* pregnancies that reached viability.
   d. *Grandmultipara*—woman who has had *six or more* viable pregnancies.

TABLE 2.4 BEHAVIORAL CHANGES IN PREGNANCY

◄ *Assessment/Characteristics*	◄ *Nursing Care Plan/Implementation*
First Trimester Emotional lability (mood swings) Displeasure with subjective symptoms of early pregnancy (nausea, fatigue, etc.) Feelings of ambivalence	Encourage verbalization of feelings, concerns Validate normalcy of feelings, behaviors *Health teaching:* diet, rest, relaxation, diversion
Second Trimester Accepts pregnancy (usually coincides with awareness of fetal movement, i.e., "quickening") Becomes introspective: resolves old conflicts (feelings toward mother, sexual intimacy, masturbation) Reevaluates self, life-style, marriage Daydreams, fantasizes self as "mother" Seeks out other pregnant women and new mothers	Encourage exploration of feelings of dependency, introspection, mood swings Discuss childbirth preparation and preparation for parenthood classes; refer, as necessary
Third Trimester Altered body image Fears body mutilation (stretching of body tissues, episiotomy, cesarean birth) Distress over loss of control over body functions (ptyalism, colostrum leakage, leukorrhea, urinary frequency, constipation, stress incontinence) Anxiety for baby (deformity, death) Fears pain, loss of control in labor Acceptance of impending labor during last 2 wk (ready to "move on")	Encourage verbalization of concerns, discomforts of late pregnancy Help meet dependency needs; reassurance, as possible *Health teaching:* Kegel's exercises; preparation for labor; anticipatory guidance and planning for needs of self, baby, and family in early postpartum

3. Methods of recording gravidity/parity—several methods of describing gravidity and parity are in common use.
   a. One method—*GTPAL*—describes the number of **G**ravida (pregnancies), **T**erm (full-term) infants, **P**reterm infants, **A**bortions, and number of **L**iving children. Examples:
      (1) A woman who is pregnant for the *first* time and is currently *undelivered* is designated as 1-0-0-0-0. *After* giving birth to a full-term living neonate, she becomes 1-1-0-0-1.
      (2) If a woman's second pregnancy ends in abortion and she has a living child from a previous pregnancy, born at term, she is designated as 2-1-0-1-1.
      (3) A woman who is pregnant for the fourth time and whose previous pregnancies yielded one full-term neonate, premature twins, and one abortion (spontaneous or induced), and who now has three living children, may be designated as 4-1-1-1-3.
   b. Others record as follows: number gravida/number para. Applying this system to the examples given above, those mothers would be designated as follows:
      (1) G1P1
      (2) G2P1
      (3) G4P2
   c. Others include recording of abortions; based on above examples:
      (1) G1P1 Ab0
      (2) G2P1 Ab1
      (3) G4P2 Ab1.

◄ **IV.** Assessment: initial *physical* aspects
   A. Height and weight.
   B. Vital signs.
   C. *Blood* work—hematocrit (Hct) and hemoglobin (Hgb) for anemia; type and Rh factor; tests for sickle cell trait, syphilis, and rubella antibody titer (see also Table 2.2)
   D. Urinalysis—glucose, protein, acetone, signs of infection, and pregnancy test (HCG).
   E. Breast examination.
   F. Pelvic examination.
      1. Signs of pregnancy.
      2. Adequacy of pelvis and pelvic structures.
      3. Size and position of uterus.
      4. Papanicolaou smear.

〰 **5.** Smears for monilial and trichomonal infections.

6. Signs of pelvic inflammatory disease.

〰 **7.** Tests for sexually transmitted diseases (STD): gonorrhea/chlamydia.

G. *Validation of pregnancy*—physician or midwife makes differential diagnosis between presumptive/probable signs/symptoms of early pregnancy and other signs.

    1. Presumptive symptoms—subjective experiences.

      a. Amenorrhea—more than 10 days past missed menstrual period.

      b. Breast tenderness, enlargement.

      c. Nausea and vomiting ("morning sickness").

      d. Quickening (week 16–18).

      e. Urinary frequency.

      f. Fatigue.

      g. Constipation (50% of women).

    2. Presumptive signs

      a. Striae gravidarum, linea nigra, chloasma (after week 16).

      b. Increased basal body temperature (BBT).

    3. Probable signs—examiner's objective findings

〰   **a.** Positive pregnancy test.

      b. Enlargement of abdomen/uterus.

      c. Reproductive organ changes (after sixth week)

        (1) *Goodell's sign*—cervical softening.

        (2) *Hegar's sign*—softening of lower uterine segment.

        (3) Vaginal changes (*Chadwick's sign*): purple hue in vulvar/vaginal area.

      d. Ballottement (after 16–20 wk).

      e. *Braxton Hicks* contractions.

    4. Positive signs

〰   **a.** Fetal heart tones.

      (1) Doptone: week 10–12.

      (2) Fetoscope: week 18–20.

      b. Examiner visualizes and feels fetal movements (usually after week 24).

〰   **c.** Sonographic examination (after week 14) when fetal head is sufficiently developed for accurate diagnosis.

◀ **V.** Assessment: *nutritional status*

A. Physical findings suggesting poor nutritional status

    1. Skin: rough, dry, scaly.

    2. Lips: lesions in corners.

    3. Hair: dull, brittle.

    4. Mucous membranes: pale.

    5. Dental caries.

B. *Risk factors* at *onset* of pregnancy

    1. Age: 15 yr or younger or 35 yr or older.

    2. Weight: less than 85% of standard weight for height or more than 120% of standard weight.

    3. Frequent pregnancies: three or more during a 2-yr period.

    4. Therapeutic diet required for a chronic disorder.

    5. Abuse of nicotine, alcohol, or drugs.

    6. Poverty.

C. *Risk factors* occurring *during* pregnancy

    1. Low hemoglobin and/or hematocrit

      a. Hemoglobin less than 11 g.

      b. Hematocrit less than 33 mg/dL.

    2. Inadequate or excessive weight gain (see discussion, p. 39).

D. Nutrition history.

◀ **E.** Analysis/nursing diagnosis

    1. *Altered nutrition: less than body requirements* related to anemia, vitamin/mineral deficit.

    2. *Altered nutrition: more than body requirements* related to obesity.

◀ **F.** Nursing care plan/implementation: goal: *health teaching.* Nutritional counseling for diet in pregnancy and/or lactation.

◀ **G.** Evaluation/outcome criteria

    1. Woman's weight gain and pattern of weight gain are within normal limits.

    2. Woman's hemoglobin and hematocrit remain within normal limits.

◀ **VI.** Assessment: *psychosocial aspects*

A. Pregnancy: planned or not; desired or not.

B. Present plans:

    1. Carry pregnancy, keep baby.

    2. Carry pregnancy, adopt baby out.

    3. Elective abortion.

C. Cultural, ethnic influences on decisions: will influence range of activities, types of safeguarding actions, diet, and health-promotion behaviors.

D. Parenting potential: actively seeking medical care and information about pregnancy, childbirth, parenthood.

E. Family readiness for childbearing/child rearing

    1. Physical maintenance.

    2. Allocation of resources: identify support system.

    3. Division of labor.

    4. Socialization of family members.

    5. Reproduction, recruitment, launching of family members into society.

    6. Maintenance of order (relationships within family).

F. Perceptions of present and projected family relationships.

G. Review life-style for smoking, drugs, ETOH (alcohol), attitudes to pregnancy, and health care practices.

◀ **VII.** Analysis/nursing diagnosis

A. *Altered role performance* related to stress imposed by developmental tasks.

B. *Ineffective coping: individual, family* related to stress caused by developmental tasks/crises.

C. *Altered family process* related to developmental tasks. First baby may precipitate individual or family developmental crisis.

VIII. Nursing care plan/implementation
  A. Goal: *anticipatory guidance/support.*
    1. Discuss mood swings, ambivalent feelings, negative feelings.
    2. Reinforce "normalcy" of such feelings.
  B. Goal: *increase individual/family coping skills, reduce intrafamily stress.*
    1. Reinforce family strengths (both partners), sense of family identity.
      a. Encourage open communication between partners; share feelings and concerns.
      b. Increase understanding of mutual needs, encourage mutuality of support.
      c. Increase tendency of mother to turn to partner as most significant person (as opposed to physician).
      d. Enhance bond, success of childbirth preparation classes.
    2. Promote understanding/acceptance of role change.
      a. Facilitate/support achievement of developmental tasks.
      b. Reduce probability of postpartal psychological problems.
      c. Promote family bonding.
  C. Goal: *health teaching*
    1. *Siblings:*
      a. Alert parents to sibling needs for security, love.
      b. Include sibling in pregnancy experience.
      c. Provide clear, simple explanations of happenings.
      d. Continue demonstrations of love.
      e. Describe increased status ("big sister/brother").
      f. Discuss possible misbehavior to gain attention.
    2. *Relatives:* alert parents to possible negative feelings of in-laws.
    3. Referral to childbirth preparation/parenting classes.
    4. Appropriate community referrals for financial relief to decrease stress and provide aid.
IX. Evaluation/outcome criteria: The woman
  A. Actively participates in pregnancy-related decision making.
  B. Expresses satisfaction with decisions made.
  C. Demonstrates growth and development in parenting role.
  D. Prepares for the birth and for early parenthood.

Antepartal Experience and Management

I. General aspects of prenatal management
  A. *Scheduled visits*
    1. Once monthly—until week 32.
    2. Every 2 wk—weeks 32–36.
    3. Weekly—week 36 until labor.
  B. Assessment
    1. General well-being, signs of deviations, concerns, questions.
    2. Weight gain pattern.
    3. Blood pressure (right arm, sitting).
      a. By midpregnancy, diastolic and systolic blood pressure normally falls by 10–15 mm Hg. If diastolic blood pressure is 75 mm Hg or more in the second trimester and 85 mm Hg or more in the third trimester, statistical increase in fetal mortality occurs.
      b. NOTE: For obese woman, use thigh cuff or ultrasound to obtain accurate readings.
    4. Abdominal palpation
      a. Fundal height; tenderness, masses, hernia.
      b. Fetal heart rate (FHR).
      c. *Leopold's* maneuvers for presentation (after week 32).
    5. Laboratory tests
      a. *Urinalysis*—for protein, sugar, signs of asymptomatic infection.
      b. *Venous blood*—for Hgb, Hct (done initially: VDRL, anti-Rh titer, sickle cell). Human immunodeficiency virus (HIV) testing recommended for high-risk groups.
      c. Cultures (vaginal discharge; cervical scrapings, for *Chlamydia trachomatis*) prn.
      d. Tuberculosis screening.
      e. Maternal alpha-fetoprotein screen, 16–18 wk optimum time.
      f. Serum glucose screen, 24–28 wk.
    6. Follow-up on medications (vitamins, iron) and nutrition.
II. Common minor discomforts during pregnancy
  (For **Assessment,** see Table 2.3.)
  A. Etiology: normal maternal physiologic/psychological alterations in pregnancy.
  B. Nursing care plan/implementation
    1. Goal: *anticipatory guidance.* Discuss the importance of adequate rest, exercise, diet, and hydration in minimizing symptoms.
    2. Goal: *health teaching* (see Table 2.3).
  C. Evaluation/outcome criteria: avoids, minimizes, and/or copes effectively with minor usual discomforts of pregnancy.
III. Nutrition during pregnancy and lactation
  A. Nutrient needs (Table 2.5 and Figure 2.1).
    1. Milk group—important for calcium, protein of high biologic value, and other vitamins and minerals.
      a. *Pregnancy*—three to four servings.
      b. *Lactation*—four to five servings.
      c. *Count as one serving*—1 cup milk, ½ cup undiluted evaporated milk, ¼ cup dry milk, 1¼ cups cottage cheese, 2 cups low-fat cottage cheese, 1½ cups cheddar or Swiss cheese, or 1½ cups ice cream.

TABLE 2.5 NUTRIENT NEEDS DURING PREGNANCY

Nutrient	Maternal Need	Fetal Need	Food Source
Protein	Maternal tissue growth: uterus, breasts, blood volume, storage	Rapid fetal growth	Milk and milk products; animal meats—muscle, organs; grains, legumes; eggs
Calories	Increased BMR	Primary energy source for growth of fetus	Carbohydrates: 4 Kcal/g Proteins: 4 Kcal/g Fats: 9 Kcal/g
Minerals			
Calcium (and phosphorus)	Increase in maternal Ca^{2+} metabolism	Skeleton and tooth formation	Milk and milk products, especially Swiss cheese°
Iron	Increase in RBC mass Prevent anemia Decrease infection risk	Liver storage (especially in third trimester)	Organ meats—liver, animal meat; egg yolk, whole or enriched grains; green leafy vegetables; nuts
Vitamins			
A	Tissue growth	Cell development—tissue and bone growth and tooth bud formation	Butter, cream, fortified margarine; green and yellow vegetables
B's	Coenzyme in many metabolic processes	Coenzyme in many metabolic processes	Animal meats, organ meats; milk and cheese; beans, peas, nuts; enriched grains
Folic acid	Meet increased metabolic demands in pregnancy Production of blood products	Meet increased metabolic demands, including production of cell nucleus material	Liver; deep-green, leafy vegetables
C	Tissue formation and integrity Increase iron absorption	Tissue formation and integrity	Citrus fruit, berries, melons; peppers; green, leafy vegetables; broccoli; potatoes
D	Absorption Ca^{2+}, phosphorus	Mineralization of bone tissue and tooth buds	Fortified milk and margarine
E	Tissue growth; cell wall integrity; RBC integrity	Tissue growth; cell integrity; RBC integrity	Widely distributed: meat, milk, eggs, grains, leafy vegetables

°Swiss cheese contains twice the amount of calcium as 8 oz. of whole milk but only 0.09 as much lactose; therefore, it is a good source for those with lactose intolerance. Tofu (soybean curd) is also high in calcium, and contains *no* lactose.

2. **Meat group**—important for protein, iron, and many B vitamins.
   a. *Pregnancy*—three servings.
   b. *Lactation*—two servings.
   c. *Count as one serving* (12–14 g protein)— 6–8 ounces lean meat, fish, or poultry; two eggs; two frankfurters; 4 tbsp peanut butter; or 1 cup cooked dry beans, dry peas, or lentils.
3. **Vegetable and fruit groups**—vitamins and minerals (especially A and C) and roughage.
   a. *Pregnancy*—five to six servings.
   b. *Lactation*—five to six servings.
   c. *Count as one serving*—one-half medium grapefruit; one medium apple, banana, or orange; ¾ cup fruit juice.
   d. *Good sources (vitamin C)*—citruses, cantaloupe, mango, papaya, strawberries, broccoli, and green and red bell peppers.
   e. *Fair sources (vitamin C)*—tomatoes, honeydew melon, asparagus tips, raw cabbage, collards, kale, mustard greens, potatoes (white and sweet), spinach, and turnip greens.
   f. *Good sources (vitamin A)*—dark green or deep yellow vegetables and a few fruits (apricots, broccoli, pumpkin, sweet potato, spinach, cantaloupe, carrots, and winter squash).
   g. *Good sources of folic acid*—dark-green foliage-type vegetables.
4. **Bread and cereal group**—good for thiamine, iron, niacin, and other vitamins and minerals.
   a. *Pregnancy*—10 servings.
   b. *Lactation*—10 servings.

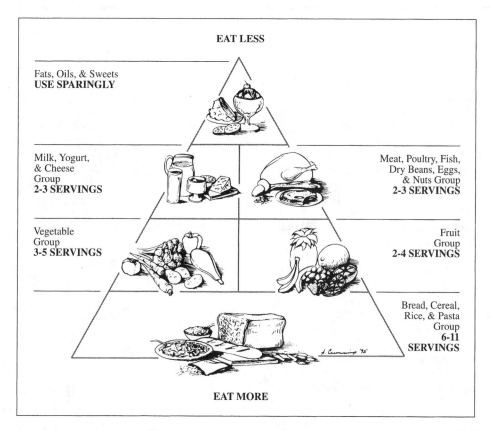

FIGURE 2.1 **FOOD GUIDE PYRAMID, A GUIDE TO DAILY FOOD CHOICES** (United States Department of Agriculture).

   c. *Count as one serving*—one slice bread, 1 ounce ready-to-eat cereal, ½ to ¾ cup cooked cereal, cornmeal, grits, macaroni, noodles, rice, or spaghetti.

5. Water (fluids)—six to eight 8 oz. glasses (1500–2000 mL)/d.

6. Energy—increase per day
   a. Pregnancy—300 calories (e.g., 1 C low-fat milk, 2 slices bread, and an orange).
   b. Lactation—500 calories (for each child).

7. Weight gain
   a. Average overall gain: 24–30 pounds; total of gain depends on prepregnancy weight for height (body mass index [BMI]), nutritional state (Table 2.6).
   b. Pattern:

Trimester	Gain	Site
1	1–2 kg (2–4 pounds)	Maternal tissues
2	Almost 0.4 kg (1 pound) per wk	Primarily in mother
3	Almost 0.4 kg (1 pound) per wk	Primarily in fetus

   c. *Consequences* of deviations from expected weight gain

TABLE 2.6 **RECOMMENDED TOTAL WEIGHT GAIN RANGES FOR PREGNANT WOMEN**[*]

Prepregnancy Weight-for-Height Category	Recommended Total Gain	
	Pounds	*kg*
Low (BMI < 19.8)	28–40	12.5–18
Normal (BMI 19.8–26)	25–35	11.5–16
High (BMI > 26.0–29.0)	15–25	7.0–11.5
Obese (BMI > 29.0)	≥15	≥7.0

BMI = body mass index.

[*] For singleton pregnancies. The range for women carrying *twins* is 35–45 pounds (16–20 kg). Young *adolescents* (<2 yr after menarche) and *African-American* women should strive for gains at the upper end of the range. *Short* women (<62 in. or <157 cm) should strive for gains at the lower end of the range.

Source: Nutrition During Pregnancy and Lactation: An Implementation Guide. Copyright © 1992 by the National Academy of Sciences. Courtesy National Academy Press, Washington, DC.

(1) *Underweight before* pregnancy: low-birth-weight (LBW) infant.
(2) *Inadequate* gain: LBW infants and intrauterine growth retardation (IUGR).
(3) *Overweight before* pregnancy: gestational diabetes, large baby, hypertension, and preeclampsia.
(4) *Excessive* gain: may indicate fluid retention and development of pre-eclampsia.

B. Assessment: (see also discussion, p. 36.)
  1. Interview—history including diet history and evaluation, food practices, living situation; access to food; inclusion or exclusion of any foods that could be problematic, such as adherence to a strict vegetarian diet, cultural, ethnic, religious food practices, or fad diets.
  2. Physical examination
    a. General appearance, including height and weight, posture, muscle tone, nervous control, general vitality.
    b. Signs of *malnutrition:* Dull, dry, brittle hair that is thin and sparse; rough, dry, scaly, pale skin; spongy, bleeding, or receding gums; unfilled caries, absent teeth; eye membranes dull; enlarged thyroid; rapid heart beat, abnormal heart rhythm; spoon-shaped, brittle nails.
    c. *Laboratory* tests—hemoglobin and hematocrit, serum folacin and B_{12}, serum albumin and total serum protein, glucose (urine and serum).

C. Analysis/nursing diagnosis
  1. *Altered nutrition:* more than body requirements related to a poor understanding of nutritional needs and optimal weight gain, cultural patterns, use of unneeded dietary supplements.
  2. *Altered nutrition:* high risk for more than body requirements related to same factors as for preceding diagnosis.

D. Nursing care plan/implementation
  1. Discuss dietary needs and assist in developing a dietary plan with input relating to preferences.
    a. *Ethnic* food patterns: Table 2.7.
    b. *Religious* considerations in meal planning.
      (1) Orthodox Jews
        (a) Kosher meat and poultry.
        (b) *No* shellfish or pork products.
        (c) Milk and dairy products *cannot* be consumed with meat or poultry; requires separate utensils.
      (2) Conservative and Reform Jews: dietary practices may vary from religious laws.
      (3) Muslims: no pork or alcohol.
      (4) Hindus: vegetarians (cows are sacred).
      (5) Seventh-Day Adventists
        (a) Vegetarianism is common (lacto-ovo).
        (b) *No* shellfish or pork products.

        (c) *Avoid* stimulants (coffee, tea, other caffeine sources).
        (d) *No* alcohol.
      (6) Mormons: *no* coffee, tea, or alcohol.
  c. Food list for ready reference in menu planning
    (1) High-cholesterol foods—over 50 mg/100-g portion: beef, butter, cheese, egg yolks, fish, kidney, liver, pork, veal.
    (2) High-sodium foods—over 500 mg/100-g portion: bacon—cured, Canadian; baking powder; beef—corned, cooked, canned, dried, creamed; biscuits, baking powder; bouillon cubes; bran, added sugar and malt; bran flakes with thiamine; raisins; breads—wheat, French, rye, white, whole wheat; butter, cheese—cheddar, parmesan, Swiss, pasteurized American; cocoa; cookies, gingersnaps; corn flakes; cornbread; crackers—graham, saltines; margarine; milk—dry, skim; mustard; oat products; olives—green, ripe; peanut butter; pickles, dill; popcorn with oil and salt; salad dressing—blue, Roquefort, French, thousand island; sausages—bologna, frankfurters; soy sauce; tomato catsup; tuna in oil.
    (3) High-potassium foods—more than 400 mg/100-g portion: almonds; bacon, Canadian; baking powder, low-sodium; beans—white, lima; beef, hamburger; bran with sugar and malt; cake—fruitcake, gingerbread; cashew nuts; chicken, light meat; cocoa; coffee, instant; cookies, gingersnaps; dates; garlic; milk—skim, powdered; peanuts, roasted; peanut butter; peas; pecans; potatoes, boiled in skin; scallops; tea, instant; tomato puree; turkey, light meat; veal; walnuts, black; yeast, brewer's.
    (4) Foods high in B vitamins
      (a) *Thiamine:* pork, dried beans, dried peas, liver, lamb, veal, nuts, peas.
      (b) *Riboflavin:* liver, poultry, beef, oysters, tongue, fish, cottage cheese, veal.
      (c) *Niacin:* liver, fish, poultry, peanut butter, lamb, veal, beef, pork.
    (5) Foods high in vitamin C: oranges, strawberries, dark green leafy vegetables, potatoes, grapefruit, tomato, cabbage, broccoli, melons, liver.
    (6) Foods high in iron, calcium, and residue
      (a) *Iron:* breads—brown, corn, ginger; fish, tuna; poultry; organ meats; whole-grain cereals; shell-

TABLE 2.7   ETHNIC FOOD PATTERNS — SELECTED EXAMPLES

Ethnic Group	Cultural Food Patterns	Dietary Excesses or Omissions
Mexican (native)	Basic sources of protein—dry beans, flan, cheese, many meats, fish, eggs; chili peppers and many deep-green and yellow vegetables; fruits include zapote, guava, papaya, mango, citrus; tortillas (corn, flour); sweet bread; fideo; tacos, burritos, enchiladas	*Limited* meats, milk, and milk products; some are using flour tortillas more than the more nutritious corn tortillas; *excessive* use of lard (manteca), sugar; tendency to boil vegetables for long periods of time
Filipino (Spanish-Chinese influence)	Most meats, eggs, nuts, legumes; many different kinds of vegetables; large amounts of rice and cereals	May *limit* meat, milk, and milk products (the latter may be due to lactose intolerance); tend to prewash rice; tend to fry many foods
Chinese (mostly Cantonese)	Cheese, soybean curd (tofu), many meats, chicken and pigeon eggs; nuts; legumes; many different vegetables, leaves, bamboo sprouts; rice and rice-flour products; wheat, corn, millet seed; green tea; mixtures of fish, pork, and chicken with vegetables—bamboo shoots, broccoli, cabbage, onions, mushrooms, pea pods	Tendency among some immigrants to use *excess* grease in cooking; may be *low* in protein, milk, and milk products (the latter may be due to lactose intolerance); often wash rice before cooking; large amounts of soy and oyster sauces, both of which are *high in salt*
Puerto Rican	Milk with coffee; pork, poultry, eggs, dried fish; beans (habichuelas); viandas (starchy vegetables; starchy ripe fruits); avocados, okra, eggplant, sweet yams; rice, cornmeal	Utilize *large* amounts of lard for cooking; *limited* use of milk and milk products; *limited* amounts of pork and poultry
African American	Milk with coffee; pork, poultry, eggs; fish; fruit: strawberries, watermelons; okra, collard greens, turnip greens, mustard greens, kale; sweet potatoes; cereals (including grits, hominy); corn breads; hot breads; molasses (dark molasses is especially good source of calcium, iron, vitamins B_1 and B_2, and niacin)	*Limited* use of milk group (lactose intolerance); extensive use of frying, "smothering," simmering for cooking; *large* amounts of fat: salt pork, bacon drippings, lard, gravies; may have *limited* use of citrus and enriched breads
Middle Eastern (Greek, Syrian, Armenian)	Yogurt; predominantly lamb, nuts, dried peas, beans, lentils; deep-green leaves and vegetables; dried fruits; dark breads and cracked wheat	Tend to use *excessive* sweeteners, lamb fat, olive oil; tend to fry meats and vegetables; *insufficient* milk and milk products (almost no butter—use olive oil, which has no nutritive value except for calories); deficiency in fresh fruits
Middle European (Polish)	Many milk products; pork, chicken; root vegetables (potatoes); cabbage; fruits; wheat products; sausages, smoked and cured meats; noodles, dumplings; bread; cream with coffee	Tend to use *excessive* sweets and to overcook vegetables; *limited* amounts of fruits (citrus), raw vegetables, and meats
Native American (American Indian—much variation)	If "Americanized," use milk and milk products; variety of meats: game, fowl, fish; nuts, seeds, legumes; variety of vegetables, some wild; variety of fruits, some wild, rose hips; roots; variety of breads, including tortillas, cornmeal, rice	*Nutrition-related problems:* obesity, diabetes, dental problems, iron-deficiency anemia; alcoholism; *limited* quantities of high-protein foods depending on availability (flocks) and economic situation; *excessive* use of sugar
Italian	Staples are pasta with sauces; bread; eggs; cheese; tomatoes and vegetables such as artichokes, eggplant, greens, and zucchini; only small amount of meat is used	*Limited* use of whole grains; *insufficient* servings from milk group; tendency to overcook vegetables; enjoy sweets

fish; egg yolk; fruits—apples, berries; dried fruits—dates, prunes, apricots, peaches, raisins; vegetables—dark-green leafy, potatoes, tomatoes, rhubarb, squash; molasses; dried beans and peas; peanut butter; brown sugar; noodles; rice.

(b) *Calcium:* milk—dry, skim, whole, evaporated, buttermilk; cheese—American, Swiss, hard; vegetables—kale; turnip greens; mustard greens; collards.

(c) *Residue:* whole-grain cereals—oatmeal, bran, shredded wheat; breads—whole-wheat, cracked wheat, rye, bran muffins; vegetables—lettuce, spinach, Swiss chard, raw carrots, raw celery, corn, cauliflower, eggplant, sauerkraut, cabbage; fruits—bananas, figs, apricots, oranges.

2. Make referrals as necessary—WIC (women, infants, and children) program or food stamps, etc.

3. Teach regarding supplementation, if ordered, e.g., take iron with vitamin C (citrus fruits, tomatoes, melons) when stomach is empty (take between meals); *avoid* bran, tea, coffee, milk, oxalates (in spinach and Swiss chard) and egg yolk when taking iron; keep this and all medications in a childproof container out of the reach of any children in the household. *Caution* against taking excessive amounts of vitamins.

✠ **E.** Evaluation/outcome criteria
  1. Woman remains healthy during pregnancy, shows adequate weight gain, and carries the pregnancy to term.
  2. Fetus is of adequate weight for age and shows no signs of maternal malnutrition.

IV. Childbirth preparation/parent education
  A. Methods
    1. *Grantly Dick-Read:* Childbirth is viewed as a natural event; education decreases fear and tension, and therefore pain; exercises improve muscle tone, increase relaxation; emphasis is on slow breathing, muscle relaxation, and pushing techniques.
    2. *Lamaze method (psychoprophylactic childbirth):* Focus is on developing a conditioned response to stimuli that then occupies nerve pathways, dulling pain perception; this is known as the **gate control theory.** This conditioned response combines relaxation, concentration on a focal point, and complex breathing patterns.
    3. *Bradley ("father-coached"):* Similar to the Dick-Read method with the addition of a coach; emphasis is on slow breathing and deep relaxation.

B. Content
  1. General: prenatal care, nutrition, labor and birth including cesarean birth, postpartum care, coping strategies: self-care, relaxation, breathing, and exercise. Most include asking the expectant parent(s) to develop a birth plan, which includes choice of attendant at labor and birth, birthing environment, type of pain control desired, etc.
  2. Relaxation methods
    a. Imagery, aroma therapy, music therapy, effleurage, biofeedback, hypnosis, yoga.
    b. **Kegel's exercises:** Woman locates the correct (pubococcygeal) muscles by stopping her flow of urine. Then she can perform the exercises in one of the following ways. *Slow:* tighten the muscle, hold it for the count of three, and relax it. *Quick:* tighten the muscle, and relax it as rapidly as possible. *Push out, pull in:* Pull up the entire pelvic floor as though trying to suck up water into the vagina. Then bear down as if trying to push the imaginary water out. This version uses abdominal muscles as well. Exercises should be practiced 10 times in a row, at least 3 times or more per day.
  3. Programs offered during different trimesters
    a. *First:* anatomy/physiology, fetal development, nutrition, sexuality, early discomforts.
    b. *Second* and *third:* same as above, and preparation for labor and birth, infant care, parenting.
  4. Family programs: siblings and grandparents.
  5. Birthing environments
    a. Hospital: traditional; LDR (labor-delivery-recovery) rooms and/or LDRP (labor-delivery-recovery-postpartum rooms), with homelike accommodations and technology available if needed.
    b. Freestanding birth center.
    c. Home birth.

✠ **C.** Assessment
  1. Knowledge of available resources, prenatal care, nutrition.
  2. Available support system: who will coach?
  3. Cultural and ethnic variations that apply.

✠ **D.** Analysis/nursing diagnosis
  1. *Knowledge deficit* related to resources available, self-care during pregnancy and labor and birth.
  2. *Ineffective individual coping* related to lack of knowledge of childbirthing environment, comfort measures available.

✠ **E.** Evaluation/outcome criteria
  1. Parent(s) verbalizes satisfaction with information given regarding available childbirthing methods and environments.
  2. Parent(s) verbalizes satisfaction with choices she/he made.

3. Parent(s) learn relaxation techniques, breathing patterns.
4. Parent(s) express feeling more confident and having less anxiety about the coming experiences.

V. Warning signs of potential problems
  A. Etiology: Specific disease processes are discussed in Chapter 3.
  ⋈ B. Nursing care plan/implementation: Goal: *health teaching*—to safeguard status. Signs to report *immediately:*

⋈ *Signs/Symptoms*	*Possible Causes*
Persistent vomiting beyond first trimester, or severe vomiting any time	Hyperemesis gravidarum
Fluid discharge from vagina—bleeding or amniotic fluid (anything other than leukorrhea)	Placental problem, rupture of membrane (ROM)
Severe or unusual pain: abdominal	Abruptio placentae
Chills or fever	Infection
Burning on urination	UTI
Absence of fetal movements after quickening	Intrauterine fetal death
Visual disturbances (blurring, double vision, "spots before eyes")	Preeclampsia
Swelling of fingers or face	Preeclampsia
Severe, frequent, or continual headache	Preeclampsia
Muscle irritability or convulsions	Preeclampsia
Uterine contractions every 10 min for 1 hr, or menstrual-like cramping, pelvic pressure, low backache, or bloody spotting or leaking of fluid from vagina	Preterm labor

⋈ C. Evaluation/outcome criteria: The woman/family
  1. Actively participates in own health maintenance/pregnancy management.
  2. Identifies early signs of potentially serious complications during the antepartal period.
  3. Promptly reports signs/symptoms and seeks medical attention.

Summary

The prenatal period is one of growth and change in the woman and the fetus. Prenatal visits are scheduled to provide the maximum supervision during this critical period. The woman (family) needs to learn about the *alterations* in the body sys-

tems, some *common discomforts* and how to cope with them, *emotional changes, warning signs* that need to be reported immediately to the physician/midwife/nurse practitioner, *nutrition,* and *childbirth preparation resources.* This period presents the nurse with an ideal time to teach health maintenance because of the parents' heightened readiness to learn.

💡 Study and Memory Aids

Sex Determination Chromosomes

Female	XX
Male	YY

Stages of Prenatal Development

Ovum
↓
Embryo
↓
Fetus

Prenatal Development by Trimester

1st	Organogenesis
2nd	Growth
3rd	Storage

Laboratory Values—General Effects of Pregnancy

↓ Blood values (dilution due to ↑ blood volume)
↑ Sedimentation rate
↑ WBC

Recording Gravidity/Parity

G—gravida
T—term
P—preterm
A—abortions
L—living children

Validation of Pregnancy

Presumptive signs and symptoms
Probable signs
Positive signs

Questions

1. The nurse is assessing the adequacy of the diet of a 30-year-old gravida 3, para 2, who is 4 wk pregnant. The woman has been a vegan-vegetarian (eats no eggs or dairy products) for 8 yr. To which food group(s) should the nurse pay particular attention?
   1. Grains.
   2. Protein foods.
   3. Vitamin C–rich foods.
   4. Fruits and vegetables.

2. The nurse is planning diet teaching for a 17-year-old primigravida at 30 wk gestation, who is diagnosed with iron-deficiency anemia. She takes her iron and vitamin supplements sporadically because of unacceptable gastrointestinal side effects, but eats many foods that are high in iron. Which nutrient will the nurse emphasize to promote heme production?
   1. Niacin.
   2. Vitamin A.
   3. Vitamin D.
   4. Folic acid.

3. The nurse knows additional nutrition counselling is needed when a woman states that her need for additional vitamin C intake increases if she:
   1. Smokes.
   2. Drinks more than 2 cups of caffeinated coffee each day.
   3. Uses oral hormonal contraceptives.
   4. Drinks more than 8 oz. of alcohol every day.

4. The nurse's health teaching for self-care related to "morning sickness" during pregnancy should include instructions to:
   1. Eat dry carbohydrates.
   2. Use antiemetics per physician's directions.
   3. Eat three large meals per day.
   4. Eat highly seasoned foods to increase taste appeal.

5. At midpregnancy, the nurse expects a pregnant woman's blood pressure (BP) to:
   1. Fall by 10–15 mm Hg.
   2. Increase by 10–15 mm Hg.
   3. Remain the same.
   4. Fall below her baseline, then rise above her baseline by the end of pregnancy.

6. During which time period should the nurse first expect a pregnant woman to experience physiologic anemia, relaxation of the ureters, linea nigra, and increasing introspection?
   1. First trimester.
   2. Second trimester.
   3. Third trimester.
   4. Postpartum.

7. In planning care with a pregnant woman, the nurse needs to consider that normal cardiovascular adaptations to pregnancy include:
   1. A 30–50% increase in blood volume.
   2. A decrease in sedimentation rate.
   3. A gradual increase in blood pressure.
   4. An immediate increase in hematocrit.

8. During a parent education class, a woman in her 6th month of pregnancy expresses concern that she is "short of breath," feels her uterus up under her ribs, and wonders if she gets enough air for herself and her baby. To ease her anxiety, the nurse bases a response on knowledge that maternal adaptation allows for an increase in volume of tidal air, because:
   1. The diaphragm is displaced upward by about 3 cm.
   2. The heart is displaced upward and to the left of the midclavicular line.
   3. Expansion of lower ribs increases.
   4. Blood volume is increased by about one-third.

9. In preparing prenatal parent education classes, the nurse knows that one characteristic of the third trimester of pregnancy is that:
   1. Quickening occurs.
   2. The uterus becomes an abdominal organ.
   3. It is the best time to learn relaxation and breathing for labor.
   4. The mother experiences increased concern about acceptance of coming baby by husband and other children.

10. In the tenth week of pregnancy, a woman is concerned about her dark nipples and the dark line beginning from her symphysis pubis in the midline. The nurse explains that these pregnancy changes are temporary and are due to hyperactivity of the:
    1. Ovaries.
    2. Pituitary gland.
    3. Adrenal gland.
    4. Thyroid gland.

11. Ferrous sulfate, 300 mg every day, has been ordered for a pregnant adolescent. The nurse can best evaluate patient compliance by:
    1. Asking her if her stools are black.
    2. Asking her if she is taking it as ordered.
    3. Assessing fundal height for fetal growth.
    4. Assessing hemoglobin and hematocrit.

12. The nurse instructs an expectant couple that travel during pregnancy is safest during which trimester(s)?
    1. First.
    2. Second.
    3. Third.
    4. All trimesters, equally.

13. The nurse is planning a preconception counseling class for a group of women who enjoy an active life-style that includes a great deal of exercise, such as jogging. The nurse needs to include in the plan teaching that maximal exercise during pregnancy has been associated with:
    1. Maternal arrhythmia.
    2. Maternal bradycardia.
    3. Fetal bradycardia.
    4. Fetal tachycardia.

14. To plan care for a pregnant adolescent, the nurse should ask her:
    1. "How are your parents taking your being pregnant?"
    2. "Did you get along with your mother when you were growing up?"
    3. "When did you become sexually active?"
    4. "Why did you become pregnant?"

15. An expectant couple request prenatal classes because they want "everything to go just right with this pregnancy."' The nurse knows that the primary purpose of prenatal classes is to:
    1. Prepare for childbirth.
    2. Experience childbirth without tension or fear in order to decrease the perception of pain.
    3. Minimize amount of analgesia and/or anesthesia the mother will need.
    4. Minimize the possibility of dystocia and/or medical/surgical intervention.

16. A prenatal nurse's intake interview must include an obstetric history as a basis for risk management. A pregnant woman whose history reveals one pregnancy that ended in a miscarriage at 11 wk should be recorded as a:
    1. Primigravida.
    2. Multipara.
    3. Gravida 1, para 1.
    4. Gravida 2, para 0.

17. A woman has had her initial clinic visit for a pregnancy of 8 wk duration. Before she leaves, the nurse tells her that at each prenatal visit she can expect to have:
    1. Finger stick for hemoglobin and hematocrit.
    2. Measurement of fundal height.
    3. Collection of urine for culture.
    4. An ultrasound test.

18. While giving her diet history, a pregnant woman indicates she cannot tolerate milk and does not eat meat. The nurse can suggest alternate protein-rich foods, such as:
    1. Pasta, cereal, and bread made with fortified flour.
    2. Broccoli, green beans, potatoes.
    3. Cooked dry beans, tofu, and peanut butter.
    4. Eggs, yogurt, nuts.

19. At the end of a prenatal class, the nurse evaluates the women's (couples') understanding of warning signs/symptoms of pregnancy. Which statement by a woman would indicate a need for further evaluation/intervention?
    1. "I will report any burning on urination and urinary frequency to my midwife."
    2. "I will see my eye doctor if I have a bad headache and blurred vision."
    3. "I will report severe vomiting to my doctor."
    4. "If I cough and have to sit up to breathe, I will call the doctor."

20. A woman's LMP started March 23; she "spotted a little" on April 23. The nurse tells her that she can expect to give birth on:
    1. January 16.
    2. January 30.
    3. December 16.
    4. December 30.

21. The nurse notes the following physiologic changes in the chart of a pregnant woman. Which changes are abnormal?
    1. Hgb ↑, sedimentation rate ↓, respirations 28, BMR ↓ 25%.
    2. Hct ↓, glucosuria, BP ↓, palpitations.
    3. Vaginal pH 6.5, pulse 92, urinary frequency, leukorrhea.

4. Montgomery's tubercles, audible S_1–S_2 split, slightly ↓ clotting time, funic souffle.

22. The nurse knows intervention is required when a pregnant woman states that she relieves:
    1. Morning sickness by eating dry toast before getting out of bed.
    2. Leg cramps by plantar-flexing her foot to point her toes.
    3. Heartburn by bending at the knees instead of leaning over.
    4. Constipation by eating raw fruits, vegetables, and wheat bread.

23. To prevent heartburn, the nurse advises the pregnant woman to:
    1. Sleep lying flat in a lateral position.
    2. Eat dry, unsalted carbohydrates at bedtime.
    3. Bend from the waist.
    4. Avoid coffee or cigarette smoke.

24. A woman of standard weight for height (BMI [body mass index] 19.8–26) at the start of her pregnancy is encouraged by the nurse to gain:
    1. No more than 10 pounds.
    2. 10–20 pounds.
    3. 25–35 pounds.
    4. Just enough to keep her Hgb at a minimum of 12 g.

25. The nurse should counsel a pregnant woman that the lunch menu that provides the most calcium is:
    1. One cup low-fat yogurt, rhubarb pie.
    2. Turkey on white toast, orange juice.
    3. Bagel with peanut butter, one ear of corn.
    4. Spaghetti and meatballs with tomato sauce.

26. The nurse should advise a pregnant woman that the snack that provides the most iron is:
    1. One ounce cheddar cheese and crackers.
    2. One cup tapioca pudding.
    3. One-half cup tuna salad and water wafers.
    4. One-half cup dried peaches or apricots.

27. A pregnant woman's obstetric history reveals one elective abortion and one child at home. The nurse determines her gravidity and parity to be:
    1. G-2, P-1001.
    2. G-3, P-1011.
    3. G-3, P-1111.
    4. G-3, P-0121.

28. During a parent education class for expectant parents, a spouse/partner of a pregnant woman asks how to be of most assistance during the pregnancy. The nurse-led discussion identifies that the most helpful response would be to:
    1. Give sympathy regarding the discomforts of pregnancy.
    2. Assist with household duties.
    3. Meet the expectant mother's needs for affection and support.
    4. Encourage the expectant mother to keep her weight within prescribed limits.

29. In planning the care of a pregnant 16-year-old, the nurse should set goals based on the knowledge that the teen will most likely be:
    1. Self-centered.
    2. In need of instant gratification.

3. Realistic in coping with stress.

4. Emotionally independent from her parents.

30. Which finding needs further assessment to rule out cardiac decompensation in a pregnant woman?

1. Exaggerated splitting of the first heart sound.

2. Heart rate increased by 10–15 beats/min.

3. Respirations: 25/min.

4. Occasional shortness of breath at rest.

31. The nurse knows intervention is required when a pregnant woman states that she relieves:

1. Morning sickness by eating dry toast before going to bed at night.

2. Leg cramps by dorsiflexing her foot to point her heel.

3. Heartburn by assuming the knee-to-chest position.

4. Backache by wearing a maternity bra and low-heeled shoes.

32. A pregnant woman states that she has lactose intolerance and cannot drink milk, but knows how important calcium is during pregnancy. The nurse counsels her that a food source high in calcium and low in lactose is:

1. Cottage cheese.

2. Swiss cheese.

3. Eggs.

4. Yogurt.

Answers/Rationale

1. **(2)** Vegetarians who omit dairy foods may be unable to meet the requirement for an additional 30 g protein per day over their nonpregnant needs. Individuals who have been vegetarians for some time usually have evolved diets adequate in grain intake **(1)**, along with a wide variety of vitamin C–rich fruits and vegetables **(3 and 4)**, which meet pregnancy requirements not only for vitamin C, but also for fiber and other nutrients. **AS, 4, PhI**

2. **(4)** Folic acid (folacin) is essential for increased heme production for hemoglobin and prevention of megaloblastic anemia. Niacin **(1)** has no direct or indirect role in erythropoiesis or heme production. Vitamin A **(2)** is essential for *fetal bone growth* and tooth development. Vitamin D **(3)** is essential for *mineralization of bone tissue* and calcium and phosphorus absorption. **PL, 4, PhI**

3. **(2)** Since coffee does not increase one's need for additional vitamin C, additional counseling is needed. The actions in options **1, 3,** and **4** *do* increase one's need for additional vitamin C. **EV, 4, HPM**

4. **(1)** Eating dry carbohydrates, such as unbuttered toast, crackers, or popcorn, before arising slowly is one preventive measure. Others include avoiding unpleasant odors or greasy foods. Medications **(2)** are generally not prescribed for this discomfort of pregnancy. She should eat six small meals, rather than three large meals **(3)**. Highly seasoned foods **(4)** can contribute to this discomfort. **IMP, 4, HPM**

5. **(1)** At midpregnancy, the healthy woman's BP drops by about 10–15 mm Hg. If it remains at her baseline, she is observed for possible preeclampsia in her third trimester. The BP decreases *rather than* increasing **(2)** or remaining the same **(3)**. The BP should rise to the woman's normal range, *not* above **(4)**, by term. **EV, 5, HPM**

6. **(2)** Physiologic anemia, relaxation of ureters, linea nigra, and increasing introspection are usually seen first in the second trimester. The time periods in options **1, 3,** and **4** are all incorrect: The maternal adaptations listed all appear first during the *second* trimester. **AN, 5, HPM**

7. **(1)** There is a 30–50% increase in blood volume during pregnancy; therefore, the nurse can expect physiologic anemia, altered laboratory test results, altered response to blood loss, and increased stress on the cardiovascular system. An increase, not a decrease **(2)** is seen in the sedimentation rate, due to the increase in globulins and fibrinogen products. There is a small *drop* in BP, not increase **(3)**, at midpregnancy, with a gradual rise to within the woman's normal range at term pregnancy. Initially, there seems to be a *drop* in hematocrit, not an increase **(4)**, due to physiologic anemia. **PL, 6, HPM**

8. **(3)** The lower ribs expand; thus, tidal air volume can increase. Women can be reassured that although respiratory rate increases only slightly (2/min), they do breathe deeper. A feeling of shortness of breath is normal. Because of rib expansion plus breast development, a maternity bra is needed. Although the diaphragm is displaced upward by 3 cm **(1)**, that adaptation does *not* result in an increase in volume of tidal air. Although the heart is displaced upward and to the left of the midclavicular line **(2)**, that adaptation does *not* result in an increase in volume of tidal air. Although the blood volume is increased **(4)**, that adaptation does *not* result in an increase in volume of tidal air. **IMP, 6, HPM**

9. **(3)** The third trimester is the best time to learn relaxation and breathing for labor. The expectant mother experiences ambivalence in trimester one and introspection in trimester two. Thoughts of labor become foremost as the expected date of birth approaches (e.g., she becomes ready to learn). Quickening, or feeling of life **(1)**, is characteristic of the *second* trimester. The uterus becomes an abdominal organ **(2)** between the end of *first* and start of the *second* trimester. The feelings in option **4** usually surface during the *second* trimester. **AN, 5, HPM**

10. (2) The melanotropin from the anterior pituitary gland increases during pregnancy; this hormone is responsible for increased pigmentation. Because of the feedback mechanism, the ovaries **(1)** are *quiescent* during pregnancy. Hyperactivity of the adrenal gland **(3)** results in symptoms of Cushing's syndrome, which are not seen during pregnancy. Hyperactivity of the thyroid gland **(4)** would manifest as increased temperature, pulse, and respirations. **IMP, 5, HPM**

11. (4) Assessing hemoglobin and hematocrit provides evidence of compliance with prescribed therapy. Black stools **(1)** may or may not mean that she is taking the medication; they could also indicate internal GI bleeding. If asked about compliance **(2)**, the adolescent will probably answer the way she thinks the nurse wants her to; in addition, she may feel threatened if asked whether she has "obeyed." Assessing fundal height **(3)** does not provide the data needed to evaluate patient compliance with the medication. **EV, 6, HPM**

12. (2) Travel during pregnancy is safest during the second trimester. If traveling to high altitudes or flying in unpressurized airplanes (some private planes), susceptible women may experience spontaneous abortion in the first trimester **(1)** and preterm labor in the third trimester **(3)**. Therefore, travel is safest during the *second* trimester, not all trimesters **(4)**. **IMP, 1, HPM**

13. (3) Maximal exercise during pregnancy has been associated with fetal bradycardia. Maternal arrhythmia **(1)** is not associated with maximal exercise. Maternal exercise is safe up to 148 beats/min (approximately 70% of maximal aerobic power); at this level there is little risk of fetal bradycardia **(2)**. Fetal bradycardia, not tachycardia **(4)**, follows maximal exercise. **IMP, 3, HPM**

14. (1) To develop a therapeutic plan of care for the pregnant adolescent, it is important to know how the parents are reacting to the pregnancy. In addition, this tells the adolescent that the nurse understands that this is an emotionally charged area. The questions in options **2, 3,** and **4** are irrelevant and may sound judgmental and condescending to the adolescent. **IMP, 7, HPM**

15. (1) Prenatal classes prepare parents for labor and childbirth, and possible unexpected outcomes. They also clarify misconceptions, and suggest various means of self-help (e.g., relaxation techniques). No one type of method can guarantee that all tension or fear will be *eliminated* **(2)**, although the perception of pain may be decreased. Childbirth preparation does help the woman to cope better with the labor and may be one factor in minimizing the amount of pharmacologic pain relief she will need **(3)**, but that is *not* the *primary* purpose of childbirth classes. Childbirth preparation may have a positive effect on the course of labor and the ability to cope with dystocia **(4)**, but it *cannot* eliminate dystocia for some women, and *cannot* guarantee a labor/birth without medical/surgical intervention. **PL, 5, HPM**

16. (4) This is her second pregnancy; she is gravida 2. She has carried no pregnancy past the age of viability; she is para 0. She is a secunda gravida (pregnant for the second time), not a primigravida (**1** and **3**). She is a nullipara since she has not yet retained a pregnancy past the age of viability at 22 wk, *not* a multipara **(2)** or primipara **(3)**. NOTE: Using the five-digit system (GTPAL), this woman is 2-0-0-1-0. This is her second pregnancy **(2)**, she has carried no pregnancy to term (T), she has had no preterm births (P), she has had one abortion (A), and she has no living children (L). **AN, 5, HPM**

17. (2) She can expect fundal height to be measured at each clinic visit as one means of assessing the growth of the fetus. Hgb and Hct **(1)** are done at the initial visit and then repeated at about 30–32 wk in most cases. Urine cultures **(3)** are done only if there is an indication of urinary tract infection. An ultrasound **(4)** is not done for every woman. Some women may have one to determine fetal age and growth and development, or to rule out possible hydramnios, etc. **EV, 5, HPM**

18. (3) Cooked dry beans, tofu (a soybean product), and peanut butter all contain vegetable protein. Bread products alone **(1)** do *not* provide sufficient protein. The vegetables in option **2** are *not* high in protein. Yogurt **(4)** is a milk product, which she *cannot* tolerate. **IMP, 4, HPM**

19. (2) The nurse will need to intervene if the woman thinks that headache with blurred vision is reportable to an *eye* doctor; these symptoms may be indicative of preeclampsia, and should be reported to the woman's health care provider (physician/midwife). Women *should* report possible UTIs **(1)**, hyperemesis gravidarum **(3)**, or cardiac decompensation **(4)** to the physician or midwife, and therefore no intervention is needed. **EV, 2, HPM**

20. (4) To determine the expected date of birth (EDB), identify the start of the LMP, count forward 9 mo, and add 7 days. March 23 is the correct LMP, since about 25% of women "spot" during the time of their first missed period following conception. (Nagele's rule is used to calculate the due date; however, counting forward 9 mo from the LMP and adding 7 days is the easier method.) Options **1, 2,** and **3** are all incorrect: None follows the known methods of calculating the expected date of birth. NOTE: If the woman's cycles are extremely short or extremely long, the EDB is adjusted accordingly. **IMP, 5, HPM**

21. (1) This list includes abnormal changes. Hgb normally *decreases* in pregnancy secondary to increased plasma volume (physiologic anemia); sedimentation rate normally *increases* (therefore, it cannot be used in evaluating for infection); respirations usually remain at the same rate; BMR *increases* by 25%. The other options list *normal* changes. Option **2:** Hct *does* decrease as a result of physiologic anemia during pregnancy; glucosuria is *normal;* BP *does* decrease by 10–15 mm Hg during the second trimester; palpitations are *normal.* Option **3:** Vaginal pH *is* less acidic (6.5) during pregnancy (making the woman more vulnerable to vaginal infections); pulse *does* increase about 10 beats/min; urinary frequency *is* common; leukorrhea (whitish, watery vaginal discharge in increased amounts) *is* common. Option **4:** Montgomery's tubercles *do* become more prominent around the areola during pregnancy; the increased cardiac output and plasma volume *do* result in the audible S_1–S_2 split; the tendency to coagulate increases; the funic souffle is the sound of blood in the fetal umbilical cord (the souffle is the same as the FHR). **AN, 5, HPM**

22. **(2)**   The nurse must intervene because plantar-flexing the foot will aggravate the cramp; the woman should *dorsiflex* her foot to point the *heel*, thus stretching the gastrocnemius muscle and relieving the cramp. For the other options, the nurse does not need to intervene; the pregnant woman *is* using the *correct* methods to prevent/relieve morning sickness **(1)**, heartburn **(3)**, and constipation **(4)**. **EV, 3, HPM**

23. **(4)**   Coffee and cigarette smoke can increase the risk for heartburn because of their irritating effect on the stomach lining. She should sleep propped up on pillows, not flat **(1)**; this position helps to keep the stomach from being compressed by the growing uterus, thus preventing stomach contents from entering the esophagus through the pregnancy-caused relaxed pyloric sphincter. Eating dry unsalted carbohydrates **(2)** before getting *out* of bed is a preventative measure for "*morning sickness.*" Bending from the waist **(3)** encourages stomach contents to re-enter the esophagus through the relaxed pyloric sphincter; she should bend at the *knees*, not from the waist. The question asks for an intervention that *prevents* heartburn, not one that *treats/relieves* it **(4)**. **IMP, 3, HPM**

24. **(3)**   To meet energy needs for normal pregnancy, an adequate weight gain is necessary: for this woman, 25–35 pounds. The amounts in options **1, 2** and **4** are not within the range of weight gain recommended by the National Academy of Sciences (1992). **IMP, 4, HPM**

25. **(1)**   One cup yogurt has 415 mg calcium; rhubarb pie has 211 mg. Calcium needs during pregnancy increase from 800 mg/d to 1200 mg/d. The other menus provide less calcium. Option **2**: Turkey = 7 mg; orange juice = 27 mg. Option **3**: Bagel = 9 mg; peanut butter = 9 mg; one ear of corn = 2 mg. Option **4**: Spaghetti and meatballs with tomato sauce = 20 mg. NOTE: Calcium, HCl, and ascorbic acid are needed for the absorption of iron. **IMP, 4, HPM**

26. **(4)**   Dried peaches have 5 mg iron; apricots have 3.6 mg. The other foods contain less iron: 1 ounce cheddar cheese **(1)** = 0.2 mg, 1 cup tapioca pudding **(2)** = 0.7 mg, and ½ cup tuna salad **(3)** = 1.4 mg. NOTE: The iron effect in the body is increased with vitamin C, and is decreased with milk (and other dairy foods), eggs, whole-grain bread and cereal, and tea. Iron supplements are to be taken 1 hr before or 2 hr after meals, with liquid (water, orange juice—but not with milk or tea). The nurse should caution women that their stools may appear black. **IMP, 4, HPM**

27. **(2)**   This woman has been pregnant three times; therefore, she is a G3; she has had one full-term pregnancy, no preterm births, one elective abortion, and one living child. The numbers in options **1, 3,** and **4** do not match her status. **AN, 5, HPM**

28. **(3)**   The expectant mother needs affection and support to assist her transition to the mothering role. Although expressing sympathy **(1)** may help somewhat, it is a less active form of support than meeting her needs for affection. Assisting with household duties **(2)** is a definite "plus," but meeting her needs for affection and support takes priority at this time. Encouraging her about her weight **(4)** can be seen as controlling or scolding, and could be construed by her as nonsupportive. **IMP, 7, PsI**

29. **(1)**   Self-centeredness is characteristic of adolescence. Option **2** reflects a characteristic of a younger age (e.g., toddlers), although some adults may occasionally demonstrate this trait. Option **3** is incorrect since at this stage of psychosocial development, she has not developed cognitively to the point of being realistic in coping with stress. Option **4** is incorrect since she is only now learning how to become independent from her parents; pregnancy interrupts this developmental phase. **PL, 6, PsI**

30. **(3)**   Rapid respirations, 25 breaths per minute or more, may suggest cardiac decompensation; further assessment is needed. The findings in options **1, 2,** and **4** are *normal* manifestations of adaptations to pregnancy. NOTE: The woman should also be assessed for other symptoms of cardiac decompensation (increasing fatigue or dyspnea, or both, with usual activities; frequent coughing and feeling of smothering; palpitations), and for other signs (irregular, weak, rapid pulse [100 beats/min or more]; progressive, generalized edema; crackles [rales] at base of lungs; orthopnea; moist, frequent cough; cyanosis of lips and nail beds). **EV, 6, PhI**

31. **(1)**   The nurse must intervene since a dry, unsalted carbohydrate (toast, cracker, popcorn) should be taken before getting *out* of bed in the *morning*. For the other options, the nurse will *not* have to intervene because the pregnant woman is using the correct methods to prevent/relieve leg cramps **(2)**, heartburn **(3)**, and backache **(4)**. NOTE: The knee-to-chest position also helps to expel burps and flatus. **EV, 4, HPM**

💡 Read the *entire* option.

32. **(2)**   Swiss cheese is high in calcium and low in lactose, and therefore an excellent food source during pregnancy. The foods in options **1, 3,** and **4** are high in calcium *and* lactose. **IM, 4, HPM**

High-Risk Conditions and Complications During Pregnancy

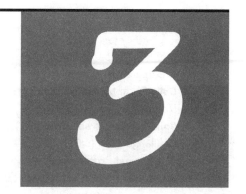

Chapter Outline

- Diagnostic Tests To Evaluate Fetal Growth and Well-Being
  - Daily Fetal Movement Count (DFMC)
  - Nonstress Test (NST)
  - Contraction Stress Test (CST); Oxytocin Challenge Test (OCT)
  - Biophysical Profile (BPP)
  - Ultrasound
  - Amniocentesis
  - Analysis of Amniotic Fluid
  - Chorionic Villous Sampling (CVS)
- Summary
- Study and Memory Aids
- Questions
- Answers/Rationale

🔑 KEY POINTS

- Risk factors affecting the pregnancy and fetus/neonate include *anatomic, physiologic, therapeutic, environmental,* and *idiopathic* events.
- Hypertensive disorders, infections, and hemorrhage are leading causes of maternal and perinatal morbidity and mortality worldwide.
- Effects of alcohol and substance abuse, sexually transmitted diseases (STDs), and genital and perigenital infections are biologic events, for which all individuals have a right to expect objective, compassionate, and effective health care.
- Preexistent and concurrent endocrine, cardiovascular, and medical-surgical problems are *affected* by pregnancy, and *affect* the pregnancy and its outcome.
- Nurses skilled in home care can significantly affect the outcome of the pregnancy and the newborn.

Key Words

Cardiac decompensation
Cerclage
Cullen's sign
Fomites
Gestational trophoblastic disease (GTD)
Glycosylated hemoglobin (Hgb$_{Alc}$)
Kehr's sign
Learned helplessness
Phosphatidylglycerol
Rape trauma syndrome
Rh incompatibility
  Isoimmunization
  Coombs test

High-Risk Conditions

I. General aspects
  A. Etiology
    1. Normal alterations and increasing physiologic stress of pregnancy affect status of coexisting medical disorders.
    2. Conditions affecting mother's general health also affect ability to adapt successfully to normal physiologic stress of pregnancy.
    3. Aberrations of normal pregnancy.
  B. Goal: *reduce incidence of health problems affecting maternal/fetal health and pregnancy outcome*
    1. Identify presence of risk factors and signs and symptoms of complications early.
    2. Treat emerging complications promptly and effectively.
    3. Minimize effects of complications on pregnancy outcome.
  ▶ C. **Assessment:** risk factors
    1. *Age*
      a. Adolescent, ≤17 yr.
      b. Primigravida, age 35 or older.
      c. Multigravida, age 40 or older.
    2. *Socioeconomic* level: lower.
    3. *Ethnic group/race:* higher perinatal/newborn mortality and morbidity among nonwhite groups.
    4. Previous pregnancy *history*
      a. Habitual abortion.
      b. Multiparity greater than 5.
      c. Previous stillbirths.
      d. Previous cesarean birth.
      e. Preterm labor.
    5. *Multifetal pregnancy.*
    6. *Prenatal* care
      a. Enters health care system late in pregnancy.
      b. Irregular/episodic prenatal care visits.
      c. Noncompliance with medical/nursing recommendations.
    7. *Pre- or coexisting medical disorders*
      a. Cardiovascular: hypertension, heart disease (e.g., women who have taken methyldopa for hypertension for more than 1 yr may have direct and indirect *Coombs*-positive hemolytic anemia).
      b. Diabetes.
      c. Other: renal, respiratory, infections, acquired immunodeficiency syndrome (AIDS).
    8. Substance abuse.
  ▶ D. **Nursing care plan/implementation**

1. Goal: *health teaching* (discussed under specific health problem).
2. Goal: *early identification/treatment of emerging health problems* (if any).
   a. Monitor status and progress of pregnancy.
   b. Refer for medical management, as necessary.
3. Goal: *emotional support.*

E. Evaluation/outcome criteria: the woman (family)
1. Understands present health status, interactions of coexisting disorder and pregnancy.
2. Accepts responsibility for own health maintenance.
3. Makes informed decisions regarding pregnancy.
4. Minimizes potential for complications of coexisting disorder/pregnancy.
   a. Avoids factors predisposing to health problems.
   b. Understands and implements therapeutic management of coexisting disorder/pregnancy.
   c. Increases compliance with medical/nursing recommendations.
5. Carries uneventful pregnancy to successful termination.

II. Disorders affecting fluid-gas transport: *cardiac disease*
   A. Pathophysiology: cardiac overload → cardiac decompensation → right-sided failure → pulmonary edema.
   B. Etiology
   1. Congenital heart defects.
   2. Valvular damage—due to rheumatic fever; most common lesion is mitral stenosis, which can lead to pulmonary edema and emboli.
   3. Increased circulating-blood volume and cardiac output—exceeds cardiac reserve. Greatest risk: *after 28 wk gestation*—reaches maximum (30–50%) volume increase; *postpartum*—due to diuresis.
   4. Secondary to treatment (e.g., tocolysis and betamethasone)
   5. Pregnancy after valve replacement.
   C. Normal physiologic alterations during pregnancy that *mimic cardiac disorders*
   1. Systolic murmurs, palpitations, tachycardia, and hyperventilation with some dyspnea on normal moderate exertion.
   2. Edema of lower extremities.
   3. Cardiac enlargement.
   4. Elevated sedimentation rate near term.
   D. Assessment
   1. Medical evaluation of cardiac status. Classification of severity of cardiac involvement:
      a. *Class I*—least affected; asymptomatic with ordinary activity.
      b. *Class II*—activities somewhat limited; ordinary activities cause fatigue, dyspnea, angina.
      c. *Class III*—moderate/marked limitation of

activity; common activities result in severe symptoms of fatigue, etc.
      d. *Class IV*—most affected; symptomatic (dyspnea, angina) at rest; should avoid pregnancy.
   2. **Emergency: cardiac decompensation**
      a. **Subjective Symptoms**
         (1) Palpitations; feeling that her heart is "racing."
         (2) Increasing fatigue or difficulty in breathing, or both, with her usual activities.
         (3) Feeling of smothering and/or frequent cough.
         (4) Periorbital edema; edema of face, fingers (e.g., rings do not fit anymore), feet, legs.
      b. **Objective Signs**
         (1) Irregular, weak, rapid pulse (≥100 beats/min).
         (2) Rapid respirations (≥25 breaths/min).
         (3) Progressive, generalized edema.
         (4) Crackles (rales) at base of lungs, after two inspirations and exhalations.
         (5) Orthopnea; increasing dyspnea on minimal physical activity.
         (6) Moist, frequent cough.
         (7) Cyanosis of lips and nail beds.
   E. Analysis/nursing diagnosis
   1. *Fluid volume excess* related to inability of compromised heart to handle increased workload (decreased cardiac reserve → heart failure).
   2. *Impaired gas exchange* related to pulmonary edema secondary to heart failure (HF).
   F. Nursing care plan/implementation
   1. **Medical management**
      a. *Diuretics*, electrolyte supplements.
      b. **Digitalis**
         (1) Dose may need to be higher because of dilution in the increased blood volume of pregnancy.
         ! (2) Alert: shortens the length of labor.
      c. *Antibiotics:* prophylaxis against rheumatic fever; treatment of bacterial infections during pregnancy.
      d. *Anticoagulants:* **Heparin** is preferred since its large molecule cannot easily cross placenta. Occasionally, sequelae may include
         ! maternal hemorrhage, preterm birth, stillbirth.
      e. **Naloxone hydrochloride (Narcan) or naltrexone hydrochloride (Trexan):**
         ! Physical and emotional stress stimulate the production of endorphins, which have a depressive effect on the cardiovascular system and blood pressure; therefore, narcotics-antagonists may be needed.
      f. Oxygen, as needed.

g. Mitral valvotomy for mitral stenosis often brings dramatic relief.

h. If woman is a transplant recipient:

(1) Transplant recipients can become pregnant, but they need to postpone conception for 1–2 yr so that graft function stabilizes and immunosuppressive agents can be given at maintenance levels.

(2) Women with cardiac transplantation can have a successful pregnancy, but they are at increased risk for complications such as heart failure.

2. Nursing management: *home care*

a. Goal: *health teaching*

(1) Need for compliance with therapeutic regimen, medical/nursing recommendations.

(2) Drug actions, dosage, necessary self-care actions (how to take own pulse, reportable signs/symptoms).

(3) Methods for *decreasing work of heart*:

(a) Adequate *rest*—minimum 10 hr sleep each night; half-hr nap after each meal.

(b) *Avoid* heavy physical *activity* (including housework), fatigue, excessive weight gain, emotional stress, infection.

(c) *Avoid situations* of reduced ambient oxygen, such as smoking, exposure to pollutants, flight in unpressurized small planes.

b. Goal: *nutritional counseling*

(1) Well-balanced *diet;* adequate protein, fresh fruits and vegetables, water.

(2) *Avoid* "junk food," stimulants (caffeine), excessive salt intake.

c. *Anticipatory planning:* **management of labor**

(1) Goal: *minimize physiologic and psychological stress.*

(2) *Medical management:*

(a) Reevaluation of cardiac status before estimated date of birth (EDB) and labor.

(b) Regional anesthesia for labor/birth.

(c) Low-outlet forceps birth; episiotomy.

(3) **Assessment:** continuous

(a) Physiologic response to labor stimuli—frequent vital signs (*heart rate* most sensitive and reliable indicator of impending HF).

(b) Color, respiratory effort, diaphoresis.

(c) Contractions, etc.—same as for any laboring mother.

(4) **Nursing care plan/implementation:** *labor*

(a) Goal: *safeguard status*

(i) Report *promptly:* pulse rate over 100; respirations ≥25 between contractions.

(ii) Oxygen at 6 liters, as needed.

(b) Goal: *emotional support*—to reduce anxiety, facilitate cooperation

(i) Encourage verbalization of feelings, fears, concerns.

(ii) Explain all procedures.

(c) Goal: *promote cardiac function.* Position—semirecumbent; support arms and legs.

(d) Goal: *promote relaxation/control over labor discomfort.* Encourage Lamaze (or other) breathing/relaxation techniques.

(e) Goal: *reduce stress on cardiopulmonary system.* Discourage bearing-down efforts.

(f) Goal: *relieve stress of pain, eliminate bearing-down.* Prepare for regional anesthesia.

(g) Goal: *maintain effective cardiac function.* Administer medications, as ordered (e.g., digitalis, diuretics, antibiotics).

d. *Anticipatory planning:* **postpartal management**

(1) Factors increasing risk of cardiac decompensation:

(a) Birth → rapid, decreased intra-abdominal pressure → vasocongestion and rapid rise in cardiac output.

(b) Loss of placental circulation.

(c) Normal diuresis increases circulating blood volume.

(2) **Assessment**

(a) Observe for tachycardia and/or respiratory distress.

(b) Monitor blood loss, I&O—potential hypovolemic shock, cardiac overload due to diuresis.

(c) Pain level—potential neurogenic shock.

(d) Same as for any postpartum mother (fundus, signs of infection, etc.).

(3) **Nursing care plan/implementation:** *postpartum*

(a) Goal: *minimize stress on cardiopulmonary system.*

(b) Methods:

(i) Rest, dangle, ambulate with aid.

(ii) Gradual increase in activity—as tolerated without symptoms.

(iii) *Position,* semi-Fowler's if needed.

(iv) Extra help with newborn care.

✏ **G. Evaluation/outcome criteria:** The woman:
  1. Successfully carries uneventful pregnancy to term.
  2. Experiences no cardiopulmonary embarrassment during labor, birth, or postpartum.

III. Disorders affecting fluid-gas transport in fetus: *Rh incompatibility*
  A. Pathophysiology—in an *Rh-negative mother:* Rh-positive fetal red blood cells enter the maternal circulation → maternal antibody formation → antibodies cross placenta and enter fetal bloodstream → attack fetal red blood cells → hemolysis → anemia, hypoxia.
    1. The *pregnant Rh-positive mother* carries her infant (Rh negative *or* positive) without incident.
    2. The *pregnant Rh-negative mother* carries an *Rh-negative infant* without incident.
    3. The *pregnant Rh-negative mother usually* carries her *first Rh-positive child* without problems *unless* she has been sensitized by inadvertent transfusion with Rh-positive blood. NOTE: Fetal cells do not usually enter the maternal bloodstream until placental separation (at abortion, abruptio placentae, amniocentesis, or birth).
  B. Etiology
    1. The Rh factor is an antigen on the red blood cells of some people (these people are *Rh positive*); the Rh factor is dominant; a person may be homozygous or heterozygous for Rh factor.
    2. An *Rh-negative* person is homozygous for this recessive trait—does *not* carry the antigen; develops antibodies when exposed to Rh-positive red blood cells (**isoimmunization**) via transplacental (or other) transfusion.
    3. Following birth of an Rh-positive infant, if fetal cells enter the mother's bloodstream, maternal antibody formation begins; antibodies remain in the maternal circulation.
    4. At time of next pregnancy with Rh-positive fetus, antibodies cross placenta → hemolysis. NOTE: *Degree* of hemolysis depends on amount (titer) of maternal antibodies present.
  C. Possible serious complication (fetal)—rare today. **Hydrops fetalis**—most severe hemolytic reaction: severe anemia, cardiac decompensation, hypoxia, edema, ascites, hydrothorax; may be stillborn.
✏ **D. Assessment**
  〰 1. *Prenatal*—diagnostic procedures:
    a. Maternal blood type and Rh factor.
    b. **Indirect Coombs test**—to determine presence of Rh sensitization (titer indicates amount of maternal antibodies).
    c. **Amniocentesis**—as early as 26 wk gestation—amount of bilirubin by-products indicates severity of hemolytic activity.
    💊 d. Rh$_o$ (D antigen) immune globulin (Rh$_o$GAM) given between 28 and 32 wk to prevent maternal antibody formation.

  〰 2. *Intrapartal* observation of amniotic fluid (on membrane rupture)
    a. Straw-colored fluid—mild disease.
    b. Golden fluid—severe fetal disease.
    3. *Postnatal*—see III.A. Rh Incompatability, in Chapter 9.
✏ **E. Nursing care plan/implementation**
  1. Goal: *prevent isoimmunization* in *Coombs-negative women.*
    💊 a. *Postabortion*—if no evidence of Rh sensitization (antibody formation) in the Rh-negative mother, administer Rh$_o$GAM.
    b. *Prenatal*—if no evidence of sensitization, administer Rh$_o$GAM at 28 wk gestation, as ordered, to all Rh − women.
    c. *Postpartum*—if no evidence of sensitization, administer Rh$_o$GAM to Rh − mother within 72 hr of birth of Rh + baby.
    d. An injection of Rh$_o$GAM results in artificial passive immunity; it contains high concentrations of antibodies produced by another person. The new mother will have temporary benefit for as long as these antibodies are present.
  2. Goal: *health teaching*
    a. Explain, discuss that Rh$_o$GAM suppresses antibody formation in susceptible Rh-negative women carrying Rh-positive fetus. NOTE: Cannot reverse sensitization if already present.
    b. RhoGAM required during and after each pregnancy, with Rh + fetus.
✏ **F. Evaluation/outcome criteria:** The woman:
  1. Successfully carries pregnancy to term.
  2. Shows no evidence of Rh isoimmunization.
  3. Gives birth to viable infant.

IV. Disorders affecting nutrition: *diabetes mellitus*
  A. Pathophysiology—increased demand for insulin exceeds pancreatic reserve → inadequate insulin production; enzyme (insulinase) activity breaks down circulating insulin → further reduction in available insulin; increased tissue resistance to insulin; glycogenolysis/gluconeogenesis → ketosis.
  B. Etiology—increased metabolic rate; action of placental hormones (see below), enzyme (insulinase) activity.
  C. Normal physiologic alterations during pregnancy that may affect management of the *diabetic* woman, or *precipitate gestational diabetes* in susceptible women
    1. Hormone production:
      a. Human placental lactogen (hPL).
      b. Progesterone.
      c. Estrogen.
      d. Cortisol.
    2. *Effects of hormones and insulinase:*
      a. Decreased glucose tolerance.
      b. Increased metabolic rate.
      c. Increased production of adrenocortical and pituitary hormones.
      d. Decreased effectiveness of insulin (in-

creased resistance to insulin by peripheral tissues).

   e. Increased gluconeogenesis.

   f. Increased size and number of islets of Langerhans to meet increased maternal needs.

   g. Increased mobilization of free fatty acids.

   h. Decreased renal threshold, increased glomerular filtration rate; glycosuria common.

   i. Decreased carbon dioxide combining power of blood; higher metabolic rate increases tendency to acidosis.

  3. *Effect of pregnancy on diabetes:*

   a. Nausea and vomiting—predispose to ketoacidosis.

   b. Insulin requirements—relatively stable or may decrease in first trimester; rapid *increase* during second and third trimesters; rapid *decrease* in postpartum to prepregnant level.

   c. Pathophysiologic progression (nephropathy, retinopathy, and arteriosclerotic changes) may appear; existing pathology may worsen.

  4. *Effect of poorly controlled diabetes on reproduction/pregnancy*—increased incidence of:

   a. Infertility.

   b. Urinary tract infection (UTI).

   c. Vaginal infections (moniliasis).

   d. Spontaneous abortion.

   e. Congenital anomalies (3 times as prevalent).

   f. Preeclampsia/eclampsia.

   g. Hydramnios.

   h. Preterm labor and birth.

   i. Fetal macrosomia—cephalopelvic disproportion (CPD).

   j. Stillbirth.

D. Assessment: *gestational diabetes mellitus*

  1. History:

   a. Family history.

   b. Previous infant 4200 g or more.

   c. Unexplained fetal wastage—abortion, stillbirth, or early neonatal death.

   d. Obesity with very rapid weight gain.

   e. *Hydramnios* (excessive amniotic fluid).

   f. Previous infant with congenital anomalies.

   g. Increased tendency for intense vaginal and/or urinary tract infections.

  2. Symptoms: *three "Ps"—polydipsia, polyphagia, polyuria*—and weight loss.

  3. *Abdominal assessment:*

   a. Fetal heart rate.

   b. Excessive fundal height

    (1) Hydramnios.

    (2) Large-for-gestational-age (LGA) fetus. *Note:* With vascular pathology, small-for-gestational-age (SGA) fetus.

  4. *Medical diagnosis*—procedures:

   a. Abnormal glucose tolerance test (GTT): two or more of the following findings are

not within normal limits (normal values follow).

    (1) Fasting blood sugar (FBS)—60–80 mg/dL (90 mg/dL may be normal during first trimester).

    (2) One hr—under 200 mg/dL.

    (3) Two hrs—under 150 mg/dL (~120).

    (4) Three hrs—under 150 mg/dL (~120).

   b. *Diabetic classification criteria*

    (1) *Class A*—gestational or chemical diabetes (abnormal GTT).

    (2) *Class B*—overt diabetes, onset after age 20, duration less than 10 yr, no vascular involvement.

    (3) *Class C*—overt diabetes, onset before age 20, duration 10–20 yr, no vascular involvement.

    (4) *Class D*—overt diabetes, onset before age 10, duration longer than 20 yr, vascular involvement, benign retinopathy, calcification of leg vessels.

    (5) *Class F*—renal impairment.

   c. *Glycosylated hemoglobin* (Hgb_{A1c}) provides a measurement of glycemic control over time, e.g., for the previous 4–6 wk: good diabetic control—2.5–5.9%; fair diabetic control—6.0–8.0%; poor diabetic control—over 8%. High levels are associated with spontaneous abortion and congenital anomalies.

  5. *Woman with known diabetes*—all classes

   a. Knowledge and acceptance of disease and its management

    (1) Signs and symptoms of hyperglycemia/hypoglycemia (see Table 3.1, p. 56).

    (2) Appropriate behaviors (e.g., skim milk for symptoms of hypoglycemia).

   b. Skill and accuracy in monitoring serum glucose;

   c. Skill and accuracy in preparing and administering insulin dosage; site rotation; subcutaneous injection.

   d. Close monitoring—prenatal status assessment every 2 wk until 30 wk, then weekly until birth. Alert to signs of emerging problems (need for insulin adjustment, hydramnios, macrosomia).

   e. Other—as for any pregnant woman.

E. Analysis/nursing diagnosis

  1. *Knowledge deficit* related to pathophysiology, interactions with pregnancy, management (e.g., insulin administration).

  2. *Altered nutrition, more or less than body requirements*, related to weight gain.

  3. High-risk pregnancy: high risk for infection, ketosis, perinatal wastage, fetal macrosomia, cephalopelvic disproportion, hydramnios, preterm labor and birth, congenital anomalies.

F. Nursing care plan/implementation

  1. Goal: *health teaching*

a. Pathophysiology of diabetes, as necessary; effect of pregnancy on management.

b. Signs and symptoms of hyperglycemia, hypoglycemia; appropriate management of symptoms.

c. Hygiene—to reduce probability of infection.

d. Exercise—needed to control serum-glucose levels, regulate weight gain, and for feeling of well-being.

e. Need for close monitoring during pregnancy.

f. Insulin regulation:

(1) Requirements vary through pregnancy: *first trimester*—may decrease with some periods of hypoglycemia due to fetal drain; *second trimester*—increased need for insulin; *third trimester*—needs may be triple prepregnant dose; acidosis more common in late pregnancy (precipitated by emotional stress, infection).

(2) Serum-glucose testing—dextrometer, acucheck, or other.

(3) Preparation and self-administration of insulin injection, as necessary.

(4) Prompt reporting of fluctuating serum-glucose levels.

g. Diagnostic testing/hospitalization:

(1) Nonstress test.

(2) Sonography.

(3) Amniocentesis.

2. Goal: *dietary counseling*

a. Optimal weight gain—about 24 pounds.

b. Needs 35 calories/kg of ideal body weight.

c. Protein—20% (2 g/kg, or about 70 g/d).

d. Carbohydrates: 30–45% in complex form (milk, bread).

e. Fats—unsaturated.

f. Appropriate exchanges.

3. *Medical management:* hospitalize woman for:

(1) Regulation of insulin (oral hypoglycemics [Glucotrol] *contraindicated* in pregnancy, due to teratogenicity).

(2) Control of infection.

(3) Determination of fetal jeopardy and/or indications for early termination of pregnancy.

G. **Evaluation/outcome criteria:** The woman:

1. Understands and accepts diagnosis of diabetes.

2. Actively participates in effective management of diabetes and pregnancy.

3. Maintains serum-glucose levels within acceptable parameters (e.g., 60–90 mg/dL after fasting; 2 hr postprandial, less than 120 mg/dL).

a. Monitors serum-glucose levels accurately (dextrometer, acucheck, urine testing).

b. Prepares and self-administers insulin appropriately.

c. Demonstrates compliance with dietary regimen.

Antepartal Hospitalization

I. **Assessment**

A. *Medical evaluation—procedures*

1. Serum-glucose levels (≤120 mg).

2. Sonography for fetal growth: biophysical profile (BPP) evaluates fetal physical well-being and volume of amniotic fluid.

3. Nonstress testing/contraction stress testing.

4. Amniocentesis for fetal maturity (NOTE: lecithin-sphingomyelin [L/S] ratio may be elevated in diabetic women); *phosphatidylglycerol (PG)* more accurate for diabetic women.

B. *Nursing assessment*

1. Daily weight, vital signs, fetal heart rate (FHR) q4h, I&O.

2. Fundal height and Leopold's maneuvers on admission.

II. **Nursing care plan/implementation:** goal: *emotional support*—to reduce anxiety and tension, which contribute to insulin imbalance

A. Explain all procedures.

B. Assist with tests for fetal status.

C. Prepare for possibility of preterm or caesarean birth.

Anticipatory Planning—Management of Labor

I. **Assessment:** continuous

A. Signs and symptoms of hypoglycemia, ketoacidosis (hyperglycemia) (Table 3.1).

B. Electronic fetal monitoring—to identify signs of fetal distress.

C. Other—as for any laboring woman.

II. **Nursing care plan/implementation:** goal: *safeguard maternal/fetal status. Position:* lateral Sims'—to reduce compression of inferior vena cava and aorta due to hydramnios or LGA baby. (*Supine hypotensive syndrome* results from compression; reduced placental perfusion increases incidence of fetal hypoxia/anoxia.)

III. *Medical management of labor*—varies widely

A. Timing—amniocentesis to determine PG (phosphotidyglycerol) and phosphotidilynosital levels (estimate fetal pulmonary surfactant).

B. Insulin added to intravenous infusion of 5–10% dextrose in water (D/W), and titrated to maintain serum glucose between 100 and 150 mg/dL. D/W needed to prevent hypoglycemia that may lead to maternal ketoacidosis; hyperglycemia may result in newborn hypoglycemia.

C. Ultrasound or X-ray pelvimetry to identify cephalopelvic disproportion (CPD).

Anticipatory Planning—Management of Postpartum Period

I. Factors influencing serum-glucose levels

A. Loss of placental hormones that degrade insulin.

TABLE 3.1   COMPARISON OF DIABETIC COMPLICATIONS

	Hypoglycemia	*Ketoacidosis/Hyperglycemia*
Pathophysiology	Major metabolic complication when too little food or too large dose of insulin or hypoglycemic agents administered; interferes with oxygen consumption in nervous tissue	Major metabolic complication in which there is insufficient insulin for metabolism of carbohydrates, fats, and proteins; seen most frequently with patients who are *insulin dependent*; precipitated in the known diabetic by stressors (such as infection, trauma, major illness) that increase insulin needs
Risk factors	Too little food Emotional or added stress Vomiting or diarrhea Added exercise	Insufficient insulin or oral hypoglycemics Noncompliance with dietary instructions Major illness/infections Therapy with steroid administration Trauma, surgery Elevated blood sugar: >200 mg/100 mL
▶ **Assessment**	**Behavioral change:** *Subjective data*—nervous, irritable, anxious, confused, disoriented *Objective data*—abrupt mood changes, psychosis	**Behavioral change:** *Subjective data*—irritable, confused *Objective data*—drowsy
	Visual: *Subjective data*—blurred vision, diplopia *Objective data*—dilated pupils	**Visual:** *Objective data*—eyeballs: soft, sunken
	Skin: *Objective data*—diaphoresis, **pale, cool, clammy,** goose bumps (piloerection), tenting	**Skin:** *Objective data*—loss of turgor, **flushed face,** pruritus vulvae
	Vitals: *Objective data*—tachycardia; palpitations, thready pulse	**Vitals:** *Objective data*—respirations-Kussmaul's breath: fruity; BP: hypovolemic shock
	Gastrointestinal: *Subjective data*—hunger, nausea *Objective data*—diarrhea, vomiting	**Gastrointestinal:** *Subjective data*—increased thirst and hunger, abdominal pain, nausea *Objective data*—vomiting, diarrhea, dry mucous membrane; lips, tongue: red, parched
	Neurologic: *Subjective data*—headache; lips/tongue: tingling, numbness *Objective data*—fainting, yawning; speech: incoherent; convulsions; coma	**Neurologic:** *Subjective data*—headache; irritability; confusion; lethargy, weakness
	Musculoskeletal: *Subjective data*—weak, fatigue *Objective data*—trembling	**Musculoskeletal:** *Subjective data*—fatigue; general malaise. **Renal:** *Objective data*—polyuria
	Blood sugar: <80 mg/100 mL	Blood sugar: >130 mg/100 mL

    B. Lower metabolic rate. Woman requiring large doses of insulin may need to triple caloric intake and decrease insulin by one-half.

▶ **II. Assessment**
    A. Observe for
        1. Hypoglycemia.
        2. Infection.

        3. Preeclampsia/eclampsia (higher incidence in diabetic women).
        4. Hemorrhage (associated with hydramnios, macrosomia, induction of labor, forceps birth, or cesarean birth).
    B. Monitor healing of episiotomy/abdominal incision.

TABLE 3.1   COMPARISON OF DIABETIC COMPLICATIONS (*Continued*)

	Hypoglycemia	*Ketoacidosis/Hyperglycemia*
✉ **Analysis/nursing diagnosis**	*Risk for injury* related to deficit of needed glucose *Knowledge deficit* related to proper dietary intake or proper insulin dosage *Altered nutrition, less than body requirements,* related to glucose deficiency	*Risk for injury* related to glucose imbalance *Knowledge deficit* related to proper balance of diet and insulin dosage
✉ **Nursing care plan/ implementation**	Goal: *provide adequate glucose to reverse hypoglycemia:* administer simple sugar **stat,** PO or IV; glucose paste absorbed in mucous membrane; monitor blood sugar levels: identify events leading to complication	Goal: *promote normal balance of food and insulin:* **regular** insulin as ordered; IV saline, as ordered; bicarbonate and electrolyte replacements, as ordered; potassium replacements once therapy begins and urine output is adequate
	Goal: *health teaching:* to prevent further episodes; importance of careful monitoring of balance between glucose levels and insulin dosage	Goal: *health teaching:* diet instructions; desired effects and side effects of prescribed insulin or hypoglycemic agent (onset, peak, and duration of action); importance of recognizing signs of imbalance
✉ **Evaluation/outcome criteria**	Adheres to diet and correct insulin dosage Adjusts dosage when activity is increased Glucose level 80–120 mg/dL	Avoids serious complications Accepts prescribed diet Takes medication (correct dose and time) Glucose level 80–120 mg/dL

Source: SL Lagerquist (ed). *Little, Brown's NCLEX-RN Examination Review.* Boston: Little, Brown, 1996. P 127.

✉ **III. Nursing care plan/implementation**
  A. *Medical management:* insulin calibration—requirement may drop to one-half or two-thirds pregnant dosage on first postpartum day if woman is on full diet (due to loss of human placental lactogen and conversion of serum glucose to lactose).
  B. *Nursing management*
  ☞ **1.** Goal: *euglycemia.* Acucheck, insulin as ordered.
  2. Goal: *avoid trauma, reduce risk of UTI. Avoid* catheterization, where possible.
  ☞ **3.** Goal: *health teaching.* Nipple care—to prevent fissures and possible mastitis.
  4. Goal: *reduce serum-glucose and insulin needs.* Encourage/support breastfeeding → antidiabetogenic effect. NOTE: If *acetonuria* occurs, stop breastfeeding while physician readjusts diet/insulin balance; may pump breasts to maintain lactation. If *hypoglycemic,* adrenaline level rises → decreased milk supply and letdown reflex.
  C. *Anticipatory guidance*—**discharge planning**
  1. Goal: *counseling.* Reinforce recommendations of physicians/genetic counselors.
    a. Risk of infant inheriting gene for diabetes is greater if mother has early-onset disease.
    b. Increased risk of congenital disorders.

  2. Goal: *family planning*
    a. Oral contraceptives **contraindicated** since they decrease carbohydrate tolerance; intrauterine device (IUD) **contraindicated**—due to impaired response to infection. Barrier contraceptives (diaphragm or condoms with spermicides) recommended.
    b. Tubal ligation: if mother has vascular involvement, i.e., retinopathy or nephropathy, increased risk with later pregnancies.
  3. Goal: *health teaching*
    a. Self-care measures.
    b. Importance of eating on time, even if infant must wait to breast- or bottlefeed.
    c. Importance of adequate rest and exercise to maintain insulin/glucose balance.
    d. Organize schedule to care for infant, other children, and her diabetes. Allow time for self.
  ✉ **4. Evaluation/outcome criteria:** The woman:
    a. Successfully completes an uneventful pregnancy, labor, and birth of a normal, healthy newborn.
    b. Makes informed judgments regarding parenting, family planning, management of her diabetes.

Disorders Affecting Psychosocial-Cultural Behaviors: Substance Abuse

▶ **I. Assessment:** pregnant substance abuser
  A. *Medical history*
    1. Infections: human immunodeficiency virus (HIV)-positive status, AIDS, STDs, hepatitis, cirrhosis of liver, cellulitis, endocarditis, pancreatitis, pneumonia.
    2. Psychiatric illness: depression, paranoia, irritability.
    3. Trauma related to violence.
  B. *Obstetric history*
    1. Spontaneous abortions.
    2. History of abruptio placentae.
    3. Preterm labor.
    4. Premature rupture of membranes.
    5. Fetal death.
    6. Low-birth-weight (LBW) infants.
  C. *Current pregnancy*
    1. Preterm labor contractions.
    2. Hypoactivity—hyperactivity in fetus.
      a. Maternal withdrawal from cocaine puts fetus at risk for intrauterine *asphyxia.* Its significant and agonizing withdrawal is felt as violent movements in utero.
      b. Maternal episodes of vasospastic hypertension cause numerous small strokes in the fetus.
    3. Poor or decreased weight gain.
    4. Sexually transmitted disease.
    5. Undiagnosed vaginal bleeding.
    6. Drugs being used and methods of self-administration.
  D. *Psychosocial history*
    1. Attitudes re: pregnancy.
    2. Current support system: lacking.
    3. Current living arrangements; life-style.
    4. History of psychiatric illness.
    5. History of physical, sexual abuse.
    6. Involvement with legal system.
  E. *Physical examination.*
  ▬ **F.** *Commonly abused substances*
    1. Nicotine.
    2. Alcohol (fetal alcohol syndrome [FAS] or fetal alcohol effects [FAE]).
    3. Marijuana.
    4. Stimulants—cocaine, crack, ice.
    5. Opiates—heroin, methadone, propoxyphene hydrochloride (Darvon), acetaminophen (Tylenol).
    6. Sedatives, hypnotics.
    7. Caffeine.
  G. *Neonatal outcomes*
    1. LBW (low birth weight), small heads.
    2. Irritable, difficult to console.
    3. Disorganized suck-swallow reflex.
    4. Impaired motor development.
    5. Congenital anomalies: genitourinary, gastrointestinal, limb anomalies.
    6. Cerebral infarctions (CVAs).

    7. Breastfeeding contraindicated unless mother is drug free for 3 mo.
    8. Poor, slow weight gain; failure to thrive.
▶ **II. Analysis/nursing diagnosis**
  A. *Altered nutrition: more than body requirements—*weight gain related to poor nutrition.
  B. *Altered nutrition: less than body requirements—*slow fetal growth related to slow gain in weight.
  C. *Altered placental function* related to high risk for abruptio placentae.
  D. *Noncompliance* with health care protocols related to persistent drug use.
  E. *Altered parenting* related to psychological illness (substance dependence).
▶ **III. Nursing care plan/implementation**
  A. Early identification of substance abuser.
  B. Stabilize physiologic status.
  C. Fetal surveillance.
  D. Urge consistent obstetric care.
  E. Refer for social services.
▶ **IV. Evaluation/outcome criteria:** The woman:
  A. Seeks out and utilizes social services and drug treatment program.
  B. Abstains from illicit substances during pregnancy.
  C. Successfully completes an uneventful pregnancy, labor, and birth of normal healthy infant.

Disorders Affecting Protective Function: Infections

Vaginitis—Inflammation of Vagina

  I. Pathophysiology—local inflammatory reaction (redness, heat, irritation/tenderness, pain).
  II. Etiology
  A. Common causative organisms
    1. Bacteria—streptococci, *Escherichia coli,* gonococci, chlamydia.
    2. Viruses—herpes type II, cytomegalovirus (CMV), human papillomavirus (HPV).
    3. Protozoa—*Trichomonas vaginalis.*
    4. Fungi—*Candida albicans.*
  B. Atrophic changes—due to declining hormone level (postmenopausal women).
▶ **III. Assessment:** differentiate among common vaginal infections:
  A. Vulvovaginal erythema.
  B. Pruritus, dysuria, dyspareunia.
  C. Vaginal discharge.
  〰 **D.** Evaluate Papanicolaou (Pap) smear results, e.g., to aid in identifying HPV.
  〰 **E.** Evaluate enzyme-linked immunosorbent assay (ELISA) test results.
▶ **IV. Analysis/nursing diagnosis:** *pain* related to inflammation, discharge.
▶ **V. Nursing care plan/implementation**
  A. Goal: *emotional support.*
  B. Goal: *health teaching.* Instruct woman in self-care measures to promote comfort and healing
    ☞ **1.** Perineal care.
    2. Sitz baths.

3. Douching (as ordered). *Not* recommended during pregnancy.
4. Exposure of vulva to air.
5. Cotton briefs.
6. Medication: dosage/administration, action, side effects, expected outcomes.
7. Proper insertion of vaginal suppository.
8. Possible sequelae: e.g., abnormal Pap smear results, cervical intraepithelial neoplasia (CIN), pelvic inflammatory disease (PID), and infertility.

C. Goal: *prevent reinfection*
1. Suggest sexual partner use condom until infection is eliminated—or abstain from intercourse.
2. Recommend sexual partner seek examination and treatment.

D. Goal: *medical consultation/treatment.* Refer for diagnosis and treatment.

VI. Evaluation/outcome criteria
A. Woman is asymptomatic; unable to recover organism from body fluids or tissue.
B. Woman avoids reinfection.

Gonorrhea

I. Pathophysiology
A. *Men*—early infection usually confined to urethra, vestibular glands, anus, or pharynx. Untreated: ascending infection may involve testes, causing sterility.
B. *Women*—early infection usually confined to vestibular glands, endocervix, urethra, anus (vagina is resistant). May ascend to involve pelvic structures, e.g., PID: fallopian tubes, ovaries; scarring may cause sterility.
C. *Pregnant* women—may result in premature rupture of membranes (PROM), amnionitis, preterm labor, postpartum salpingitis.
D. Sequelae (untreated)
1. May develop carrier state (asymptomatic; organism resident in vestibular glands).
2. Systemic spread may result in gonococcal
   a. Arthritis.
   b. Endocarditis.
   c. Meningitis.
   d. Septicemia.
3. Pelvic inflammatory disease (PID) and impaired fertility.
E. Newborn—*ophthalmia neonatorum* (gonococcal conjunctivitis). Untreated sequelae: blindness.

II. Etiology: gram-negative diplococcus (*Neisseria gonorrhoeae*).

III. Epidemiology
A. Portal of entry—oral or genitourinary mucous membranes.
B. Mode of transmission—usually sexual contact; or via *fomites* (nonliving material on which disease-producing organisms may be conveyed, e.g., bed linens).
C. Incubation period: 2–5 d; may be asymptomatic.

D. Communicable period—as long as organisms are present; to 4 d after antibiotic therapy begun.
E. In the United States, adolescents have the highest prevalence of gonorrhea (and of *Chlamydia trachomatis*) infection.

IV. Assessment
A. History of known (or suspected) contact.
B. *Men*
1. Complaint of mucoid or mucopurulent discharge.
2. Medical diagnosis—procedure: urethral discharge Gram stain.
C. *Women*
1. Often asymptomatic; acute infection: severe vulvovaginal inflammation, venereal warts, greenish-yellow vaginal discharge.
2. Medical diagnosis—procedure: endocervical culture.
D. *Gonococcal urethritis* (men and women)—sudden severe dysuria, frequency, burning, edema.
C. *Salpingitis/oophoritis*—severe, sudden abdominal pain, fever (with or without vaginal discharge).

V. Analysis/nursing diagnosis: *impaired tissue integrity* related to tissue inflammation.

VI. Nursing care plan/implementation
A. Goal: *emotional support.*
B. Goal: *health teaching* to prevent transmission, sequelae, reinfection.
1. Need for accurate diagnosis and effective treatment, follow-up examination in 7–14 d, and culture.
2. All sexual partners need examination treatment.
3. *Avoid* spread via fomites.
4. Possible sequelae/complications (sterility, carrier state).
5. *Avoid* multiple sex partners.
6. Employ "safer sex" practices.
C. Goal: *medical consultation/treatment*
1. Determine allergy to *penicillin, erythromycin, probenecid.*
2. Refer for diagnosis and treatment.
   a. Diagnosis.
   b. Treatment—*aqueous penicillin* G, 2.4 million units in each buttock (4.8 million units total dose), and *probenecid,* 1 g PO.
   c. Follow-up culture before birth.
   d. Notification of sexual partners.

VII. Evaluation/outcome criteria: The woman:
A. Verbalizes understanding of mode of transmission, prevention, importance of examination treatment of sexual contacts.
B. Informs sexual contacts of need for examination.
C. Returns for follow-up examinations.
D. Successfully treated; weekly follow-up cultures: negative on two successive visits.
E. Avoids reinfection.

Chlamydia Trachomatis

I. Pathophysiology

A. Most common sexually transmitted disease in U.S.; highest prevalence in adolescents.

B. Initial infection mild in females; inflammation of cervix with discharge.

C. If untreated, may lead to urethritis, dysuria, PID, tubal occlusion, infertility.

II. Etiology

A. *Chlamydia trachomatis* has maternal-fetal effects.

B. Bacteria can exist only within living cells.

C. Transmission is by direct contact from one person to another.

III. **Assessment**—maternal

A. Inflamed cervix (may be asymptomatic).

B. Cervical congestion, edema.

C. Mucopurulent discharge.

IV. **Assessment**—fetal-neonatal

A. Increased incidence of stillbirth.

B. Preterm birth may result.

C. Contact with infected mucus occurs during birth.

D. Newborn may be asymptomatic.

E. Conjunctivitis may lead to scarring.

F. Respiratory problems—tachypnea, dyspnea, apnea. Pneumonia may result.

V. **Analysis/nursing diagnosis**

A. *Pain* related to inflamed reproductive organs.

B. *Fatigue* related to inflammation.

C. *Knowledge deficit* related to mode of treatment, disease transmission.

VI. **Nursing care plan/implementation**

A. Treatment with antibiotics, generally *erythromycin, tetracycline. Ophthalmic erythromycin* instilled into newborn's conjunctival sac.

B. Provide pain relief (e.g., sitz baths), analgesics.

C. Counsel regarding use of condoms (even during pregnancy) and spermicidal agents (containing *nonoxynol-9*) to prevent reinfection.

VII. **Evaluation/outcome criteria**

A. Woman understands treatment and shows compliance.

B. Woman understands portal of entry and risk for reinfection.

Herpes Genitalis

I. Pathophysiology—initial infection: varies in severity of symptoms, may be local or systemic; duration: prolonged; morbidity: severe.

II. Etiology—herpes virus type II.

III. Epidemiology

A. Portal of entry—skin, mucous membranes.

B. Mode of transmission—usually sexual.

C. Incubation: 3–14 days.

D. Communicable period—while organisms are present.

IV. **Assessment**

A. Lesions—painful, red papules; pustular vesicles that break and form wet ulcers that later crust; self-limiting (3 wk).

B. Severe itching and/or pain.

C. Discharge—copious; foul-smelling.

D. Dysuria.

E. Lymph nodes—enlarged, inflammatory, inguinal.

F. Pregnant woman—vaginal bleeding, spontaneous abortion, fetal death.

G. May shed virus for 7 wk.

H. Medical diagnosis: multinucleated giant cells in microscopic examination of lesion exudate; culture for herpes simplex virus (HSV).

V. **Analysis/nursing diagnosis**

A. *Pain* related to inflammation process.

B. *Fear* related to longevity of disease, no cure for disease.

C. *Knowledge deficit* related to transmission to future partners.

VI. **Nursing care plan/implementation**

A. Goal: *emotional support.*

B. Goal: *health teaching*

1. Virus remains in body for life (dormant, non-infectious) in 25–30% of population; small percentage have symptoms.

2. Recurrence probable; usually shorter and milder.

3. Annual Pap smear important—associated with later development of cervical cancer.

4. Need for close surveillance during pregnancy; cesarean birth may be indicated if active lesions.

5. *Avoid* multiple sex partners; practice "safer sex."

C. Goal: *promote comfort.*

D. Goal: *accurate definitive treatment.* Refer for diagnosis and treatment.

1. Diagnosis—cervical smears.

2. Treatment—*acyclovir* ointment (Zovirax, but not in pregnancy).

VII. **Evaluation/outcome criteria**

A. Woman remains asymptomatic.

B. Pregnancy continues to term with no newborn effects.

Syphilis

I. Pathophysiology

A. *Primary stage:* nonreactive VDRL

1. *Men:* 3–4 wk after contact, painless, localized penile/anal ulcer (chancre); lymph nodes—enlarged, regional.

2. *Women:* often asymptomatic; labial, vaginal, or cervical chancre.

3. Medical diagnosis—procedure: dark-field microscopic examination of lesion exudate.

B. *Secondary stage:* reactive VDRL

1. Six to eight wk after infection.

2. Rash—macular, papular; on trunk, palms, soles.

3. Malaise, headache, sore throat, weight loss, low-grade temperature.

C. *Latent stage;* reactive serologic test for syphilis (STS). Asymptomatic; noninfectious.

D. *Tertiary stage*

1. Gumma formation in skin, cardiovascular or central nervous system.
2. Psychosis.
II. Etiology: *Treponema pallidum* (spirochete).
III. Epidemiology
   A. Portal of entry—skin, mucous membranes.
   B. Mode of transmission—usually sexual.
   C. Incubation period—9 d–3 mo.
   D. Communicable period—primary and secondary stages.
 IV. **Assessment**
   A. *Primary*—chancre, when detectable. Medical diagnosis—procedure: dark-field examination of lesion exudate.
   B. *Secondary*
      1. Malaise, lymphadenopathy, headache, elevated temperature.
      2. Macular, papular rash on palms and soles; may be disseminated.
      3. Medical diagnosis—see *D.* below.
   C. *Tertiary*
      1. Subcutaneous nodules (gumma).
      2. NOTE: Gumma formation may affect any body system; symptoms associated with area of involvement.
   D. Medical diagnosis—procedures: stages other than primary—STS: VDRL, rapid plasma reagin (RPR), *Tr. pallidum* immobilization (TPI), fluorescent treponemal antibody absorption (FTA). *False-positive STS* in: collagen diseases, infectious mononucleosis, malaria, systemic tuberculosis.
V. **Analysis/nursing diagnosis**
   A. *Pain* related to inflammation process.
   B. *Knowledge deficit* related to treatment and transmission of the disease.
VI. **Nursing care plan/implementation**
   A. Goal: *emotional support*
      1. Nonjudgmental.
      2. Caring, supportive manner.
   B. Goal: *health teaching*
      1. Need for accurate diagnosis and treatment, follow-up examinations.
      2. All sexual partners need examination and treatment.
      3. *Avoid* multiple sex partners; practice "safer sex."
   C. Goal: *medical consultation/treatment*
      1. Refer for diagnosis and treatment. NOTE: In pregnancy—treatment by 18th gestational week prevents congenital syphilis in neonate; however, treat at time of diagnosis.
      2. Treatment
         a. Primary, secondary—*benzathine penicillin G*, 2.4 million units.
         b. Other stages—7.2 million units over 3-wk period.
         c. *Erythromycin* for penicillin-allergic patients.
VII. **Evaluation/outcome criteria**
   A. If treated by 18th week of pregnancy, congenital syphilis is prevented.

B. Appropriate treatment after 18th week cures both mother and fetus; however, any fetal damage occurring before treatment is irreversible.
C. Follow-up VDRL: nonreactive at 1, 3, 6, 9, and 12 mo.
D. *Tertiary*—cerebrospinal fluid examination negative at 6 mo and 1 yr following treatment.
E. Woman verbalizes understanding of mode of transmission, potential sequelae without treatment, importance of examination/treatment of sexual contacts, preventive techniques.
F. Woman informs contacts of need for examination.
G. Woman returns for follow-up visit.
H. Woman avoids reinfection.

Pelvic Inflammatory Disease (PID)

I. Pathophysiology—ascending pelvic infection; may involve fallopian tubes (*salpingitis*), ovaries (*oophoritis*); may develop pelvic *abscess* (most common complication), pelvic *cellulitis,* pelvic *thrombophlebitis, peritonitis.*
II. Etiology
   A. *Chlamydia trachomatis.*
   B. Gonococci.
   C. Streptococci.
   D. Staphylococci.
III. Assessment
   A. Pain: acute, abdominal.
   B. Vaginal discharge: foul-smelling.
   C. Fever, chills, malaise.
   D. Elevated white blood cell count.
   E. Number of sex partners.
   F. Sex practices, e.g., consistent use of "safer sex" practices.
IV. Analysis/nursing diagnosis
   A. *Pain* related to occluded tubules.
   B. *Infertility* related to permanent block of tubes.
   C. *Knowledge deficit* related to transmission of disease.
   D. *Altered urinary elimination* related to dysuria.
V. Nursing care plan/implementation—for hospitalized woman:
   A. Goal: *emotional support.*
   B. Goal: *limit extension of infection*
      1. Bedrest—*position:* semi-Fowler's, to promote drainage.
      2. *Force fluids* to 3000 mL/d.
      3. Administer antibiotics, as ordered.
   C. Goal: *prevent autoinoculation/transmission*
      1. Strict aseptic technique (handwashing, perineal care).
      2. Contact-item isolation.
      3. *Health teaching:* if untreated: high risk of tubal scarring, sterility, or ectopic pregnancy; pelvic adhesions; transmission of disease.
   D. Goal: *promote comfort*
      1. Analgesics, as ordered.
      2. External heat, as ordered.
VI. Evaluation/outcome criteria
   A. Woman responds to therapy; uneventful recovery.
   B. Woman avoids reinfection.

HIV-Positive Status and AIDS

I. *General aspects*—AIDS is a serious condition affecting the immune system. It is the fourth leading cause of death among reproductive-aged women in the U.S. Heterosexual females are considered at risk if they or their sexual partners:
  - **A.** Are HIV positive.
  - **B.** Are IV drug users (50%).
  - **C.** Received blood between 1977 and 1985 (9%).
  - **D.** Are homosexual or bisexual males (39%).
  - **E.** Are hemophiliacs.

II. Assessment—general symptoms:
  - **A.** Malaise.
  - **B.** Chronic cough; possible tuberculosis.
  - **C.** Chronic diarrhea.
  - **D.** HIV positive.
  - **E.** Weight loss: 10 pounds in 2 mo.
  - **F.** Night sweats; lymphadenopathy.
  - **G.** Skin lesions; thrush.
  - **H.** PID; STDs; vulvovaginitis—usually yeast (*candidiasis*), often refractory and severe.
  - **I.** Cervical cytologic abnormalities; often infected with HPV.

III. Analysis/nursing diagnosis
  - **A.** *Altered nutrition, less than body requirements*, related to general malaise.
  - **B.** *Fatigue*, related to altered health status, weight loss.
  - **C.** *Fear* related to progressively debilitating disease.
  - **D.** *Knowledge deficit* related to disease progression, treatment, life expectancy.
  - **E.** *Ineffective individual coping* related to disease progression.

IV. Nursing care plan/implementation
  - **A.** Identify women at risk.
  - **B.** Protect confidentiality.
  - **C.** Implement universal precautions.
  - **D.** Use proper gloves, gown, handwashing.
  - **E.** Use protective eyewear and mask in labor, birth.

V. Evaluation/outcome criteria
  - **A.** Further transmission of virus is avoided.
  - **B.** Woman's confidentiality maintained.
  - **C.** Universal precautions implemented.
  - **D.** Emotional support implemented.
  - **E.** Supportive groups contacted.

HIV-Positive Women

I. *Antepartum*
  - **A.** Increased incidence of other STDs (gonorrhea, syphilis, herpes, HPV, candidiasis).
  - **B.** Increased incidence of CMV.
  - **C.** Differential diagnosis for all pregnancy-induced complaints.
  - **D.** Counsel regarding nutrition.
  - **E.** Advise about risk to infant.
  - **F.** Counsel regarding safer sex (e.g., using condoms even during pregnancy).

II. *Intrapartum*
  - **A.** Focus on prevention of transmission (use universal precautions).
  - **B.** External electronic fetal monitoring (EFM) preferred.
  - **C.** *Avoid* use of fetal scalp electrodes or sampling.
  - **D.** Mode of birth not based on disease.

III. *Postpartum*
  - **A.** No remarkable alteration in disease progression.
  - **B.** Breastfeeding contraindicated.
  - **C.** Implement universal precautions for mother and infant.
  - **D.** Refer to specialists in AIDS care and treatment.

IV. *Nurse with needle-stick injury* should receive *zidovudine* (ZDV) *STAT*.

V. Health teaching—an effective disinfectant against HIV is household bleach (*sodium hypochlorite*) 1:10.

Newborn or Neonate with AIDS

I. *General aspects*: neonatal AIDS—exact mode of transmission unknown, but possibly transplacental, contact with maternal blood at birth, and/or postnatal exposure to infected parent (i.e., breastfeeding). Classic signs evident in adult often not present. *Common signs*: lymphadenopathy, hepatosplenomegaly, oral candidiasis, bacterial infections, failure to thrive.

II. If a new mother is HIV positive, newborn has an *ELISA test* for presence of HIV antibodies at 6 mo of age. (About 30–50% of infants of HIV+ mothers are HIV+.) A positive test indicates only that antibodies from the mother have passed to the fetus.

III. *Zidovudine* (ZDV) is the first-line therapy for HIV; it can reduce the rate of transmission during pregnancy from over 25% to just over 8%. Women can be offered the option of this medication starting at 14 wk gestation if they have not had it before and if their CD4 count is less than 200/μL.

IV. Nursing care plan/implementation
  - **A.** Provide supportive nursing care (thermoregulation, respiratory).
  - **B.** Encourage parent-infant contact.
  - **C.** Provide opportunities for sensory stimuli and touch.
  - **D.** Monitor intake and weight gain.
  - **E.** Observe for signs of infection.
  - **F.** Initiate social service consultation.

Other Infections

I. TORCH infections (see Table 3.2).

II. Other infections of concern: Coxsackie virus B, *varicella* (*chickenpox*), influenza, listeriosis, Lyme disease, mumps (parotitis), parvovirus B-19, rubeola, *tuberculosis, human papillomavirus* (genital warts). Brief comments follow regarding selected infections.
  - **A.** *Chickenpox (varicella-zoster virus). Maternal consequences:* pneumonia, which could be life-threatening, and encephalitis with long-term neurologic sequelae. Therefore, exposed women who are not immune can receive *varicella-zoster immune globulin* (VZIG), which is considered safe to administer during pregnancy. The woman with varicella-zoster pneumonia is given *acyclovir*. Women with chickenpox at the time of birth should *not* have contact with their newborns until

TABLE 3.2   TORCH INFECTIONS

Infection	Maternal Effects	Fetal Effects	Teaching/Nursing Implications
Toxoplasmosis	Flulike symptoms	Parasitemia	*Avoid* raw meat and litter from infected cats
Other **H**epatitis A (infectious)	Abortion, fever	Anomalies, preterm birth	*Transmission:* droplet and hand contact ⊂ Tx: gamma globulin
Hepatitis B (serum)	Symptoms variable: fever, aching, etc.	Infected during birth	*Transmission:* contaminated needles, blood, etc. ⊂ Tx: hepatitis B vaccine (series of 3)
Group B streptococcus (GBS)	Miscarriage, preterm birth, fever, puerperal infection	Life-threatening perinatal infection	*Transmission:* from mother to infant during birth; transmission rate: 50 to 75%
Rubella	Usually mild infection	*First 2 mo:* malformations: heart, cataracts, damaged cranial VIII nerve (deafness), mental retardation	Vaccinate susceptible women after birth; woman signs informed consent to avoid pregnancy for 3 mo following vaccination
Cytomegalo-virus (CMV)	Mononucleosislike syndrome	Fetal or neonatal death; hydrocephaly, etc.	*Transmission:* transplacental infection or during birth; disease progresses through infancy/childhood
Herpes genitalis, type 2	See discussion, p. 60		

Tx = treatment.

all vesicles have crusted. *Newborns* with varicella lesions should be *strictly isolated* from other hospitalized infants. The nurse must remember that transmission of this virus occurs through aerosol spray (sneezes) or through contact with vesicular fluid and cells from fresh skin lesions.

B. *Tuberculosis.* Pregnancy is not jeopardized by pulmonary tuberculosis, but spontaneous abortion does occur in one of five infected women. Following birth, the mother will *not* have close contact with her baby until contagion is *no longer* a problem. A woman who has had tuberculosis needs to wait 1½–2 yr after she is declared free of the disease before attempting pregnancy.

C. *Human papillomavirus (HPV)*, responsible for venereal or genital warts, can have serious consequences for the woman and for her fetus/newborn. It is the *most* common viral sexually transmitted infection—3 times greater than genital herpes. Having multiple sex partners increases the likelihood of HPV infection; other risk factors include smoking and use of oral contraceptives. Smoking and substance abuse impair the immune system.

1. *Women:* Several strains (e.g., 16, 18, 31, 33, and 35) are associated with cervical neoplasia, cervical intraepithelial neoplasia (CIN). At-risk women need frequent Pap smears for early identification. Coexistence of herpes and chlamydia infection may play a role in development of CIN or invasive cervical cancer. In women under 18 yr of age, the metaplastic condition of the adolescent cervix, plus the other risk factors, may also increase the risk of cervical cancer.

2. *Children:* congenitally-derived respiratory papillomatosis.

Age-Related Risk Factors
The Pregnant Adolescent

I. *General aspects*

A. Pregnancy in female between 12 and 17 yr old.

B. Incidence increasing dramatically; approximately one-third of all births are to adolescents.

C. *Predisposing factors:* early menarche, early experimentation with sex (vaginal and cervical mucosa is not mature before age 18 yr), poor family relationships, poverty, late or no prenatal care.

D. *Associated health problems:* preeclampsia/eclampsia, preterm labor, SGA infants, anemia, bleeding disorders, infections, cephalopelvic disproportion (CPD).

E. *Social problems:* poorly educated mothers, child abuse, single-parent families, mothers who are unemployed or working at minimum wage, or who lack support system.

II. Assessment
    A. Present physical/health status.
    B. Feelings toward pregnancy.
    C. Plans for the future.
    D. Factors influencing decisions related to self, pregnancy, baby.
    E. Signs and symptoms of complications of pregnancy (see I.D. *Associated health problems,* p. 63).
    F. Potential for gestational diabetes.
    G. Need/desire for health maintenance information (family planning)
        1. Adolescents become sexually active an average of 15 mo before starting regular contraception.
        2. Most discontinue use within first year after starting contraception.
        3. Adolescents frequently romanticize boyfriends' decisions not to use contraceptives as an affirmation of love or commitment.

III. Analysis/nursing diagnosis
    A. *Ineffective coping, individual/family,* related to need to alter life-style, plans, expectations.
    B. *Altered family processes,* related to unexpected/unwanted pregnancy.
    C. *Altered parenting* related to intrafamily stress secondary to unexpected pregnancy, developmental tasks.
    D. *Self-esteem disturbance* related to altered self-concept, body image, role performance, personal identity.
    E. *Knowledge deficit* related to family planning, health maintenance, risk factors, pregnancy options.
    F. *Altered nutrition* related to life-style.

IV. Nursing care plan/implementation
    A. Goal: *emotional support*
        1. Assure confidentiality.
        2. Establish acceptant, supportive environment.
        3. Encourage verbalization of feelings, concerns, fears, desires, etc.
        4. Maintain continuity of care—consistency of nursing approach, to establish trust, confidentiality.
    B. Goal: *facilitate informed decision making.* Discuss available options; aid in exploring implications of possible decisions.
    C. Goal: *nutritional counseling* (anemia)
        1. Needs for own growth and that of fetus.
        2. High-quality diet—value for character of skin, return to prepregnant figure.
        3. Include pizza, hamburgers, milkshakes as acceptable—to minimize anger at being "different."
    D. Goal: *health teaching*
        1. Rest, exercise, hygiene—as for other women.
        2. Prevention of infection—STD, UTI, etc.

        3. Breast self-examination; Pap smear.
        4. Future family planning options (see Table 1.2, pp. 10–13).
    E. Goal: *assist in achievement of normal developmental tasks.* Developmental tasks of adolescence are interrupted by those of pregnancy. Encourage exploration of new role and responsibilities.
    F. Goal: *referral to appropriate resources*
        1. Abortion.
        2. Preparation for childbirth and parenting classes that respect adolescents' needs and developmental level: use concrete examples, creativity, flexibility, humor.
        3. Family counseling.
        4. Social services.
    G. Goal: *assist in facilitating continuing/completing basic education*
        1. Communicate with school nurse.
        2. Explore other options available in community.

V. Evaluation outcome criteria
    A. Adolescent makes informed decisions appropriate to individual and family needs, desires.
    B. Adolescent actively participates in own health maintenance.
        1. Complies with medical/nursing recommendations.
        2. Minimizes potential for complications of pregnancy.
    C. Adolescent copes effectively with normal physiologic and psychosocial alterations of pregnancy.
    D. Both adolescent and baby's father express satisfaction with decision and management of this pregnancy. If parenthood is chosen and pregnancy is successful, accepts parenting role.

Older Mothers: Primigravida Over Age 35

I. *General aspects*—higher incidence of congenital anomalies (e.g., *Down syndrome*), increased possibility of complications of pregnancy; however, generally it is a conscious decision to have postponed childbearing. Individuals are usually used to making own decisions regarding career and health care.

II. Assessment
    A. Same as for other pregnant women.
    B. Reaction to reality of pregnancy.
    C. Family response to pregnancy.

III. Analysis/nursing diagnosis
    A. *Fear* related to threat to pregnancy.
    B. *Knowledge deficit* related to aspects of pregnancy care.

IV. Nursing care plan/implementation
    A. Goal: *anticipatory guidance.* Preparation for parenthood, altered life-style, potential change of career. Assist with realistic expectations. Refer to "over 30" parents' support group.
    B. Goal: *health teaching.* Explain, discuss special diagnostic procedures. See *Amniocentesis,* p. 80.
    C. Other—same as for other pregnant women.

V. Evaluation/outcome criteria
    A. Woman experiences normal, uncomplicated preg-

nancy, labor, and birth of normal, healthy newborn.
 B. Woman expresses satisfaction with decision and outcome of this pregnancy.

Older Mothers: Multipara Over Age 40

 I. *General aspects*
 A. Increased incidence of pre- and coexisting medical disorders (hypertension, diabetes, arthritis).
 B. Increased incidence of complications of pregnancy (preeclampsia/eclampsia, hemorrhage).
 C. Smoking is major risk factor.
 II. **Assessment**
 A. Same as for other pregnant women.
 B. Reaction to pregnancy (varies from pleasure at still being "young enough," to despair, if facing decision to abort).
 C. History, signs and symptoms of coexisting disorders.
 D. Indications of reduced physical ability to cope with normal physiologic alterations of pregnancy.
 E. Family constellation: stage of family developmental cycle, responses to this pregnancy (especially adolescents' reaction to mother's pregnancy).
 III. **Analysis/nursing diagnosis:** same as for over-35 age group.
 IV. **Nursing care plan/implementation**
 A. Goal: *emotional support.* Encourage verbalization of feelings, fears, concerns.
 B. Goal: *referral to appropriate resource*
  1. Genetic counseling.
  2. Abortion/support groups.
  3. Preparation for childbirth and parenthood classes.
 C. Goal: *facilitate/support effective family process.* Involve family in preparation for birth and integration of newborn into family unit.
 D. Other—same as for other pregnant women.
 V. **Evaluation/outcome criteria**
 A. Woman makes informed decisions related to pregnancy.
 B. Woman expresses satisfaction with decision and outcome of this pregnancy.
 C. Woman experiences uncomplicated pregnancy, labor, and birth of normal, healthy newborn.

Other Medical-Surgical Conditions Placing Pregnancy at Risk

Asthma: Medical Management

 I. Effect on pregnancy is unpredictable.
 ! II. Woman with preexisting asthma has an increased possibility of: hyperemesis, hemorrhage, preeclampsia, and complicated labor. Other dangers are: prematurity, low birth weight, and neonatal hypoxia.
 III. Asthma status can be monitored by a *pulmonary flow test* using a portable peak-flow meter to assess the greatest flow velocity during forced expiration from fully inflated lungs.

 IV. Most asthma medications are safe to take during pregnancy—for up to 4 doses/d; inhaled medications are preferable.
 A. *Theophylline,* one of the mainstays of asthma therapy during pregnancy, may exacerbate gastroesophageal reflux (severe heartburn).
 B. Inhaled *glucocorticoids.*
 C. Inhaled β_2 agonists (e.g., *terbutaline,* [*Brethaire, Brethine, Bricanyl*]) are useful in managing acute asthma during pregnancy.
 D. Inhaled *Altrovent* (ipratropium bromide) may be beneficial in presence of mucus-producing cough.
 E. Acute episodes may require *steroids, aminophylline, oxygen,* and correction of fluid-electrolyte imbalance.
 F. *Labor*
  1. Meperidine (*Demerol*) relieves bronchospasm; *morphine* is *not* used in labor because it may cause bronchospasm.
  2. Vaginal birth with local or regional anesthesia is method of choice.
 G. Breastfeeding is possible if medications are inhaled, because of their low systemic bioavailability.
 V. Teratogenic effects, if they occur, do so during the first trimester, the period of organogenesis.

Sickle Cell Disease (Hemoglobin Type SS): Management

 I. Heart failure is a potential problem: Assess vital signs, auscultate for rales (crackles) frequently, place in *semirecumbent* position, prevent bearing down (pushing) with second-stage labor.
 II. Control asthma, because it can promote sickling crises by shifting the oxygen-hemoglobin dissociation curve to the right.
 III. Prevent infection—pneumococcal pneumonia (but also salmonella osteomyelitis, and urinary tract infections) can promote sickling crises by shifting the oxygen-hemoglobin dissociation curve to the right.
 IV. Ensure adequate hydration to prevent/treat infection. *Crisis is caused by:* hypoxia, hypotension, acidosis, dehydration, exertion, sudden cooling, and low-grade fever. Thrombophlebitis may occur from increased blood viscosity.
 V. For crises: Analgesia is administered, prn.
 VI. Blood transfusions given to maintain hemoglobin at ≥8 mg/dL, hemoglobin A at over 40%, and hematocrit at ≥30%.
 VII. Prepare for birth with forceps assistance under local or regional anesthesia.
 VIII. Assess for pseudopreeclampsia (hypertension and proteinuria, but with *no* weight gain) that often accompanies bone pain crisis.

Systemic Lupus Erythematosus (SLE): Health Teaching

 I. Maternal complications correlate with degree of cardiac or renal involvement.

II. SLE should be in remission at least 6 mo *before* pregnancy is attempted.

III. If SLE has been controlled well on low doses of corticosteroids for 2 yr, pregnancy may be considered. *Prednisone* and *azathioprine* can be continued during pregnancy; they do not appear to be teratogenic. Many other medications used in treating SLE are not recommended during pregnancy.

IV. While planning for pregnancy, the woman with SLE needs to know:
   A. Risk of miscarriage is higher than in normal pregnancy.
   B. She is twice as likely to suffer a flare-up during pregnancy.
   C. Hypertension is a major problem.

V. Contraception
   A. Oral contraceptives are *contraindicated*.
   B. Condoms and diaphragms are the preferred methods if pregnancy is desired in the future.

Women Who Have Had Phenylketonuria (PKU): Health Teaching

I. Strict adherence to a *phenylalanine-restricted diet before* and *during* pregnancy is essential; phenylalanine is teratogenic.
   A. A restricted diet during pregnancy has only questionable preventive value.

II. Fetal damage (microcephaly, mental retardation, cardiac defects) and intrauterine growth retardation (IUGR) *can* be largely prevented, but even careful management of phenylalanine levels does *not ensure* the birth of a normal infant.

Cystic Fibrosis: Woman with Both Recessive Genes

I. Pathophysiology
   A. Most women are infertile, but pregnancy is not uncommon.
   B. *Pulmonary* function: unable to maintain vital capacity, so that there is decreased oxygen to the myocardium, decreased cardiac output, and an increase in hypoxemia. Severe pulmonary infection is associated with increased maternal and perinatal mortality.
   C. Amount of *sodium* lost through sweat can be significant; *hypovolemia* can occur.

II. Medical management
   A. In the presence of any degree of *cor pulmonale*, she must be guarded against fluid overload.
   B. Oxygen is given freely during labor; epidural or local anesthesia is given for birth.

III. Health teaching
   A. Genetics
      1. Child will carry at least one gene for cystic fibrosis, since this is an *autosomal-recessive* disorder.
      2. If the father of the child also carries the gene and passes it on, this child *will* exhibit the disease; if the father contributes a normal

gene, the child will carry one gene for cystic fibrosis.
   B. Breastfeeding is deferred until after the sodium content of the woman's breast milk has been estimated; it may be as high as 280 mmole/liter. Breastfeeding is encouraged if levels of sodium are acceptable.
   C. Formula feeding is encouraged if this is the woman's choice, even if her breast milk has an acceptable amount of sodium.

Hyperthyroidism: Medical Management

I. Affects approximately 1 to 2/1000 pregnancies.

II. May be responsible for anovulation and amenorrhea; not a recognized cause of spontaneous abortion or fetal malformation.

III. Surgical treatment of hyperthyroidism (subtotal thyroidectomy) may be performed during the second and third trimesters.

IV. Controlled with *propylthiouracil* (PTU).
   A. Readily crosses the placenta.
   B. May induce fetal hypothyroidism and goiter; at birth, a *free T_4 index determination* on cord blood is needed to assess newborn status.

Epilepsy

I. Risk of congenital anomalies: 2 to 3 times greater than general population.

II. *Valproic acid* associated with 1–2% incidence of neural tube defects; *not* recommended during pregnancy.

III. Phenytoin (*Dilantin*): anticonvulsant
   A. Can cause *fetal hydantoin syndrome:* microcephaly, mental retardation, developmental delay, intrauterine growth retardation, facial clefts, and nail hypoplasia.
   B. Interferes with normal *folate* absorption from GI tract; 1 mg/d ordered.
   C. Interferes with normal *vitamin D* production; supplementation recommended.

Spinal Cord Injury (SCI): Management

I. Although individuals with SCI are physiologically the same as other women, some normal *adaptations* do require *special consideration:* urinary frequency, urinary tract infection, constipation, and need to relieve pressure on ischial spines and gluteal muscles and to straighten body, since pregnancy precludes lying prone.

II. *Oxytocin*, if needed, is used cautiously and only when personnel are versed in the recognition and treatment of autonomic dysreflexia. The headache and hypertension must *not* be confused with preeclampsia.

III. Although women with SCI do *not* experience labor as other women do, they are in tune with their bodies and know when something is happening.

IV. The woman with SCI experiences no trouble with a vaginal birth even though she has no ability to push. Uterine contractions, plus a relaxed perineum, facilitate a vaginal birth.

☼ *Life-Threatening Situations: Nursing Management*

I. Cardiopulmonary resuscitation (CPR)
  A. Done with woman *supine* with *lateral uterine tilt*.
  B. Maintain 5 : 1 ratio; pause at end of every fifth compression. Total: 12 breaths/min.
  C. If mother is resuscitated, the fetus will be too.

II. Heimlich maneuver
  A. If *conscious:* Encircle her chest and provide chest thrusts.
  B. If *unconscious:* Give chest compressions as for women without a pulse.

III. Anaphylaxis (an immediate hypersensitivity reaction)
  A. *Local* reactions: angioedema (redness and swelling).
  B. *Systemic* reactions: cardiovascular collapse; nausea, vomiting, diarrhea; asthmalike symptoms.
  C. Therapy: *epinephrine* by injection is the drug of choice. It dilates the bronchi, constricts blood vessels, increases blood pressure, and increases rate/strength of heartbeat (and, therefore, the circulation of oxygen throughout body).

☼ *Surgical Emergencies*

I. Acute suppurative appendicitis—*medical aspects*
  A. The appendix is carried high and to the right, away from McBurney's point, by the enlarged uterus, complicating diagnosis. Increased *sedimentation rate* is normal during pregnancy, and therefore *cannot* be used in diagnosis.
  B. Therapeutic abortion is *never* indicated.
  C. Maternal mortality: increases to about 10% in the third trimester; 15% if it occurs during labor.
  D. Perinatal mortality: approximately 10% with unruptured appendicitis; 35% if complicated with peritonitis.
  E. Rupture and peritonitis: 2–3 times more often than in nonpregnant women.

II. Intestinal obstruction (adynamic ileus)—*management*
  A. Not common during pregnancy.
  B. Assess *signs/symptoms*
    1. Persistent cramplike abdominal pain.
    2. Auscultatory rushes within the abdomen and "laddering" of the intestinal shadows on x-ray films aid in diagnosis.
  C. Immediate surgical intervention to release the intestinal obstruction (adynamic ileus) rarely adversely affects pregnancy.

III. Nonobstetric preoperative care
  A. *Antacids* are given *before* surgery because the hydrochloric acid in the stomach (if aspirated) may cause an asthmalike syndrome with necrotizing bronchitis.
    1. *Cimetidine:* a histamine blocker; decreases production of gastric acid.
    2. Metoclopramide (*Reglan*) increases gastric emptying.
  B. Prolonged NPO can lead to ketosis and hypoglycemia; IV fluids with dextrose are given to prevent them.
  C. Greater risk of postoperative atelectasis and pulmonary complications because of the decreased respiratory excursion associated with the enlarged uterus.
  D. Stress of surgery may stimulate the onset of labor.

Cancer and Pregnancy

I. For each 1800 pregnant women, 1 will also have cancer. In order of frequency, the types are: breast cancer, leukemia and lymphomas as a group, melanomas, gynecologic (cervical and ovarian) tumors, and bone tumors.
II. With diagnosis, many complex issues and reactions arise:
  A. Decision to continue or terminate pregnancy.
  B. Selection of therapies: surgery, chemotherapy, radiation.
  C. Moral and philosophic dilemmas.
III. Key points: cancer therapy and pregnancy
  A. Chemotherapy and radiation are specific against rapidly growing cells. Therefore, the embryo/fetus is most at risk during the *first* trimester, the period of organogenesis and tissue growth.
  B. After the first trimester, live births with few congenital abnormalities occur following judicious use of chemotherapy. *Alkylating agents, 5-fluorouracil* and *vincristine,* are relatively safe for the fetus.
  C. Radiation can cause damage at any stage of embryonic/fetal development.
  D. Surgery may be performed safely in many cases.

Breast Cancer

I. approximately 1–2% of women are pregnant when breast cancer is diagnosed. The nurse needs to counsel women that breastfeeding is *contraindicated* because lactation increases vascularity and possible metastasis.

Malignant Melanoma (Rare in Pregnant Women)

I. Effect on *woman:* Although the effect of pregnancy on melanoma is unknown, women with melanoma are cautioned about getting pregnant because there is a natural increase in melanocyte-stimulating hormone (MSH) during pregnancy. Adrenocorticotropic hormone (ACTH) production also increases during pregnancy, which heightens MSH activity. Stage for stage, there is no significant difference in the survival of pregnant and nonpregnant women with malignant melanoma.
II. Effect on *fetus:* 50% of placental metastases and almost 90% of fetal metastases occur from maternal melanoma.

Violence

Rape: Sexual Assault

I. *Rape trauma syndrome*—characteristics
   A. *Acute phase:* fear, humiliation, anger, and self-blame; feels unclean and wants to bathe and douche despite fact she would be destroying evidence.
   B. Desire to forget the incident is characteristic of the *first* reorganization phase (*adjustment*).
   C. Urgency to change residence or phone number is characteristic of the *first* reorganization phase (*adjustment*).
   D. Nightmares and eating disorders are very common in the *second* reorganization phase (*integration*) and the *third* reorganization phase (*recovery*).

II. *Medical management*
   ☞ A. Specimens are obtained from orifices, e.g., vaginal vault.
   B. Physical injuries are treated.
   ▬ C. Prophylaxis for infection is given.
   ▬ D. Prophylaxis for pregnancy is provided.

Assault and Battery

I. General comments
   A. Violence against women respects no social, economic, racial or ethnic categories.
   B. Prevalence of abuse toward pregnant women ranges from 8–17%; violence often starts and/or becomes worse during pregnancy.
   C. Cycle of violence occurs in *three phases: building, battering, calm.*
   D. Alcohol has not been causally related to battering, but batterers do have a high rate of alcohol abuse.
   E. Abused women are 1½ times more likely to have low-birth-weight (LBW) infants and more likely to have associated risk factors for LBW, such as poor obstetric history, infections, and alcohol or drug use.

▶ II. **Assessment:** Nursing interview technique must be skillful, help the woman focus on the situation, *avoid* implication that she is somehow responsible, and be unthreatening. Example: "How safe do you feel when you are with your partner?" does not place blame on the woman or accuse the partner.

III. A woman in a battering situation is *more likely* to seek help early if she has not experienced violence in her family of origin; that is, she has not been taught "learned helplessness." Others who seek help early are those beaten frequently and severely and those who see an alternative to life in their marriages—specifically, those with jobs.

IV. Women *less likely* to seek help are those who: have just learned they are pregnant, have one or more preschool children, or are afraid that the batterer will punish them.

▶ V. **Nursing intervention:** Most therapeutic action is to assist the woman in identifying her options, which may include remaining in the relationship.

Avoid taking sides against the batterer or suggesting that the woman leave the batterer.

▶ VI. **Evaluation/outcome criteria** of nursing intervention: Goals have been met when the woman can use phrases such as "*I* am . . . ," which indicate a developing self-esteem, feelings of worth and personal adequacy, and independence. NOTE: Following the "advice" of counselors is a submissive, passive, and dependent act—a continuation of "learned helplessness."

▶ Trauma—Nursing Management

☞ I. *First* intervention: Tilt uterus off the major vessels to facilitate venous return and prevent supine hypotension and placental congestion. If on backboard, tilt entire board. If CPR needed, perform while keeping uterus tilted off vessels (see p. 67).

II. Do **not** place in Trendelenburg's position, which could severely impair maternal respirations when the heavy enlarged uterus presses up against the diaphragm.

III. Establish an *intravenous line* for fluid and electrolyte replacement.

☞ IV. Place a *central venous or Swan-Ganz catheter* to monitor fluid therapy. The woman may sustain a significant blood loss of approximately 30% without the usual signs and symptoms of hypovolemia. A rapid pulse may reflect only the usual increase of 10–15 beats/min during pregnancy, or it may be a sign of hypovolemia.

☞ V. Insert a *retention urinary catheter.* Although not the priority action, the catheter is inserted to measure hourly urine output during fluid therapy, to assess for shock, and to assess for bladder injury secondary to the trauma. (During pregnancy, the bladder is pulled up above the symphysis pubis and is more vulnerable to injury.)

☞ VI. Auscultate fetal heart rate (*FHR*) after the woman's condition is assessed and therapy is instituted. When her condition has been stabilized, attention is given to the FHR and to the possibility of preterm labor and placental abruption.

VII. Observe the maternal-fetal unit for 48 hr to rule out complications such as preterm labor and placental abruption.

Common Complications: First Trimester

Complications Affecting Fluid-Gas Transport: Hemorrhagic Disorders

General Aspects

Review Emergency Conditions, Table 3.3

▶ I. Assessment
   A. Vital signs, output, general status.
   B. Evidence of internal/external bleeding.
   C. Pain.

TABLE 3.3   EMERGENCY CONDITIONS

First Trimester

◨*Assessment/Observations*	*Possible Problem*	◨*Nursing Care Plan/Implementation*
Fluid-Gas Transport		
a. *Cramping*—with or without bleeding or passage of tissue	Abortion (before 24 wk) Threatened Imminent, incomplete, septic	• Bedrest, sedation, *avoid* coitus—if threatened; start IV fluids and draw blood for *laboratory* work: CBC, type/cross-match, electrolytes, platelets, hCG levels
b. *Passage of tissue* (products of conception; grapelike vesicles) or *brown spotting;* fundus too high for gestational age; *blood pressure* elevated; often associated with hyperemesis gravidarum and preeclampsia	Hydatidiform mole (gestational trophoblastic disease)	• Vital signs q 5–15 min, prn
c. Severe *pain, shock* out of proportion to amount of overt blood; shoulder-strap pain (*Kehr's sign*), a "referred pain" that indicates intraabdominal bleeding (or rupture of ovarian cyst); amenorrhea of 6–12 wk	Ectopic pregnancy	• Save all pads or tissue passed through vagina for physician evaluation • No rectal or vaginal examination until physician is present
d. Malodorous *discharge; hyperthermia and chills;* tender abdomen	Septic abortion (self-induced or "criminal")	• Take complete history, if possible • Convulsion precautions if hypertensive
e. *Ecchymosis or bleeding*—with a history that includes any or all of the following: had symptoms of pregnancy, but they subsided; pregnancy test negative; uterine size diminishing; no FHT	Missed abortion with possible DIC (retained dead fetus syndrome)	• Emotional support for loss of pregnancy (through nurse's manner, tone of voice, touch, use of woman's name, keep her informed of what is happening) ☞ • Oxygen, prn

(continued)

D. Emotional response.
E. Perineal pads saturated and number.
F. Speculum examination.
◨ **II.** Analysis/nursing diagnosis
   A. *Knowledge deficit* related to diagnosis, prognosis, treatment, sequelae.
   B. *Anxiety/fear* related to loss of pregnancy, surgery.
   C. *Fluid volume deficit, potential/actual,* related to excessive blood loss.
   D. *Pain.*
   E. *Ineffective coping, individual/family,* related to knowledge deficit and fear.
   F. *Anticipatory/dysfunctional grieving,* related to loss of pregnancy.
   G. *Disturbance in self-esteem, body image, role performance,* related to threat to self-image as woman and childbearer.
◨ **III.** Nursing care plan/implementation
   A. Goal: *minimize blood loss, stabilize physiologic status*
     1. Facilitate prompt medical management.
     ☞ 2. Administer IV fluids, blood, as ordered.
     💊 3. Administer analgesics, as needed.
   ☞ B. Goal: *prevent infection.* Strict aseptic technique.
   C. Goal: *emotional support*
     1. Encourage verbalization of anxiety, fears, concerns.
     2. Supportive care for grief reaction (see Loss of Pregnancy, Table 3.4).
◨ **IV.** Evaluation/outcome criteria

TABLE 3.3   EMERGENCY CONDITIONS (*Continued*)

Second Trimester

⋈*Assessment/Observations*	*Possible Problem*	⋈*Nursing Care Plan/Implementation*
Fluid-Gas Transport		
a. Cramping; passage of products of conception	Late abortion	• Same as for first trimester
b. Labor—cervical changes, "show"	Incompetent cervical os	• See MD immediately for possible cerclage
c. *Prolonged* nausea and vomiting; unexplained *hypertension* or *preeclampsia*; passage of dark blood or grapelike vesicles; *absent FHTs*; excessive fundal height for gestation	Hydatidiform mole	• Maintain hydration; assess for dehydration • Refer to MD
Sensory-Perceptual		

a. *Preeclampsia/eclampsia*
Assessment: hypertension first noted after 24 wk; followed by increased proteinuria
Symptoms: blurred or double vision; pain: headache, epigastric (late sign)
Signs: BP 160/110; 3$^+$ proteinuria
Edema: facial, digital; pulmonary
Oliguria
Hyperreflexia
	With increased severity: renal failure, circulatory collapse, CVA, coagulation defects (DIC); abruptio placentae	• Pharmacologic management of woman with hypertension
		☞*Convulsion (seizure) precautions*
		  1. Emergency tray at bedside
		  2. Oxygen/suction
		  3. Start IV
		  4. Padded siderails
		  5. Indwelling urinary catheter
		  6. Constant observation
		  7. Deep tendon reflexes
		  8. Daily weight
		  9. I&O
		  10. Note any complaints and changes
		  〰11. Prepare for *lab work* (type and cross-match, CBC, platelets, BUN, and creatinine)

b. *Convulsions* in absence of hypertension, proteinuria, or facial edema	CVA, epilepsy, drug toxicity; intracranial injury; diabetic complications; encephalopathy	☞*Convulsion (seizure) care:* see p. 76
		  1. Oxygen/mask; drugs (magnesium sulfate IV)
		  2. Observe
		    a. Uterine tone, FHRs, fetal activity
		    b. Signs of labor
		  3. Emotional support for woman and family

(continued)

A. Woman's blood loss minimized; physiologic status stable.
B. Woman (family) copes effectively with loss of pregnancy.

Spontaneous Abortion: Before Viable Age of 20–22 wk

I. Etiology
  A. Defective products of conception.

B. Insufficient production of progesterone.
C. Acute infections.
D. Reproductive system abnormalities, e.g., incompetent cervical os.
E. Trauma (physical or emotional).
F. Rh incompatibility.

⋈ **II. Assessment:** types
  A. *Threatened*—mild bleeding, spotting, cramping; cervix closed.

TABLE 3.3 EMERGENCY CONDITIONS (*Continued*)

Third Trimester

◁Assessment/Observations	Possible Problem	◁Nursing Care Plan/Implementation
Fluid-Gas Transport a. *Bleeding:* painless, bright red, vaginal Contractions and/or uterine tone normal	Placenta previa	• **No vaginal examination** ☞ • Apply fetal monitor; assess for labor ☞ • *Position:* semi- to high Fowler's
b. *Pain:* abdomen rigid and tender to touch Increased uterine tone; signs of shock disproportionate to visible blood loss; may have loss of FHTs; associated with: pre-eclampsia, multiparity, precipitous labor, oxytocin induction, trauma, cocaine use	Abruptio placentae	• As for placenta previa; *position:* Sims'

FHR = fetal heart rate; DIC = disseminated intravascular coagulation; CBC = complete blood count; hCG = human chorionic gonadotropin; CVA = cerebrovascular accident.

B. *Inevitable*—moderate bleeding, painful cramping; cervix dilated, positive *Nitrazine test* (membranes ruptured).

C. *Imminent*—profuse bleeding, severe cramping, urge to bear down.

D. *Incomplete*—fetal parts or fetus expelled; placenta and membranes retained.

E. *Complete*—all products of conception expelled; minimal vaginal bleeding.

F. *Habitual/recurrent*—history of spontaneous loss of three or more successive pregnancies.

G. *Missed*—fetal death with no spontaneous expulsion within 4 wk.
  1. Anorexia, malaise, headache.
  2. Fundal height—inconsistent with gestational estimate.
  3. Laboratory tests—prolonged clotting time, due to resultant concurrent hypofibrinogenemia (disseminated intravascular coagulation [DIC], a major threat to mother).

H. Elective abortions (intentionally introduced loss of pregnancy).

◁ **III. Analysis/nursing diagnosis**
  A. *Altered family processes* related to pregnancy, circumstances surrounding abortion.
  B. *Sexual dysfunction* related to compromised self-image, altered interpersonal relationship, guilt feelings.

◁ **IV. Nursing care plan/implementation**
  A. *Threatened*—goal: *health teaching.* Suggest: *avoid coitus and orgasm,* especially around normal time for menstrual period.
  B. *Incomplete, inevitable, imminent*
    1. Goal: *safeguard status*
      a. Save all perineal pads, clots, tissue for expert diagnosis.

      b. Report immediately any change in status, excessive bleeding, signs of infection, shock.
      c. Prepare for surgery.
    2. Goal: *comfort measures*
      a. Administer analgesics, as necessary.
      b. *Bedrest,* quiet diversional activities.
    3. Goal: *emotional support*
      a. Encourage verbalization of fear, concerns.
      b. Reduce anxiety, as possible.
      c. If pregnancy terminates, facilitate grieving process; assist in working through guilt feelings (see Table 3.4).
      d. Supportive care for grief reaction (see Table 3.4).
    4. Goal: *prevent isoimmunization.* See Rh incompatibility, p. 53
    5. *Medical management*
      a. Laboratory tests—blood type and Rh factor, indirect Coombs, platelets, serum fibrinogen, clotting time.
      b. Replace blood loss; maintain fluid levels with IV.
      c. Dilatation and curettage.
  C. *Habitual*—determine etiology.

◁ **V. Evaluation/outcome criteria**
  A. *Threatened abortion*—woman responds to medical/nursing regimen; abortion avoided, successfully carries pregnancy to term.
  B. *Spontaneous abortion*—after uterus emptied
    1. Woman's bleeding is controlled.
    2. Woman's vital signs are stable.
    3. Woman (family) copes effectively with loss of pregnancy.
    4. Woman (family) expresses satisfaction with care.

TABLE 3.4   LOSS OF PREGNANCY

Stage of Grief	*Possible Maternal Response*	✉ *Nursing Care Plan/Implementation*
Shock, disbelief	Pulls back, withdraws: not interested in events around her; may stay in bed, staring at wall, with shades drawn	Since mother cannot communicate effectively now, nurse demonstrates caring behaviors by *staying* with her, touching or *massaging* her; providing *physical* care; giving her opportunity to talk if she wants to; do *not* make light of her situation
Anger, fear	Verbal fault-finding and possible physical aggression, irritability, insomnia	State that it is normal to be angry; help her identify her questions and concerns (guilt); be available to her (and her family)
Helplessness, despair, guilt	Dependent behaviors—may become demanding, may cry, may exhibit regressive behaviors; may see no purpose to anything; may feel very guilty, worthless	Help her *verbalize* her actual and implied feelings: "It is hard to understand," "You probably feel you are to blame . . ."; "The way you feel may seem strange or even 'crazy' to you." Do provide *physical* care, give massage, keep her physically comfortable
Reorganization (after discharge)	Begins to be interested in events around her, to have increased amounts of energy; inquires again about events leading to the situation, the etiology, the medical and nursing management, as she tries to integrate the experience; older siblings may show regressive behavior: fear of the dark, fear of school, or behavioral difficulties	Community health or clinic nurse listens, clarifies, fills in gaps. Reexplain the grieving process—that her (their) behaviors were normal; that acute grief lasts 6 wk, while the entire process lasts about 1 yr or more. Talk about what older siblings or other family members may be feeling—a young child's return to bed-wetting may be a response to the parents' tension, etc.

C. *Habitual abortion*—cause identified and corrected; woman carries subsequent pregnancy to successful termination.

Hydatidiform Mole (Complete)

I. Pathophysiology—gestational trophoblastic disease (GTD), in which chorionic villi degenerate into grapelike cluster of vesicles; may be antecedent to **choriocarcinoma.**

II. Etiology—genetic base of complete mole (sperm enters empty egg and its chromosomes replicate; 23 pairs of chromosomes are all of paternal origin); rare complication; more common in women *over 45* yr of age and Asian women.

✉ **III.** **Assessment**
  A. Uterus—rapid enlargement; fundal height inconsistent with gestational estimate.
  B. Brownish discharge—beginning about *week 12*; may contain vesicles.
  C. Signs and symptoms of preeclampsia/eclampsia (*before* third trimester), increased incidence of hyperemesis gravidarum (see pp. 73, 75).

D. *Medical evaluation*—procedures
  ∿ **1.** Sonography, X-ray, amniography—no fetal parts present; "snow storm."
  2. *Laboratory test*—for elevated human chorionic gonadotropin (hCG) levels.
  3. Follow-up surveillance of hCG levels for at least one year; persistent hCG level is consistent with choriocarcinoma; x-ray.

✉ **IV.** **Analysis/nursing diagnosis**
  A. *Anxiety/fear* related to treatment, possible sequelae of hydatidiform mole (choriocarcinoma).
  B. *Potential for injury* related to hemorrhage, perforation of uterine wall, preeclampsia/eclampsia.
  C. *Fluid volume deficit* related to injury.

✉ **V.** **Nursing care plan/implementation**
  A. *Medical management*
  1. Monitor for preeclampsia/eclampsia.
  2. Evacuate the uterus—hysterectomy may be necessary.
  3. *Strict* contraception for at least 1 yr to enable accurate assessment of status.
  ☞ **4.** Choriocarcinoma—chemotherapy (*metho-*

trexate plus *dactinomycin*) and/or radiation therapy.

B. *Nursing management*
1. Goal: *safeguard status.* Observe for hemorrhage, passage of retained vesicles and abdominal pain, or signs of infection (because woman is at-risk for perforation of uterine wall).
2. Goal: *health teaching*
   a. Explain, discuss diagnostic tests; prepare for tests.
   b. Discuss contraceptive options.
   c. Discuss importance of follow-up.
3. Goal: *preoperative and postoperative care.*
4. Goal: *emotional support.* Facilitate grieving (see Table 3.4).

VI. Evaluation/outcome criteria
A. Woman verbalizes understanding of diagnosis, tests, and treatment.
B. Woman complies with medical/nursing recommendations.
C. Woman tolerates surgical procedure well
   1. Bleeding controlled.
   2. Vital signs stable.
   3. Urinary output adequate.
D. Woman copes effectively with loss of pregnancy.
E. Woman returns for follow-up care/surveillance.
F. Woman selects and effectively implements method of contraception; avoids pregnancy for 1 yr or more.
G. Tests for hCG remain negative for 1 yr; no evidence of malignancy.
H. Woman achieves a pregnancy when desired.
I. Woman successfully carries pregnancy to term; normal, uncomplicated birth of viable infant.

Ectopic Pregnancy

I. Pathology—implantation outside of uterine cavity.
II. Types:
A. Tubal (most common).
B. Cervical.
C. Abdominal.
D. Ovarian.
III. Etiology
A. Pelvic inflammatory disease (PID)—pelvic salpingitis and endometritis.
B. 43% caused by sexually transmitted disease (STD)—related factors: 25%, chlamydial; 20%, previous STD.
C. Tubal or uterine anomalies, tubal spasm.
D. Adhesions from PID or past surgeries.
E. Presence of intrauterine device (IUD).
IV. Assessment: dependent on implantation site
A. *Early signs*—abnormal menstrual period (usually following a missed menstrual period), spotting, some symptoms of pregnancy; possible dull pain on affected side.
B. *Impending or posttubal rupture*—sudden, acute, lower abdominal pain; nausea and vomiting; signs of shock; referred shoulder pain (*Kehr's sign*) or

neck pain—due to blood in peritoneal cavity; blood in cul-de-sac may → rectal pressure.
C. *Cullen's sign:* ecchymotic blueness of umbilicus, indicative of hematoperitoneum. Sharp, localized pain when cervix is touched during vaginal examination; shock and circulatory collapse in some, usually *following* vaginal examination.
D. Positive pregnancy test in many women.
V. Analysis/nursing diagnosis
A. *Fear* related to abdominal pain and pregnancy status.
B. *Grief* related to pregnancy loss.
VI. Nursing care plan/implementation
A. *Medical management:* surgical removal/repair.
B. *Nursing management*
   1. Goal: *preoperative and postoperative care, health teaching.*
   2. Goal: *supportive care for grief reaction;* encourage verbalization of anxiety and concerns of further pregnancies.
VII. Evaluation/outcome criteria
A. Woman experiences uncomplicated postoperative course.
B. Woman copes effectively with loss of pregnancy.

Complications Affecting Nutrition/Elimination

Hyperemesis Gravidarum

I. Pathophysiology—pernicious vomiting during first 14–16 wk (peak incidence around 10 wk gestation); excessive vomiting at any time during pregnancy. Potential hazards include:
A. Dehydration with fluid and electrolyte imbalance.
B. Starvation, with loss of 5% or more of body weight; protein and vitamin deficiencies.
C. *Metabolic acidosis*—due to breakdown of fat stores to meet metabolic needs.
D. Hypovolemia and hemoconcentration; *increased* blood urea nitrogen (BUN); *decreased* urinary output.
II. Etiology
A. *Physiologic*—secretion of hCG, decrease in free gastric HCl, decreased gastrointestinal motility. Increased incidence in hydatidiform mole and multifetal pregnancy (due to high levels of hCG).
B. *Psychological*—thought to be related to rejection of pregnancy and/or sexual relations.
III. Assessment
A. Intractable vomiting.
B. Abdominal pain.
C. Hiccups.
D. Marked weight loss.
E. Dehydration—thirst, tachycardia, skin turgor.
F. Increased respiratory rate (metabolic acidosis).
G. Laboratory—elevated BUN.
H. *Medical evaluation:* rule out other causes (infection, tumors).
IV. Analysis/nursing diagnosis

A. *Altered nutrition, less than body requirements,* related to inability to retain oral feedings.

B. *Fluid volume deficit* related to dehydration.

C. *Ineffective individual coping* related to symptoms, insecurity in role, psychological stress of unwanted pregnancy.

D. *Personal identity disturbance* related to symptoms and/or perception of self as inadequate in role, sick, socially unpresentable.

✄ **V. Nursing care plan/implementation**

   A. Goal: *physiologic stability*

☞   1. Rest GI tract (keep NPO), e.g., maintain IV fluids, parenteral nutrition.

     2. Progress *diet,* as ordered; present small feedings attractively.

     3. Weigh daily, assess hydration; note weight gain.

   B. Goal: *minimize environmental stimuli*

     1. Limit visitors and phone calls.

     2. *Bedrest* with bathroom privileges.

   C. Goal: *emotional support*

     1. Establish accepting, supportive environment.

     2. Encourage verbalization of anxiety, fears, concerns.

     3. Support positive self-image.

✄ **VI. Evaluation/outcome criteria**

   A. Woman's signs and symptoms subside; she takes oral nourishment and gains weight.

   B. Woman's pregnancy continues to term without recurrence of hyperemesis.

Common Complications: Second Trimester

See Table 3, p. 70.

Complications Affecting Comfort, Rest, Mobility

Incompetent Cervix

  I. Pathophysiology—inability of cervix to support growing weight of pregnancy; associated with repeated spontaneous second trimester abortion.

  II. Etiology

   A. Unknown.

   B. Congenital defect in cervical musculature.

   C. Cervical trauma during previous birth, abortion; aggressive, deep, or repeated dilatation and curettage.

✄ **III. Assessment**

   A. History of habitual, second trimester abortions.

   B. Painless, progressive cervical effacement and dilatation during second trimester.

   C. Signs of threatened abortion or (early third trimester) preterm labor.

✄ **IV. Analysis/nursing diagnosis**

   A. *Pain* related to early dilatation.

B. *Fear* related to possible pregnancy loss.

✄ **V. Nursing care plan/implementation**

   A. *Medical management*

     1. Cerclage surgical procedure (*Shirodkar, McDonald*).

   B. *Preoperative nursing management*

     1. Goal: *reduce physical stress on incompetent cervix. Bedrest,* supportive care.

     2. Goal: *emotional support.* Encourage verbalization of anxiety, fear, concerns.

     3. Goal: *health (preoperative) teaching.* Explain procedure—purse-string suture encircles cervix and reinforces musculature.

     4. Goal: *preparation for surgery.*

   C. *Postoperative nursing management*

     1. Goal: *maximize surgical result. Bedrest,* supportive care.

     2. Goal: *health teaching*

       a. *Avoid:* strenuous physical activity; straining.

       b. Report promptly: signs of labor (vaginal bleeding, cramping).

       c. Need for continued, close health surveillance.

✄ **VI. Evaluation/outcome criterion:** Woman carries pregnancy to successful termination.

Complications Affecting Protective Functions

Preterm labor

Preterm birth is that which occurs *after week 20* but *before the end of week 37* of gestation. Preterm birth is responsible for almost two-thirds of infant deaths. Because of the high incidence, all pregnant women need to learn the signs and symptoms of preterm labor. See Chapter 5, pp. 122–125 for discussion.

Common Complications: Third Trimester

Complications Affecting Sensory/ Perceptual Functions

Preeclampsia/Eclampsia and HELLP Syndrome

  I. Pathophysiology

   A. Generalized arteriospasm → increased peripheral resistance, decreased tissue perfusion, and hypertension.

   B. *Kidney*

     1. Reduced renal perfusion and vasospasm → glomerular lesions.

     2. Damage to membrane → loss of serum protein (albuminuria). NOTE: Reduced serum albumin-globulin (A/G) ratio alters blood osmolarity → edema.

3. Increased tubular reabsorption of sodium → increased water retention (edema).
4. Release of angiotensin contributes to vasospasm and hypertension.
C. *Brain:* decreased oxygenation, cerebral edema, and vasospasm → visual disturbances and hyperirritability, convulsions, and coma.
D. *Uterus:* decreased placental perfusion → increased risk of SGA baby, abruptio placentae.

II. Etiology: unknown. *Risk factors:*
A. Pregnancy—occurs only when a functioning trophoblast is present; more common in *first* pregnancies; develops after week 24 of gestation.
B. Age related—*under* 17 and *over* 35 yr of age.
C. Coexisting conditions—diabetes, multifetal gestation, hydramnios.
D. *Diet*—low in protein.

III. **Assessment**—types:
A. **Preeclampsia**—*"mild"*
1. Hypertension—systolic increase of 30 mm Hg or more over baseline; diastolic rise of 15 mm Hg or more over baseline.
2. Proteinuria—1 g/d.
3. Edema—digital and periorbital; weight gain over 0.45 kg (1 pound)/wk.
B. **Preeclampsia**—*severe*
1. Increasing hypertension—systolic at or above 160 mm Hg or more than 50 mm Hg over baseline; diastolic, 110 mm Hg or more.
2. Urine: proteinuria (5 g or more in 24 hr); oliguria (400 mL or less in 24 hr).
3. Hemoconcentration, hypoproteinemia, hypernatremia, hypovolemic condition.
4. Persistent vomiting.
5. Epigastric pain—due to edema of liver capsule.
6. Cerebral or visual disturbances (*before* convulsive state)
a. Disorientation and somnolence.
b. Severe frontal headache.
c. Increased irritability; hyperreflexia.
d. Blurred vision, halo vision, dimness, blind spots.
C. **Eclampsia**
1. Tonic and clonic convulsions; coma.
2. Renal shutdown—oliguria, anuria.

IV. **Assessment—hospitalized woman**
A. Vital signs (blood pressure, pulse, respirations)—q 2–4 hr, while awake (if mild to moderate preeclampsia) and/or as necessary. NOTE: record, report persistent hypertension.
B. Fetal heart rate (FHR) at time of vital signs.
C. Deep tendon reflexes (DTR) and clonus—to identify/monitor CNS hyperirritability.
D. I&O—to identify diuresis. (NOTE: Oliguria indicates pathologic progression.)
E. Urinalysis (clean catch) for protein, daily or after each voiding, as necessary.
F. Signs of pathologic progression (see III. *Assessment*—types, above).
G. Signs of labor, abruptio placentae (NOTE: High

blood pressure, or a rapid drop, may initiate abruptio), DIC.
H. Emotional status.
I. Daily weight, amount/distribution of edema (pitting; pedal, digital, periorbital)—to identify signs of mobilization of tissue fluid, diuresis.

V. **Analysis/nursing diagnosis**
A. *Fluid volume deficit:* hemoconcentration, edema related to altered blood osmolarity (due to loss of protein from vascular compartment) and sodium/water retention. Hypovolemia results.
B. *Altered nutrition, less than body requirements:* protein deficiency related to dietary lack and/or loss through damaged renal membrane.
C. *Altered tissue perfusion* related to increased peripheral resistance and vasospasm in renal, cardiovascular system.
D. *Altered urinary elimination:* oliguria, anuria related to hypovolemia.
E. *Sensory/perceptual alterations:* visual disturbances, hyperirritability related to cerebral edema, decreased oxygenation to brain.
F. *Anxiety* related to symptoms, implications of pathophysiology.
G. *Diversional activity deficit* related to need for reduced environmental stimuli, bedrest.
H. *High risk for injury* related to seizure.

VI. Prognosis
A. *Good*—symptoms mild, respond to treatment.
B. *Poor*—convulsions (number and duration); persistent coma; hyperthermia, tachycardia (120 beats/min); cyanosis.
C. *Terminal*—pulmonary edema, heart failure, acute renal failure, cerebral hemorrhage. The *earlier* the symptoms appear, the *poorer* the outcome for the pregnancy.

VII. **Nursing care plan/implementation:** home care. Goal: *health maintenance*
A. Education—learning about the condition.
B. Education—self-care
1. Taking own blood pressure.
2. Checking for proteinuria.
3. Monitoring weight gain and stat reporting of gain of more than 1 pound/wk.
C. Fetal well-being—daily fetal movement count (DFMC).
D. Rest—frequent naps in *lateral Sims' position,* or bedrest.
E. Coping with bedrest.
1. Increasing fluid intake.
2. Using diversional activities.
3. Exercising gently—hands, feet, alternately tensing and relaxing muscles.
4. Using relaxation techniques.
F. Involve family
G. Nutrition
1. *High* protein intake to increase blood osmolarity, reduce movement of vascular fluid into interstitial space; diet should be well balanced.

2. Do *not* eliminate sodium; do *avoid* foods with *high* salt (potato chips, pickles, etc.).
3. *Avoid* alcohol and smoking.
4. *Fluids*—8–10 8-oz. glasses/d.
5. Foods with *roughage.*
H. Importance of regular prenatal visits.
I. Immediate recognition and reporting of **warning signs** indicating increasing severity:
  1. Digital and periorbital edema.
  2. Severe headache, irritability.
  3. Visual disturbances.
  4. Epigastric pain.

VIII. Nursing care plan/implementation—hospital care
A. Goal: *reduce environmental stimuli.* To minimize stimulation of hyperirritable CNS. Limit visitors and phone calls.
B. Goal: *emotional support*
  1. Encourage verbalization of anxiety, fears, concerns.
  2. Explain all procedures, seizure precautions.
C. Goal: *supportive care*
  1. Encourage bedrest in *lateral Sims' position*—to increase tissue perfusion, promote diuresis, and reduce risk of supine hypotensive syndrome.
  2. Suggest diversional activities, teach relaxation techniques to reduce stress.
D. Goal: *health teaching.* High-protein diet—to replace protein lost in urine, to retain fluid in the intravascular compartment, to reduce edema; moderate sodium—reduce intake of high-sodium foods, no added salt. *Do not eliminate* sodium from diet.
E. Goal: *administer medications as ordered and monitor effects*
  1. See Pharmacology Box 3.1.

2. Emergency: magnesium sulfate toxicity
Assess for signs/symptoms:
Respirations ≤ 12/min
DTRs: hyporeflexia, or absence (patella)
Urinary output ≤ 30 mL/hr
Toxic *serum levels* ≥ 9.6 mg/dL
Fetal distress: drop in FHRs, no fetal movement
Significant drop in maternal pulse or BP
Collaborative management:
stat: discontinue MgSO₄; open maintenance IV line
Call for assistance stat; notify attending physician
Administer *calcium gluconate* or *calcium chloride* as ordered (e.g., 1 g by IV injection **given over 3-min. period**)
Monitor frequently: DTRs, respirations, urinary output, MgSO₄ serum levels
Notify nursery nurses about possible neonatal effects

F. Goal: *seizure precautions,* to safeguard maternal-fetal health and well-being (see Table 3.3, p. 70).

1. *Environment:* nonstimulating, quiet, subdued lighting.
2. *Safety:* padded siderails; equipment for suctioning and oxygen administration, tested and ready for use; call button easily reached.
3. Emergency fluids and medication tray easily accessible
  a. *Magnesium sulfate* and *hydralazine.*
  b. *Calcium gluconate* available in a well-labeled syringe.
4. Emergency birth pack readily available.

5. Observe for warning signs and symptoms of impending seizure
  a. Frontal headache.
  b. Epigastric pain.
  c. Sharp cry.
  d. Eyes fixed; unresponsive.
  e. Facial twitching.

6. Continue close observation for 48 hr postpartum.

G. Goal: **seizure care** (of eclamptic patient)
  1. Maintain patent *airway*—prop in *lateral position;* after seizure, suction and administer oxygen by face mask.
  2. Administer medications/fluids as ordered.
  3. Assess uterine activity for labor and/or abruptio placentae.
  4. Check perineum for impending birth.
  5. Check FHR.
  6. Observe, report, and record
    a. Onset and progression of convulsion.
    b. If followed by coma and/or incontinence.

IX. **Evaluation/outcome criteria**
  1. Woman complies with medical/nursing plan of care.
  2. Woman's symptoms respond to treatment; progression halted.
  3. Woman carries uneventful pregnancy to successful termination.

X. *Severe preeclampsia/HELLP syndrome*
A. Definition: a critical complication of severe preeclampsia.
B. **Assessment**
  1. Signs and symptoms of severe preeclampsia (see III.R, p. 75), *plus* Table 3.3, p. 70.
  2. **H**emolysis, **E**levated **L**iver enzymes, and **L**ow **P**latelets.
C. **Analysis/nursing diagnosis**
  1. *High risk for injury* (**mother**) related to CNS irritability secondary to cerebral edema, vasospasm, decreased renal perfusion; seizures.
  2. *High risk for injury* (**fetus**) related to altered tissue perfusion (uteroplacental insufficiency, abruptio placentae) and/or preterm birth.
D. **Nursing care plan/implementation**
  1. Assist at birth, the only definitive treatment
    a. *Vaginal,* if cervix is favorable and fetal presentation and position are favorable.
    b. *Cesarean,* if induction for an extended period of time would be needed.

PHARMACOLOGY BOX 3.1   HYPERTENSION IN PREGNANCY AND LABOR

Drug/Dosage	*Indication/Action*	⋈ *Assessment: Side Effects*	⋈ *Nursing Management*
Anticonvulsant			
Magnesium sulfate (injection) *IM:* 1–5 g, prn *IV:* 1–4 g 1 h *Infusion:* 4 g in 250 mL 5% dextrose at ≤ 3 mL/m (loading dose) through infusion pump	Anticonvulsant activity due to inhibition of peripheral neuromuscular transmission Severe preeclampsia, eclampsia, HELLP syndrome	See Box: magnesium sulfate toxicity, p. 76.	Education: Explain procedure, rationale to woman, family Take safety precautions Provide comfort measures 🕱 *Warning*—do *not* give to women on digoxin (arrhythmias may occur); emergency artificial ventilation may be necessary
Antihypertensive			
Hydralazine (*Apresoline, Neopresol*) (arteriolar vasodilators), 50–200 mg (0)/d	Peripheral arterioles: decreases muscle tone, thereby decreasing peripheral resistance	**Mother:** Headache Flushing Palpitation Tachycardia **Fetus:** Tachycardia: late decelerations and bradycardia if maternal diastolic pressure below 90 mm Hg	Monitor effects of medications Alert mother (family) to expected effects of medications Monitor BP (precipitous drop can lead to shock and perhaps to abruptio placentae); monitor urinary output Maintain bedrest in *lateral position* with siderails for safety
Methyldopa (*Aldomet*) (used if maintenance therapy is needed): 250–500 mg orally q8h (α₂-receptor agonist)	Reduces peripheral vascular resistance CNS: sedation	**Mother:** Sleepiness Postural hypotension Constipation **Fetus:** After 4 mo of maternal therapy, 〰 *positive Coombs'* test in infant	See *Hydralazine* NOTE: 10%–20% of women receiving medication over 1 yr will have *direct* and *indirect Coombs-positive hemolytic anemia*
Labetalol hydrochloride (*Normodyne*)	Beta-blocking agent causing vasodilatation in peripheral arterioles, without significant change in cardiac output	Dizziness, drowsiness Bradycardia, postural hypotension Nausea/vomiting/diarrhea	See *Hydralazine*
Nitroglycerin	Potent vasodilator of venous system Decreases BP by decreasing cardiac output	If maternal BP drops, FHR variability may decrease	Monitor BP electronically, FHRs Needs special IV setup See *Hydralazine*

NOTE: Diuretics such as *thiazides* and *furosemide* (*Lasix*) are used only in severe situations: pulmonary edema. If used, the physician must be ready to justify the action.

 ⬤ **2.** Administer prescribed medications
   ⬤ **a.** Magnesium sulfate—seizure prophylaxis.
   ⬤ **b.** Antihypertensive agent for diastolic ≥ 110 mm Hg.
 ! **3.** Prevent/treat hypoglycemia (a major factor in maternal mortality in this disorder): ≤ 40 mg/dL.
 ☞ **4.** To permit seepage of edematous fluid, the cesarean incisional wound may be left open from the fascial layer; scrupulous *wound care* is imperative.
5. Monitor breath sound and woman's symptoms to identify and promptly treat *adult respiratory distress syndrome* (ARDS), which is one risk factor for women with the HELLP syndrome.

6. Alert nursery nurse to observe newborn for *thrombocytopenia,* a common sequel to HELLP syndrome.

✈ **E. Evaluation/outcome criteria**
   1. Woman/fetus does not suffer adverse sequelae to HELLP syndrome or its management.
   2. Family is able to cope effectively with this complication, its management, and outcomes.

Complications Affecting Fluid-Gas Transport (see Table 3.3, p. 71)
Placenta Previa

Abnormal implantation; near or over internal os. Increased incidence with smokers.

✈ **I. Assessment**
   A. Painless vaginal bleeding (may be intermittent); absence of contractions, abdomen soft.
   B. If in labor, contractions usually normal.
   C. Boggy lower uterine segment—palpated on vaginal examination. (NOTE: If placenta previa is suspected, internal examinations are *contraindicated.*)
   ⌇ **D.** *Medical diagnosis—procedure:* sonography—to determine placental site.

✈ **II. Analysis/nursing diagnosis**
   A. *Anxiety* related to bleeding, outcome.
   B. *Fluid volume deficit* related to excessive blood loss.
   C. *Altered tissue perfusion* related to blood loss.
   D. *Altered urinary elimination* related to hypovolemia.
   E. *Fear* related to fetal injury or loss.

III. Nursing care plan/implementation
   A. *Medical management*
   ⌇ 1. Ultrasound is used to locate placental site; if unavailable, a sterile vaginal examination is conducted in a surgical suite under *double setup* (i.e., physicians and patient are ready for an immediate vaginal or cesarean birth).
   2. Vaginal birth possible if: bleeding is *minimal;* placental implantation is *marginal;* this is woman's second or *later* vaginal birth; and *fetal vertex* is presenting so that presenting part acts as tamponade.
   3. Cesarean birth for complete previa.
   B. *Nursing management.* Goal: *safeguard status.*

✈ **IV. Evaluation/outcome criteria:** see Abruptio Placentae, below, and Tables 3.3 and 3.5.

Abruptio Placentae—Premature Separation of Normally Implanted Placenta

✈ **I. Assessment**
   A. Sudden onset, severe abdominal pain.
   B. Increased uterine tone—may contract unevenly, fails to relax between contractions; very tender.
   C. Shock usually more profound than expected on basis of external bleeding or internal bleeding.

D. *Medical evaluation—procedures:* DIC screening (bleeding time, platelet count, prothrombin time, activated partial thromboplastin time, fibrinogen).

✈ **II. Analysis/nursing diagnosis**
   A. *Fluid volume deficit* related to bleeding.
   B. *Risk for fetal injury* related to utero-placental insufficiency.
   C. *Fear* related to unknown outcome.

💡 **III.** *Potential complications*
   A. Afibrinoginemia and DIC.
   B. *Couvelaire* uterus—bleeding into uterine muscle.
   C. Amniotic fluid (pulmonary) embolus.
   D. Hypovolemic shock.
   E. Renal failure.
   F. Uterine atony, hemorrhage, infection in postpartum.

✈ **IV. Nursing care plan/implementation**
   A. *Medical management*
   1. Control: hemorrhage, hypovolemic shock, replace blood loss.
   2. Cesarean birth.
   💊 3. *Fibrinogen,* if necessary (*avoided* if possible, due to chance of hepatitis).
   💊 4. *IV heparin*—by infusion pump—to reduce coagulation and fibrinolysis.
   B. *Nursing management.* Goal: *safeguard status.* Implement or assist with medical management.

✈ **V. Evaluation/outcome criteria**
   A. Woman experiences successful termination of pregnancy
   1. Gives birth to viable newborn (via vaginal or cesarean method).
   2. Has minimal blood loss.
   3. Maintains assessment findings within normal limits.
   4. Retains capacity for further childbearing.
   B. Woman has no evidence of complications (anemia, hypotonia, DIC) during postpartal period.

Complications Affecting Comfort, Rest, Mobility
Hydramnios

Amniotic fluid in excess of 2000 mL (normal volume: 500–1200 mL).

I. Etiology: unknown. Risk factors:
   A. Maternal diabetes.
   B. Multifetal gestation.
   C. Erythroblastosis fetalis.
   D. Preeclampsia/eclampsia.
   E. Congenital anomalies (e.g., anencephaly, upper GI anomalies, such as esophageal atresia).

✈ **II. Assessment**
   A. Fundal height: excessive for gestational estimate.
   B. Fetal parts: difficult to palpate, small in proportion to uterine size.
   C. Increased discomfort—due to large, heavy uterus.
   D. Increased edema in vulva and legs.
   E. Shortness of breath.
   F. GI discomfort—heartburn, constipation.

TABLE 3.5 COMPARISON OF PLACENTA PREVIA AND ABRUPTIO PLACENTAE

Pathology	Etiology	✉ Assessment	✉ Nursing Care Plan/Implementation
Placenta Previa Types: *Marginal*—low lying *Partial*—partly covers internal os *Complete*—covers internal os	Unknown More common with multiparity, advanced maternal age Fibroid tumors Endometriosis Old scars Smoking	Painless vaginal bleeding Usually manifests in 8th mo **Postpartum:** signs of hemorrhage, infection	• *No* vaginal or rectal exams or enemas • Bedrest (*high Fowler's* if marginal previa) ☞ • Continuous fetal monitor • Maternal vital signs q 4 h, or as needed • Note character and amount of bleeding • Emotional support
Abruptio Placentae Types: *Partial*—small part separates *Complete*—total placenta separates *Retroplacental*—bleeding (concealed) *Marginal*—occurs at edges; external bleeding	Preeclampsia/eclampsia Before birth of second twin Traction on cord Rupture of membranes High parity Chronic renal hypertension Oxytocin induction/augmentation of labor Cocaine addiction Trauma	Pain: sudden, severe Abdomen: rigid Uterus: very tender to touch Fetal hyperactivity; bradycardia, death Shock: rapid, profound Port-wine amniotic fluid Signs of DIC **Postpartum:** signs of: atony, infection, pulmonary emboli	• *Position:* supine; elevate (R) hip • Monitor: vital signs, blood loss, fetus • I&O (anuria, oliguria; hematuria) • Prepare for surgery • Emotional support

G. Susceptibility to *supine hypotensive syndrome*—due to compression of inferior vena cava and descending aorta while in supine position.

〰 H. *Medical diagnosis—procedures:*
   1. Sonography—to diagnose multifetal pregnancy, gross fetal anomaly, locate placental site.
   2. Amniocentesis—to diagnose anomalies, erythroblastosis.

III. *Potential complications*
   A. Maternal respiratory embarrassment.
   B. Premature rupture of membranes (PROM) with prolapsed cord and/or amnionitis.
   C. Preterm labor.
   D. Postpartum hemorrhage—due to overdistention and uterine atony.

✉ IV. **Analysis/nursing diagnosis**
   A. *Pain* related to excessive size of uterus impinging on diaphragm, stomach, bladder.
   B. *Impaired physical mobility* related to increased lordotic curvative of back, increased weight on legs.
   C. *Altered tissue perfusion* related to decreased venous return from lower extremities, compression of body structures by overdistended uterus.
   D. *Potential fluid volume deficit* related to potential uterine atony in immediate postpartum, secondary to loss of contractility due to overdistention.
   E. *Sleep pattern disturbance* related to respiratory embarrassment and discomfort in side-lying position.
   F. *Anxiety* related to discomfort, potential for complications, associated with congenital anomalies.
   G. *Altered urinary elimination* (frequency) related to pressure of overdistended uterus on bladder.

V. **Nursing care plan/implementation**
   A. *Medical management*
   〰 1. Amniocentesis—remove excess fluid very slowly, to prevent abruptio placentae.
      2. Termination of pregnancy—if fetal abnormality present *and* woman desires.
   B. *Nursing management*
      1. Goal: *health teaching*
         a. Need for lateral *Sims'* position during resting; *semi-Fowler's* may alleviate respiratory embarrassment.
         b. Explain diagnostic and/or treatment procedures.
      ! c. Signs and symptoms to be *reported immediately*: bleeding, loss of fluid through vagina, cramping.

2. Goal: *prepare for diagnostic and/or treatment procedures*
   a. *Force* fluids—for sonography.
   b. Ensure that Informed Consent for amniocentesis is signed and in woman's chart.
3. Goal: *emotional support for loss of pregnancy* (if applicable)
   a. Encourage verbalization of feelings.
   b. Facilitate grieving: permit parents to see, hold infant; if desired, take photograph, footprints for them.

VI. Evaluation/outcome criteria
   A. Woman complies with medical/nursing management.
   B. Woman's symptoms of respiratory embarrassment, etc. reduced; comfort promoted.
   C. Woman experiences normal, uncomplicated pregnancy, labor, birth, and postpartum.

Diagnostic Tests to Evaluate Fetal Growth and Well-Being

Daily Fetal Movement Count (DFMC)

I. Noninvasive test done by pregnant woman.
II. Assesses fetal activity.
   A. Three movements/hr normal activity.
   B. Two movements or less/hr may indicate fetal jeopardy.
III. Assess for fetal sleep patterns; repeat after ingesting glucose.

Nonstress Test (NST)

I. Correlates fetal movement with FHR. Requires electronic monitoring.
II. *Reactive test*—acceleration of FHR 15 beats/min above baseline FHR, lasting for 15 sec or more.
III. *Nonreactive* test—acceleration less than 15 beats/min above baseline FHR. May indicate fetal jeopardy.

Contraction Stress Test (CST); Oxytocin Challenge Test (OCT)

I. Correlates fetal heart rate response to induced uterine contractions.
II. Requires electronic monitoring.
III. Indicator of uteroplacental sufficiency.
IV. Identifies pregnancies at risk for fetal compromise from uteroplacental insufficiency.
V. Increasing doses of oxytocin are administered to stimulate uterine contractions.
VI. Interpretation: *negative* results indicate absence of abnormal deceleration with all contractions.
VII. *Positive* results indicate abnormal FHR decelerations with contractions.
VIII. Nipple stimulation (*breast self-stimulation test*) may

also release enough systemic oxytocin to contract uterus to obtain indicators of fetal well-being or fetal jeopardy.

Biophysical Profile (BPP)

I. Observation by ultrasound of five variables for 30 min:
   A. Fetal body movements.
   B. Fetal tone.
   C. Amniotic fluid volume.
   D. Response to nonstress testing.
   E. Fetal breathing movements.
II. Variables are scored at 2 if present; score of *less than* 6 is associated with perinatal *mortality*.

Ultrasound

I. Noninvasive procedure involving passage of high-frequency sound waves through uterus to obtain data regarding fetal growth, placental positioning, and the uterine cavity.
II. Purpose may include:
   A. Pregnancy confirmation.
   B. Fetal viability.
   C. Estimation of fetal age.
   D. Biparietal diameter measurement (BPD).
   E. Placenta location.
   F. Detect fetal abnormalities.
   G. Confirm fetal death.
   H. Identify multifetal gestations.
III. No risk to mother with infrequent use. Fetal risk not determined on long-term basis.

Amniocentesis

I. Invasive procedure for amniotic fluid analysis to assess fetal growth and maturity; done after 14 wk gestation.
II. Needle placed through abdominal-uterine wall; designated amount of fluid is withdrawn for examination.
III. Empty bladder if gestation greater than 20 wk.
IV. Risk of complications less than 1%. Ultrasound *always* precedes this procedure.
V. *Possible complications:* onset of contractions; infections (probably amnionitis); placental, cord puncture; bladder puncture.
VI. Advise women to observe and report to physician: fetal hypo- or hyperactivity, vaginal bleeding, vaginal discharge (clear or colored), signs of labor.

Analysis of Amniotic Fluid

I. Chromosomal studies to detect *genetic* aberrations.
II. Biochemical analysis of fetal cells to detect inborn errors of *metabolism*.
III. Determination of fetal *lung maturity* by assessing *L/S* ratios.
IV. Evaluation of *phospholipids* (PG and PI); aids in determining *lung maturity;* new and accurate.
V. Determination of *creatinine* levels, aids in determining *fetal age.* (Greater than 1.8 mg/dL indicates fetal maturity and the fetal age.)
VI. Assessment of isoimmune disease.

VII. Assessment of *alpha-fetoprotein* (AFP) levels for determination of *neural tube* defects.

! VIII. Presence of meconium may indicate *fetal hypoxia*.

⟨∿⟩ Chorionic Villous Sampling (CVS)

I. Cervically invasive procedure.

II. Advantage—results can be obtained after 10 wk gestation due to fast-growing fetal cells.

III. Procedure—removal of small piece of tissue (chorionic villi) from fetal portion of placenta. Tissue reflects genetic makeup of fetus.

IV. Determines some genetic aberrations and allows for earlier decision for induced abortion (if desired) from abnormal results. Does *not* diagnose neural tube defects; CVS patients need further diagnoses with ultrasound and serum AFP levels.

V. Protects "pregnancy privacy" because results can be obtained before the pregnancy is apparent and decisions can be made regarding abortion or continuation of gestation.

VI. Risks involve: spontaneous abortion, infection, hematoma, intrauterine death.

Summary

Assessment for risk factors helps to identify the population that would benefit from timely intervention. Early identification is essential in order to plan and implement management of care throughout the childbearing cycle. This chapter focuses on diseases that may *predate the pregnancy*: cardiac disease, Rh incompatibility, diabetes, substance abuse, STDs, age-related factors, cancer, violence, and other medical-surgical conditions. In addition, *pregnancy-related conditions* are discussed: hemorrhagic disorders; metabolic disorders; preeclampsia, eclampsia, and HELLP syndrome; and hydramnios. *Diagnostic tests* to evaluate fetal growth and well-being are outlined.

⟨💡⟩ Study and Memory Aids

Insulin Requirements in Pregnancy

Trimester one: ↓
Trimester two: ↑
Trimester three: ↑
Postpartum: ↓

Gestational Diabetes Assessment—3 Ps

Polydipsia
Polyphasia
Polyuria

Heart Failure—Assessment

Heart rate is the most sensitive and reliable indicator of impending heart failure.

RH$_o$GAM

Rh$_o$Gam is given to **Rh− *woman* only!**

Indications for RH$_o$GAM—Give Rh$_o$GAM to

1. Rh− mother who gives birth to Rh+ neonate.
2. Rh− mother after spontaneous or induced abortion (>8 wk).
3. Rh− mother after amniocentesis or chorionic villous sampling (CVS).
4. Rh− mother between 28 and 32 wk gestation.

Rh$_o$GAM Rubella Titer

Since Rh$_o$GAM is an immune globulin, rubella vaccination, given at about the same time, may not "take"; rubella titer needs to be redone at 3 mo.

Assessment of Fetal Maturity

Phosphatidylglycerol is more accurate indicator of fetal lung maturity in diabetic women.

Infections

Vaginitis: Avoid douching during pregnancy.
STDs in the U.S.: highest prevalence among teens.
AIDS in the U.S.: fourth leading cause of death among reproductive-aged women.

TORCH Infections

Toxoplasmosis
Other (hepatitis A virus [HAV], hepatitis B virus [HBV], group B streptococcus [GBS])
Rubella
Cytomegalovirus (CMV)
Herpes type 2

Asthma

Avoid morphine for woman with asthma who is in labor.

Cancer

Malignant melanoma: the only cancer that crosses the placenta to the fetus.

Cycle of Violence

Phase 1—*building*: increased tension, anger, blaming, and arguing

Phase 2—*battering*: hitting, slapping, kicking, choking, use of objects or weapons; sexual abuse; verbal threats and abuse

Phase 3—*calm* state (may decrease over time): batterer may deny violence, state he was drunk, say he's sorry, and "promise it will never happen again," **returns to phase 1.**

Modified from A Helton. *A Protocol of Care for the Battered Woman.* White Plains, NY: March of Dimes Birth Defects Foundation, 1987.

Hydatidiform Mole

Complete **H. mole:** only condition that can lead to maternal cancer.

Preeclampsia

Proteinuria differentiates preeclampsia from other pregnancy induced hypertension (PIH) states.
Preeclampsia is a disorder of *hypovolemia.*
Home care eliminates the need for hospitalization for "mild" preeclampsia.

Preeclampsia Diet

Do not *eliminate* sodium from the diet.

Hypertension—Standard American College of Obstetricians and Gynecologists (ACOG) Definition

Systolic: 30+ mm Hg above baseline
Diastolic: 15+ mm Hg above baseline

HELLP Syndrome—Assessment

Hemolysis
Elevated
Liver (enzymes)
Low
Platelets

HELLP Syndrome—Complication

Hypoglycemia: ≤ 40 mg/dL
Hypoglycemia can lead to maternal mortality.

Placenta Previa

Vaginal examinations contraindicated with undiagnosed vaginal bleeding.

Questions

1. The nurse is planning to lead a seminar for young adults on violence against women, concentrating on abuse of pregnant women. Which of the following statements is accurate and would be part of the nurse's discussion?
   1. Most of these women live below poverty level.
   2. Alcohol has been causally related to battering.
   3. The prevalence of violence lessens during pregnancy, dropping to a range of 2–4%.
   4. Abused women are more likely to have low-birth-weight (LBW) infants than women not abused during pregnancy.

2. The mode of birth of children of HIV+ mothers follows obstetric indications. Which of the following is an unnecessary precaution?
   1. Avoid scalp electrodes for electronic fetal monitoring.
   2. Avoid scalp pH determinations.
   3. Remove newborn to special care nursery immediately after birth.
   4. Delay amniotomy to reduce possibility of vertical transmission of HIV.

3. A nurse is discussing sexually transmitted diseases with a class of high school seniors. The students submitted a list of what they knew. The nurse evaluated the list. The only accurate statement is that gonorrhea:
   1. Is often spread through fomites.
   2. Is only spread through promiscuous sex.
   3. Is easily cured with penicillin.
   4. Can be prevented if condoms are used for sexual encounters.

4. The nurse considers a pregnant woman's blood pressure of 120/80 as indicative of preeclampsia if:
   1. The woman has gained 2 pounds for each of the previous 2 wk.
   2. The woman is carrying a hydatidiform mole.
   3. The woman has had ankle edema each evening for the previous 2 wk.
   4. The woman's systolic pressure has increased by 30 mm Hg; the diastolic, by 15 mm Hg.

5. A nurse case manager is developing a plan of care for a 4-wk pregnant woman with a Class I functional classification of organic heart disease. The nurse knows to plan for the normal adaptation to pregnancy that can place a cardiac patient at risk, which is:
   1. Physiologic anemia.
   2. Increase in cardiac output after the 34th week.

3. Gradual increase in size and weight of the uterus.
4. Increased heart rate during the last half of pregnancy.

6. The nurse must teach the pregnant woman with cardiac disease the symptoms specific to cardiac decompensation, which include:
   1. Fatigue.
   2. Periodic shortness of breath even when at rest.
   3. Transient palpitations.
   4. Coughing or feeling of smothering with coughing attacks.

7. Managed care of a pregnant woman in sickle cell crisis needs to be reevaluated if it includes:
   1. Adequate hydration with intravenous fluids.
   2. Blood transfusion to maintain hemoglobin at more than 10 mg/dL.
   3. Analgesia, as necessary.
   4. Control of asthma symptoms.

8. A nursing plan of care for home management of "mild" preeclampsia would include a diet consisting of:
   1. High protein, high calories, no added salt.
   2. High protein, high fiber, restrict salt.
   3. Low protein, fiber, and fat; no more than four (8 oz.) glasses of water/d.
   4. Low protein, high fiber, low salt; water to eight (8 oz.) glasses/d.

9. A pregnant woman with preeclampsia is admitted to the labor unit. Magnesium sulfate therapy is ordered. The nurse reviews the woman's chart and decides to confer with the physician before giving the medication when the following data are noted in her record:
   1. Mean arterial pressure = 107.
   2. Deep tendon reflexes are +2.
   3. Diabetic condition is controlled with insulin. *Arrhythmias may occur*
   4. Cardiac condition is controlled with digitoxin.

10. A woman who is attending a clinic for asthma sufferers tells the nurse she is pregnant. The nurse knows that, during pregnancy, preexisting asthma:
   1. Can be safely medicated with up to six doses of asthma medication per day.
   2. Increases the possibility of hyperemesis gravidarum.
   3. Is best treated with oral or parenteral formulations.
   4. Cannot be treated with sympathomimetic therapy (beta-agonist medications such as terbutaline sulfate [*Brethaire, Brethine, Bricanyl*]).

11. A pregnant woman at 32 wk gestation has been severely beaten and pushed down a flight of stairs; spinal cord injury is a possibility. Although no external bleeding is noted, internal bleeding is a possibility. When clinical signs of shock due to loss of blood appear, the nurse knows that the injured pregnant woman has lost at least what percentage of her blood volume?
   1. 30%.
   2. 40%.
   3. 50%.
   4. 60%.

12. Preconception counseling should include information about the importance of vaccinations to bolster a woman's immune system. The nurse must teach potential parents that although varicella-zoster virus (VZV) infections are infrequent during pregnancy they can cause serious consequences for the mother/fetus/newborn, which include:

   1. Mother: pneumonia, encephalitis.
   2. Placenta: abruption.
   3. Fetus: spontaneous abortion.
   4. Newborn: conjunctivitis.

13. A pregnant woman is Rh negative; her husband is Rh positive. Which statement by the woman demonstrates to the nurse that the woman understands Rh isoimmunization?
   1. "A small amount of my red blood cells crosses the placenta; the baby then becomes allergic to them."
   2. "If my baby is Rh positive, I could develop antibodies against my baby's red blood cells."
   3. "The first pregnancy is most at risk; subsequent pregnancies are not nearly as dangerous."
   4. " 'Coombs positive' means that my baby and I are protected against Rh isoimmunization."

14. During a preconception class, the discussion turns to questions about drug dependence and pregnancy. The nurse's response is based on knowledge that maternal withdrawal from cocaine dependence puts the fetus/newborn at risk for: *maternal vasopastic hypertension*
   1. Intrauterine asphyxia.
   2. Facial dysmorphia.
   3. Disseminated intravascular coagulation (DIC).
   4. Bronchopulmonary dysplasia (BPD). — *long term O2 support*

15. A pregnant woman becomes frightened when she overhears a physician say she had a reactive nonstress test (NST). The nurse clarifies the physician's comment and states that a reactive NST suggests:
   1. Intrauterine asphyxia.
   2. Fetal well-being.
   3. Need for immediate cesarean birth.
   4. Need for validation with a contraction stress test (CST).

16. Digitalis preparations may be ordered to maximize ventricular contractions. The nurse can expect to administer higher doses (or more frequent doses) of digitalis for a pregnant woman because:
   1. Maternal hormones increase the effect of digitalis.
   2. Maternal hormones decrease the effect of digitalis.
   3. During pregnancy, drugs are metabolized more rapidly.
   4. Increased plasma volume may lower circulating levels of the drug.

17. To meet the standard of care for risk management of the pregnant diabetic, the nurse must develop a plan of care to maintain the target range for postprandial (2 hr after meals) blood glucose levels during pregnancy, which is:
   1. 60–90 mg/dL.
   2. 60–105 mg/dL.
   3. 60–120 mg/dL.
   4. 90–140 mg/dL.

18. During preconception counseling, the nurse's teaching plan must include information that acidosis in a pregnant diabetic woman may be precipitated if she:
   1. Limits salt in her diet.
   2. Decreases activity.
   3. Experiences nausea, vomiting, and loss of appetite.
   4. Increases intake of simple sugars.

19. A nurse case manager's plan of care for a noncompliant pregnant diabetic woman recognizes that labor may be

induced several weeks before term in the more severe, poorly controlled cases of diabetes, because early birth:
1. Prevents the baby from getting too large.
2. Improves chances for a live-born baby.
3. Keeps diabetes from developing in the baby.
4. Decreases the infant's chances of developing respiratory distress syndrome (RDS).

20. To meet the standard of care for risk management, *all* nurses must be aware of how maternal adaptations alter assessment techniques and findings, so that timely intervention is possible. Acute suppurative appendicitis complicates about 1/1000 pregnancies. Which of the following is accurate about this condition during pregnancy?
1. Appendiceal rupture and peritonitis occur rarely during pregnancy.
2. Maternal and perinatal morbidity and mortality are greatly increased when appendicitis occurs during pregnancy.
3. Therapeutic abortion is indicated in appendicitis.
4. Appendicitis is easier to diagnose during pregnancy than in the nonpregnant woman.

21. The ability to achieve pregnancy is not affected by spinal cord injury (SCI). The nurse should plan care for a pregnant woman with SCI based on knowledge that:
1. Physiologically, the woman with SCI encounters many of the same problems that pregnant women generally experience.
2. She will be assessed frequently during the last weeks of pregnancy, since she is unable to know when she is having labor contractions.
3. Since she cannot push to give birth, she will have a forceps-assisted birth.
4. Oxytocin induction of labor is warranted if she is prone to autonomic dysreflexia (sweating, flushing, pounding headache, severe hypertension).

22. A pregnant woman slipped on her front porch steps and sustained a deep cut in her leg. Her husband has picked her up, wrapped her in a blanket, and placed her in Trendelenburg's position, and is applying direct pressure over the wound with some clean linen while waiting for the ambulance. A home health nurse, going to visit a patient in the neighborhood, stops and evaluates the care her husband is providing. The nurse should:
1. Reposition her out of Trendelenburg.
2. Compliment her husband for using Trendelenburg.
3. Apply a tourniquet above the wound on her leg.
4. Continue on to visit the home health patient; the husband has everything under control.

23. All nurses must know that rectal or vaginal examinations are contraindicated for women with undiagnosed third trimester vaginal bleeding because:
1. It is undesirable to stimulate labor.
2. A low-lying placenta may be dislodged, and bleeding will follow.
3. There is danger of rupturing the membranes.
4. Cervical dilatation is of little importance in this situation.

24. The nurse develops a plan of care to incorporate physician-ordered treatment of the pregnant woman with mild preeclampsia, which would most likely include:
1. Bedrest.
2. Analgesics.
3. Thiazide diuretics.
4. Magnesium sulfate.

25. A woman in labor is experiencing increasingly severe symptoms of preeclampsia. When she complains of epigastric pain, the nurse realizes that this complaint suggests
1. Impending convulsions.
2. Impending digestive disorder.
3. Impending birth.
4. No clinical significance.

26. When providing care for a woman in labor who has severe preeclampsia (or eclampsia), the nurse must be alert constantly for increasing severity of symptoms and for a possible associated complication—the HELLP syndrome. Which finding needs to be present for a woman to be diagnosed with the HELLP syndrome?
1. Hyperglycemia.
2. Platelet count of 100,000 or more.
3. Disseminated intravascular coagulopathy (DIC).
4. Elevated liver enzymes.

27. Following a pregnant woman's eclamptic seizure, and after ensuring a patent airway, the nurse will do all of the following. Which takes priority?
1. Assess fetal status: FHR, movement.
2. Assess labor status: contractions, cervical dilatation/effacement, membranes, station.
3. Assess maternal vital signs, deep tendon reflexes, and I&O.
4. Document event.

28. Magnesium sulfate IV is ordered. Which sign would lead the nurse to suspect magnesium sulfate toxicity?
1. Increased urine output.
2. Decreased deep tendon reflexes (DTRs).
3. Increased respiratory rate.
4. Cold, clammy skin.

29. Which assessment finding would prompt the nurse to stop the intravenous infusion of $MgSO_4$ for treatment of preeclampsia?
1. Respirations at 16/min.
2. Patellar and brachial reflexes at +1.
3. Urine output at 90 mL/4 hr.
4. Pulse pressure at 30 mm Hg.

30. The clinic nurse would suggest that a woman be brought into the emergency room if she has signs/symptoms of acute rupture of a tubal pregnancy, such as
1. Profuse vaginal bleeding.
2. Referred shoulder pain.
3. Irregular fetal heart rate.
4. Elevation of temperature.

31. A woman is admitted to the labor unit with a diagnosis of partial placenta abruptio. The nurse would question the diagnosis if assessment reveals:
1. A history of multiparity or hypertension.
2. Appearance of port-wine–stained amniotic fluid.
3. Normal uterine contractions.
4. Mild uterine hypertonicity.

32. The nursing plan of care for a woman with cardiac disease who is in labor is modified to meet her special needs. Which intervention is specific for this woman?
1. Auscultate for crackles (rales) q30 min.

2. Turn from side to side qh.
3. Monitor blood pressure qh.
4. Assess bladder filling and encourage voiding as necessary.

33. A woman in active labor has a positive culture for herpes genitalis. Her membranes are intact; the cervix is 5 cm dilated. The nurse should be prepared for what type of birth?
    1. Cesarean.
    2. Vacuum assisted.
    3. Low forceps assisted.
    4. Spontaneous vaginal.

34. A woman in active labor is HIV positive. Which fetal monitoring method should the nurse choose?
    1. Leff scope or DeHillis scope.
    2. Penard's stethoscope.
    3. External electronic fetal monitor.
    4. Internal electronic fetal monitor.

35. Few pregnant women have bronchial asthma; however, the nurse must know about the disorder since the effect of pregnancy on asthma is unpredictable. The nurse's plan of care must recognize that acute episodes may require steroids, aminophylline, oxygen, and correction of fluid-electrolyte imbalance. Regarding the management of labor for a woman with bronchial asthma, the nurse anticipates that:
    1. Vaginal birth with local or regional anesthesia is the method of choice.
    2. Morphine is used in labor because it usually relieves bronchospasm.
    3. Ephedrine and corticotropin (pressor drugs) are used if preeclampsia develops.
    4. Asthma does not affect the incidence of abortion or preterm labor, or produce adverse effects on the fetus.

36. The nurse who gives anticipatory guidance related to labor anticipates the following variation(s) from the normal routine for a woman with heart disease:
    1. The woman will probably lie flat in bed, but only on her side.
    2. Assessment of pulse and respirations will be more frequent than usual.
    3. The woman will have an unmedicated second stage of labor.
    4. Low forceps assisted birth is contraindicated.

37. The woman with a known cardiac condition must be watched carefully during labor. To prevent cardiac decompensation, she should be:
    1. Maintained with oxytocin to increase contractions.
    2. Monitored more frequently.
    3. Maintained with an I.V. infusion.
    4. Positioned on her side with her shoulders elevated.

38. The nurse monitoring a pregnant woman on digitalis must be on the alert for:
    1. Delay in the onset of labor.
    2. Shortening of the length of labor.
    3. Prolonged length of labor.
    4. Secondary uterine inertia during labor.

39. If a woman in labor vomits during a convulsion, the nurse's first action is to:
    1. Quickly obtain the necessary equipment and suction her.

2. Position the woman on her side with her head lower than her shoulders.
3. Insert a padded tongue blade.
4. Start oxygen by face mask.

40. For which sign will the nurse look that distinguishes preeclampsia from gestational hypertension? ↑ proteinuria
    1. A rise in systolic pressure of at least 30 mm Hg.
    2. Edema in the ankles.
    3. A diastolic pressure of 90 mm Hg or more.
    4. Proteinuria.

41. A common disorder in those who have rheumatic heart disease (RHD) is mitral stenosis. Ventricular failure, pulmonary edema, and atrial fibrillation can occur. The nurse needs to counsel the pregnant woman with RHD that she may expect which of the following interventions?
    1. Warfarin sodium (Coumadin).
    2. Unmedicated labor and birth.
    3. Bearing down in semi-fowler's position with legs in stirrups.
    4. Digoxin and anticoagulants.

42. A clinic patient with systemic lupus erythematosus (SLE) tells the nurse that she is anticipating having a child. She asks the nurse how SLE could affect pregnancy. The nurse's response is based on the knowledge that:
    1. The risk of miscarriage is high with SLE. than in normal preg.
    2. Hypotension is a major problem during pregnancy with SLE.
    3. Many medications used in treating SLE can be used during pregnancy.
    4. The incidence of flare-ups of SLE is decreased during pregnancy.

43. A preconception conference is particularly important for women with a history of medical complications. Before collaborating with a physician to develop a teaching plan for these women, the nurse reviews a list of women for whom pregnancy with a favorable outcome is possible. This list would include:
    1. Transplant recipients.
    2. Women with Marfan's syndrome.
    3. Women with pulmonary hypertension. —mortality
    4. Diabetic women with proliferative retinopathy.—worsens

44. A nurse case manager is developing a plan of care for pregnant women considered to be at high risk. The plan for a pregnant woman with sickle cell disease must include close monitoring, especially for infection with:
    1. Pneumococcus.
    2. Streptococcus.
    3. Staphylococcus.
    4. Enterococcus.

45. The nurse analyzes the following assessment data about a woman who is receiving magnesium sulfate intravenously for severe preeclampsia: some bleeding from her gums and a small amount of blood oozing from her IV infusion site. The nurse's first action should be to:
    1. Restart the IV at another site.
    2. Provide good mouth care.
    3. Obtain an order for a stat platelet determination.
    4. Continue with routine monitoring.

46. A pregnant woman asks her home health care nurse what she needs to know about her drug therapy for asthma during pregnancy. The nurse's best response is that:
    1. Most asthma medications are safe to take.
    2. Asthma medications make it impossible for her to breastfeed.
    3. Teratogenic effects of these medications can occur well into the second trimester.
    4. Beta-agonists cannot be used during pregnancy.

47. A pregnant woman at 32 wk gestation has been severely beaten and pushed down a flight of stairs; spinal cord injury is a possibility. The emergency room nurse plans to continuously monitor the maternal-fetal unit for at least:
    1. 4 hr.
    2. 12 hr.
    3. 24 hr.
    4. 24–48 hr.

48. The nurse analyzes the following data: on admission, the hematocrit (Hct) of a woman with preeclampsia was 34%; 3 d later, it is 38%. The nurse determines that this is probably the result of:
    1. Improved diet resulting in increased hematopoiesis.
    2. Improved perfusion of the spleen, causing depressed hemolysis of red blood cells (RBCs).
    3. A shift of fluid out of the vascular compartment.
    4. Normal physiologic polycythemia of pregnancy.

49. Which assessment finding would prompt the nurse to stop IV infusion of $MgSO_4$ for treatment of severe preeclampsia?
    1. Respirations: 14/min.
    2. Patellar and brachial reflexes: 0.
    3. Urinary output: 150 mL/4 h.
    4. Blood pressure: 142/94.

50. The home health nurse advises patients that, in addition to hospital disinfectants, another substance that is effective against HIV for washable surfaces is:
    1. Normal saline solution.
    2. Household cleanser.
    3. Household bleach (sodium hypochlorite) 1 : 10 solution.
    4. Detergent (¼ C) and hot water (1 gallon).

51. The nurse should be alert to the fact that, among leading causes of death among reproductive-aged women in the United States, acquired immunodeficiency syndrome (AIDS) ranks
    1. Third.
    2. Fourth.
    3. Fifth.
    4. Sixth.

52. A 17-year-old woman comes to the woman's clinic with the chief complaint of dysuria and painful blisters on the outside of her vagina for 2 days. Her history reveals feeling feverish and achy 1 wk ago, and having sex with a new partner 3 wk ago. The clinic nurse suspects
    1. Syphilis.
    2. Venereal warts.
    3. Primary herpes.
    4. Recurrent herpes.

53. To relieve periurethral discomfort caused by vaginal in-

fection with *Chlamydia trachomatis,* the nurse recommends
    1. Douching.
    2. A perineal heat lamp.
    3. Sitz baths.
    4. Ambulation.

54. A woman's menstrual cycles are regular, lasting 31 days. Her LMP started on March 15. When can she expect to ovulate next?
    1. March 25.
    2. March 29.
    3. April 2.
    4. April 15.

Answers/Rationale

1. **(4)** Abused women are 1½ times more likely to have LBW infants than women not abused during pregnancy, and they are more likely to have associated risk factors for LBW, such as poor obstetric history, infections, and alcohol or drug usage. Violence against women respects no social, economic, or racial categories **(1)**. Alcohol **(2)** has not been causally related to battering, but batterers have a high rate of alcohol abuse. The prevalence of abuse toward pregnant women ranges from 8–17%; violence may become *worse* during pregnancy, rather than improving **(3)**. **AN, 7, PsI**

2. **(3)** Newborns do not need to be separated from their mothers on the basis of the mother's HIV status. Options **1, 2,** and **4** are all *appropriate* precautions to take when caring for HIV+ mothers and newborns. **IMP, 1, SECE**

3. **(1)** Gonorrhea can be spread through fomites, which are nonliving material, e.g., linens, on which disease-producing organisms may be conveyed. Option **2** is incorrect because even sex with *one* partner who has gonorrhea can cause infection. Option **3** is incorrect because gonorrhea is *more difficult* to cure, since some bacterial *Neisseria gonorrhoeae* have developed resistance to penicillin, which used to cure the disease with comparative speed, especially in the early stages, and some women are allergic to penicillin. (Ceftriaxone in a single dose is recommended for treatment of pregnant and nonpregnant women; spectinomycin is the preferred alternative therapy.) Option **4** is incorrect because condoms only *protect* against (*not prevent*) transmission during penile-vaginal contact; gonorrhea can be transmitted into the rectum or the oropharynx, or through fomites. **IMP, 1, SECE**

Key to Codes

Nursing process: AS, assessment; **AN,** analysis; **PL,** planning; **IMP,** implementation; **EV,** evaluation. (See Appendix I for explanation of nursing process steps.)

Category of human function: 1, protective; **2,** sensory-perceptual; **3,** comfort, rest, activity, and mobility; **4,** nutrition; **5,** growth and development; **6,** fluid-gas transport; **7,** psychosocial-cultural; **8,** elimination. (See Appendix K for explanation.)

Client need: SECE, safe, effective care environment; **PhI,** physiological integrity; **PsI,** psychosocial integrity; **HPM,** health promotion/maintenance. (See Appendix L for explanation.)

4. (4) An increase in systolic pressure by ≥ 30 mmHg and in diastolic pressure by ≥ 15 mmHg is the accepted definition of preeclampsia. A weight gain of 2 pounds in 2 wk does *not* fit the definition of preeclampsia **(1)**. While preeclampsia *can* occur before the twentieth week in the presence of a hydatidiform mole, the presence of an H. mole does *not* indicate the presence of preeclampsia **(2)**. Ankle edema can occur in *healthy* women experiencing normal pregnancy (e.g., after a long period of standing or in the evening of a hot day), not just in preeclampsia **(3)**. **EV, 6, HPM**

5. (4) The increased blood volume and cardiac output and the increase in heart rate during the last half of pregnancy can stress the heart beyond its ability to compensate. Physiologic anemia alone **(1)** does not stress the heart beyond its ability to compensate (although *true* anemia can lead to cardiac failure). The cardiac output does not continue to increase after the 34th week **(2)**; it declines to about a 20% increase at 40 weeks. Although the size and weight of the uterus **(3)** can impede venous return to the heart when the woman is supine, proper positioning (side-lying with shoulders elevated) supports cardiac functioning. **PL, 6, HPM**

6. (4) Congestion develops as the heart is increasingly unable to maintain adequate circulation. The symptoms in options **1, 2,** and **3** *may be* symptoms of cardiac decompensation, but they are *also normal* findings during pregnancy. **IMP, 6, HPM**

7. (2) Blood transfusion is given to maintain hemoglobin at more than 8 *mg/dL* and hemoglobin A at over 40%. The other options do not require reevaluation: adequate hydration **(1)** *is* essential; analgesia **(3)** *should* be administered as necessary; asthma *must* be controlled **(4)**, since it is a condition that can promote sickling crises by shifting the oxygen-hemoglobin dissociation curve to the right. **EV, 6, PhI**

Test-taking tip: Look at what is being asked; options that do *not* require reevaluation are *true.*

8. (1) Preeclamptic women especially need high protein to replace that lost in the urine. The high caloric intake is needed to meet the extra demands of stress as well as the needs of maternal/fetal growth. All protein of high biologic value has salt; however, the woman should not add extra to her food. The other diets would not be therapeutic. Option **(2)**: Salt should not be *restricted,* and she needs extra calories. (The high fiber is generally advisable, although it is not specific to this condition.) Options **3 and 4**: She needs high, not low, protein, and she *should* have plenty of water to quench her thirst (8 glasses/d is acceptable, but does not need to be stated as a limit). **PL, 4, SECE**

9. (4) Magnesium sulfate should *not* be given to preeclamptic patients with cardiac disease who are taking digitoxin. Arrhythmias may occur; emergency artificial ventilation may be necessary. A MAP of 107 **(1)** is indicative of mild preeclampsia; the patient may be a candidate for magnesium sulfate therapy. DTRs of +2 **(2)** are within *normal* range. Magnesium sulfate is not contraindicated for patients with diabetes controlled with insulin **(3). EV, 2, PhI**

10. (2) The woman with preexisting asthma has an increased possibility of hyperemesis, hemorrhage, preeclampsia, and complicated labor. Other dangers are prematurity, low birth weight, and neonatal hypoxia. She can be safely medicated with up to four doses per day; dosing in excess of 4 times/d **(1)** is a warning sign for the woman to seek medical attention immediately. *Inhaled* medications are preferable to oral or parenteral medications **(3)**. She *can* be treated with sympathomimetic therapy **(4). AN, 6, HPM**

11. (1) During pregnancy, the woman may sustain a significant blood loss, approximately 30%, without the usual signs and symptoms of hypovolemia. The blood loss in options **2, 3,** and **4** is over 30%; while signs and symptoms of hypovolemia would already have appeared, these percentages do not represent the *minimum* amount lost before they appear. **NOTE:** A rapid pulse may reflect only the usual increase of 10–15 beats/min during pregnancy, or it may be a sign of hypovolemia. **AS, 6, PhI**

12. (1) Consequences for VZV infection for the mother are pneumonia (mortality of severe varicella pneumonia is about 3%, but can be as high as 15–40% if specific antiviral therapy is not administered) and encephalitis (mortality is between 5 and 20%; long-term neurologic manifestations may occur in as many as 15% of survivors). Abruptio placentae **(2)** is *not* a consequence. Spontaneous abortion rate **(3)** is *not* higher (however, these women are more likely to give birth at or before 37 wk gestation; congenital anomalies can occur). Conjunctivitis **(4)** is *not* one of the consequences; however, newborns may develop pneumonia, disseminated intravascular coagulation (DIC), and infection (mortality 30%). **IMP, 1, SECE**

13. (2) If the fetus is Rh positive, the woman could develop antibodies against her/his red blood cells. It is the entry of Rh-positive blood into the Rh-negative *woman's* bloodstream, not into the fetus' circulation **(1)** that stimulates the formation of antibodies against the Rh factor. The first pregnancy **(3)** is at *least* risk (risk arises only if the woman had previously developed antibodies against the Rh factor due to an erroneous blood transfusion). "Coombs positive" **(4)** refers to the titer of Rh antibodies present in the woman's blood stream; the Rh-positive fetus is at great risk of hemolysis with subsequent anemia, edema formation, and cardiac decompensation. **EV, 6, HPM**

14. (1) Maternal withdrawal from cocaine puts the fetus at risk for intrauterine asphyxia. Its significant and agonizing withdrawal is felt as violent movements in utero. Maternal episodes of vasospastic hypertension during cocaine use cause numerous small strokes; withdrawal may cause sudden maternal hypotension, which can be a cause of fetal asphyxia. Facial dysmorphia **(2)** is characteristic of fetal alcohol syndrome (FAS). DIC **(3)** has not been documented as being associated with maternal dependence on cocaine and withdrawal symptoms. BPD **(4)** is characteristic of lung dysplasia that develops in preterm infants dependent on long-term oxygen and ventilator support. **AN, 6, PhI**

15. (2) A reactive NST suggests fetal well-being. The criteria for a reactive test: two or more accelerations of 15 beats/min lasting for 15 sec over a 20-min period; normal baseline rate; long-term variability amplitude of 10 or more beats/min. Because fetal *well-being* is assured by a reactive NST, there is no indication of a problem such as asphyxia (1), and there is no need for immediate cesarean birth (3). If the test were *non*reactive, a CST should be performed (4). **IMP, 5, SECE**

16. (4) 30–50% is added to the circulating plasma volume during pregnancy, which lowers the circulating levels of the drug. Options 1, 2, and 3 are not relevant to the need to increase the dose of digitalis preparations in the pregnant cardiac woman. **NOTE:** Other medications that may be ordered for the pregnant woman with cardiac disease are heparin (vs. warfarin [Coumadin]) and antibiotics. **PL, 6, PhI**

17. (3) 60–120 mg/dL is the target range. The range in option 1 is the target range for *fasting* blood sugar (before breakfast), and the range in option 2 is the target range *before* lunch, dinner, and bedtime. The range in option 4 is too high. **NOTE:** Good diabetic control is associated with good pregnancy outcome, e.g., absence of sequelae of poor control: congenital anomalies, hydramnios, macrosomia, respiratory distress syndrome (even if born at term). **PL, 4, HPM**

18. (3) When a person does not eat, the body begins to break down its own tissues; metabolic acidosis results. None of the actions in options 1, 2, and 4 would precipitate acidosis in a pregnant diabetic woman. **PL, 4, PhI**

19. (2) The incidence of intrauterine fetal death rises dramatically starting with week 37; reasons are not known.
A macrosomal infant (1) could still be born at term, vaginally or abdominally; however, in this case early birth increases the chances for the infant's *survival.* Early birth is not related to developing diabetes (3); diabetes is familial (possibly inherited) but may also be viral related. The baby of a poorly controlled diabetic woman is at risk for RDS (4) whether preterm or term, because high insulin levels in the fetus delay the production of surfactant in the lungs. **PL, 6, PhI**

20. (2) Maternal mortality increases to about 10% in the third trimester; 15% of it occurs during labor. Perinatal mortality is approximately 10% with unruptured appendicitis; 35%, with peritonitis. Rupture and peritonitis (1) occur 2–3 times *more often* than in nonpregnant women. Therapeutic abortion (3) is *never* indicated in appendicitis. The appendix is carried high and to the right away from McBurney's point by the enlarged uterus, making diagnosis more *difficult,* not easier (4). Also, increased sedimentation rate cannot be used as an indicator of infection during pregnancy. **AS, 1, SECE**

21. (1) The woman with SCI is physiologically the same as other women. Some of the normal adaptations, however, do require special consideration: urinary frequency, urinary tract infection, constipation, the need to relieve pressure on ischial spines and gluteal muscles, and to straighten (as pregnancy precludes lying prone). Although women with SCI do not experience labor as other women do (2), they are in tune with their bodies and know when something is happening.

The woman with SCI experiences *no* trouble with a vaginal birth (3) even though she has no ability to push. Uterine contractions, plus a relaxed perineum, facilitate a vaginal birth. Oxytocin (4), if needed, is used cautiously and only when personnel are versed in the recognition and treatment of autonomic dysreflexia (the headache and hypertension must not be confused with preeclampsia). **PL, 5, HPM**

22. (1) Trendelenburg's position could severely impair maternal respirations since the heavy enlarged uterus will press against her diaphragm. She must *not* remain in Trendelenburg (2); she should be repositioned on her side. Tourniquets (3) must be used with care; direct pressure is appropriate in this case. The nurse *cannot* leave (4) until the patient's safety is assured. **EV, 1, SECE**

23. (2) Third trimester bleeding suggests a low-lying placenta, which may be dislodged during examination causing further bleeding. Stimulating the cervix or actually touching the placenta during the examination can result in further separation of the placenta and life-threatening hemorrhage. Options 1 and 3 are *not* relevant to precautions for third trimester vaginal bleeding. Although the statement in option 4 is true, it is not the *reason* that rectal or vaginal examination is contraindicated. **IMP, 6, SECE**

24. (1) Bedrest in the side-lying position increases perfusion of the uterus and kidneys and often reduces stress. (Increased perfusion of the kidneys decreases their production of angiotensin-II.) Although some authors have postulated that aspirin can have a preventive/curative effect on preeclampsia (2), no definitive evidence is available. Diuretics (3) are *contraindicated* during pregnancy, except in the case of cardiopulmonary decompensation; they can cause electrolyte imbalance. Magnesium sulfate (4) is an anticonvulsant and CNS depressant; it does *not prevent* preeclampsia. **PL, 3, PhI**

25. (1) "Epigastric" pain is the subjective description of pain from the edematous liver capsule and liver infarcts; it often heralds impending convulsions. The epigastric discomfort is *not* related to a gastrointestinal tract problem (2), and it is *not* a sign of impending birth (3). It *does* have clinical significance (4), as it should alert the nurse to possible convulsive seizures. **EV, 2, PhI**

26. (4) H = hemolysis; *EL = elevated liver enzymes;* LP = low platelets. None of the findings in options 1, 2, and 3 is part of the definition of the HELLP syndrome. **AN, 6, PhI**

27. (1) This activity takes very little time, and while doing it, the nurse can also begin assessment of uterine irritability. This provides data about fetal oxygen needs so that oxygen by face mask would be in place while continuing with assessments. Labor status (2) is assessed *after* fetal status (birth may be IMMINENT!), *then* maternal status (3). Documentation (4) is essential (characteristics of seizure and aftermath; assessment findings and woman's response to interventions), but would *follow* the other steps listed. **IMP, 2, SECE**

28. (2) Magnesium sulfate acts on the myoneural junction;

reflexes must be at least at 1+ so that paralysis of muscles does not occur. Increased urine output (1), or diuresis, is a *good* prognostic sign—the magnesium sulfate therapy is effective. Respirations are *depressed* with toxicity, *not increased* (3). Cold, clammy skin (4) is a sign of *shock, not* magnesium sulfate toxicity. **AS, 2, PhI**

29. **(3)** Urinary output should be at least 120 mL/4 hr, as renal ischemia from hypertension can cause dangerous concentrations of $MgSO_4$. Respirations must be 12/min or more to continue therapy, so a rate of 16/min (1) *is* within limits. Reflexes must be at least +1 to continue therapy, so a value of +1 (2) *is* within limits. Pulse pressure (4) is unaffected by $MgSO_4$. **EV, 8, PhI**

30. **(2)** Referred shoulder pain (Kehr's sign) is a common finding with acute rupture of a tubal pregnancy. Referred pain probably occurs because pain signals from the viscera travel along the same neural pathways used by pain signals from the shoulder; the woman perceives the pain but interprets it as having originated in the shoulder, rather than in the deep-seated viscera—the fallopian tube. Bleeding (1) occurs into the *peritoneal* cavity instead of into the intrauterine cavity. FHTs (3) are *never* heard; the tube cannot sustain a pregnancy long enough for the fetus to develop enough to have audible FHTs. Elevation of temperature (4) is *not* one of the usual findings of acute rupture of a tubal pregnancy. **EV, 1, HPM**

31. **(3)** Premature separation of the placenta (placenta abruptio) is usually accompanied by *mild to severe* uterine hypertonicity; the uterus may contract unevenly, and fail to relax between contractions. Options 1, 2, and 4 *are* all associated with placental abruption. **NOTE:** The following may also be seen with placenta abruptio: history of abdominal trauma or cocaine use; pain, mild to severe, localized over one region of the uterus, or diffuse over the uterus with a boardlike abdomen. Maternal hypertension has been identified in approximately half of the cases. **EV, 5, HPM**

32. **(1)** Since these women are at risk for heart failure during labor, the nurse auscultates for crackles (rales) every 30 min. Side-lying position facilitates venous return; it is *not* necessary for her to turn from side to side (2). Blood pressure (3) and bladder filling (4) are monitored for *all* women in labor; for *this* woman, assessment for heart failure is a priority. **IMP, 6, HPM**

33. **(1)** The route of herpes simplex virus (HSV) transmission from mother to newborn is via an infected birth canal during birth. Although cesarean birth is no longer recommended for all mothers with HSV, transplacental infection can occur; mothers with clinical evidence of active lesions will likely give birth abdominally. Vaginal birth, whether assisted (2 and 3) or spontaneous (4), is likely to be *contraindicated*. **PL, 1, SECE**

34. **(3)** This woman should be monitored with an external electronic fetal monitor. Leff and DeHillis stethoscopes (1) are used for intermittent assessment of the fetal heart rate (FHR), and are *not* the method of choice during a *high-risk* labor. Penard's stethoscope (2), a small tubelike instrument, is used for *low*-risk labors (it is not commonly used in the U.S., but may be used by

some midwives). The risk of transmission of HIV is increased with any intrusive procedure, such as an internal monitor (4). **IMP, 1, SECE**

35. **(1)** Vaginal birth with local or regional anesthesia is the method of choice since respiratory reflexes remain intact and it decreases the stress of labor and birth on the respiratory tract, liver, kidney, and metabolic system. Morphine (2) is *not* used in labor because it may cause bronchospasm in the woman. Meperidine (Demerol) will usually relieve bronchospasm. Use of ephedrine and corticotropin, pressor drugs (3), is *avoided* or limited in the treatment of eclampsia. Asthma (4) *increases* the incidence of abortion and preterm labor, but the fetus itself is unaffected. **IMP, 6, PhI**

36. **(2)** She is at risk for cardiac decompensation. The woman will be positioned with her head and shoulders up, and her arms at the level of her heart. (1) This position gives the heart more room within the cavity, and also avoids compression of the vena cava, allowing for easier and better cardiac functioning. She *will* need medication (3). Pain causes stress, which compromises cardiac function, and she must not bear down. She will need to be medicated (epidural), must not bear down, and *will* need assistance to give birth (4). **PL, 6, PhI**

37. **(4)** This position places the least stress on cardiac function, and therefore serves to *prevent* decompensation. Maintaining contractions with oxytocin (1) does not prevent decompensation. Monitoring (2) does not prevent decompensation. Maintaining an IV infusion (3) does not prevent decompensation. **PL, 3, PhI**

When all options are correct, look for *key word*. In this case, the most important word in the stem is "prevent."

38. **(2)** Shortening of the length of labor is a side effect of digitalis preparations taken by the pregnant woman. Options 1, 3, and 4 do *not* describe effects of digitalis preparations on labor. **AS, 5, PhI**

39. **(2)** This position utilizes gravity drainage to keep her from aspirating. Suction equipment (1) should be readily available *at the bedside;* suctioning will need to be done *after* the convulsion, but the priority during the convulsion is a side-lying position. Insertion of a padded tongue blade (3) is almost always difficult, if not impossible, and can itself lead to injury. Oxygen (4) is started only *after* the airway is clear. NOTE: The FHR is assessed only *after* the woman is out of immediate danger. **IMP, 1, SECE**

40. **(4)** Proteinuria is characteristic *only* of preeclampsia, not of gestational hypertension. A rise in systolic pressure of 30 mm Hg or more over baseline (1), without a rise in diastolic pressure of 15 mm Hg or more over baseline, is *not* indicative of preeclampsia; also, in preeclampsia, the rise is accompanied by proteinuria. Edema in the ankles (2) occurs in many pregnant women, especially late in pregnancy, during hot humid weather, or after standing for long periods; physiologic edema is a *normal* finding in pregnant women. A diastolic pressure of 90 mm Hg or more (3) is *not specific* for preeclampsia. Diastolic pressure characteristic of preeclampsia represents a rise of 15 mm Hg over baseline, and is accompanied by a rise in systolic pressure of

30 mm Hg or more over baseline; in addition, proteinuria must be present before preeclampsia is diagnosed. **AS, 6, PhI**

41. **(4)** Digoxin and anticoagulants are given prophylactically to improve the function of the heart and to prevent emboli secondary to atrial fibrillation. If the woman needs an anticoagulant, *heparin* is the drug of choice; heparin's larger molecules are less likely to cross the placenta than are the small molecules of Coumadin **(1)**. Options **2** and **3** are incorrect because these women must be spared any stress during labor, and their hearts *cannot* tolerate the stress of pushing; stress leads to cardiac decompensation. **IMP, 6, PhI**

42. **(1)** The risk of miscarriage is higher with SLE than in a normal pregnancy. *Hyper*tension, *not* hypotension **(2)**, is a major problem during pregnancy. Many medications used in treating SLE **(3)** are *not* recommended during pregnancy. Patients with SLE are *twice* as likely to suffer a flare-up during pregnancy, *not* less likely **(4)**. **AN, 5, HPM**

43. **(1)** Transplant recipients *can* become pregnant, but they must postpone conception for 1–2 yr so that graft function stabilizes and immunosuppressive agents can be given at maintenance levels. Women with Marfan's syndrome **(2)** must be evaluated for aortic root involvement, complicated coarctation of the aorta, and dilated cardiomyopathy—conditions associated with a marked increase in maternal *mortality*. Pulmonary hypertension **(3)** is associated with a 50% maternal *mortality*. Proliferative retinopathy **(4)** often *worsens* despite advances in diagnosis and treatment. **AN, 1, HPM**

44. **(1)** Infections—especially pneumococcal pneumonia, but also salmonella, osteomyelitis, and urinary tract infections—can promote sickling crises by shifting the oxygen-hemoglobin dissociation curve to the right. It is *not* streptococcus **(2)**, staphylococcus **(3)**, or enterococcus **(4)** that places the woman most at risk. **AS, 1/6, SECE**

45. **(3)** Those signs indicate that disseminated intravascular coagulation (DIC) may be present (secondary to severe hypertension). The index of presence of DIC is the platelet count. Restarting the IV at another site **(1)** will not address the problem of possible DIC. Good mouth care **(2)** and monitoring **(4)** are warranted only *after* diagnosis and initiation of treatment for DIC, if it is the problem; the cause of the signs must be investigated and treated at this time. **IMP, 6, PhI**

46. **(1)** Most asthma medications are safe to take during pregnancy. Breastfeeding **(2)** *is* possible if medications are inhaled; inhaled asthma medications have proved to be safe for breastfeeding mothers because of their low systemic bioavailability. Teratogenic effects **(3)** occur during the period of organogenesis, the *first* trimester. Beta-agonists **(4)**, such as terbutaline, *are* used to manage acute asthma attacks during pregnancy. **IMP, 6, PhI**

47. **(4)** The complications of preterm labor or placental abruption, if they occur, usually happen within 24–48 hr. Options **1, 2,** and **3** are all incorrect because the maternal-fetal unit must be monitored for up to 48 hr,

to rule out complications such as preterm labor and placental abruption. **IMP, 1, PhI**

48. **(3)** The hemoconcentration is due to hypovolemia, following a shift of fluid out of the vascular compartment; this woman's condition is worsening. Preeclampsia is a disease of hypovolemia: Protein, which retains fluid within the vascular compartment, is lost in the urine; the fluid leaves the intravascular space and enters surrounding tissue. Options **1, 2,** and **4** are all incorrect because again, hemoconcentration due to hypovolemia is responsible for the increase in hematocrit. **AN, 6, PhI**

49. **(2)** These reflexes must be *at least at +1* to continue therapy ($MgSO_4$ suppresses reflexes by preventing nerve impulses from crossing the myoneural junction to the muscles). The first sign of $MgSO_4$ *toxicity* is the *disappearance* of the knee-jerk (patellar) reflex. Respirations of 14/min **(1)** *is* an *acceptable* value; respirations must be 12/min or more to continue therapy ($MgSO_4$ suppresses respiratory activity). Urinary output of 150 mL/4 hr **(3)** *is acceptable;* the minimum limit is 120 mL/4 hr. (the level of urinary output must be monitored since renal ischemia from hypertension can cause dangerous concentrations of $MgSO_4$ if output is not maintained.) A blood pressure of 142/94 **(4)** is still elevated, and further treatment *is needed*. **EV, 2, PhI**

50. **(3)** An effective disinfectant (for washable surfaces) against HIV is household bleach (sodium hypochlorite) 1 : 10 solution. The substances in options **1, 2,** and **4** are not effective disinfectants against HIV. **IMP, 1, SECE**

51. **(2)** AIDS is the fourth leading cause of death among reproductive-aged women in the U.S. (In many major *metropolitan* areas, it is the *leading* cause of death for that age group.) Options **1, 3,** and **4** are all incorrect because AIDS ranks fourth. **AN, 1, HPM**

52. **(3)** Dysuria, painful blisters, and her history support the diagnosis of primary herpes. Other symptoms include malaise, anorexia, painful lymphadenopathy, and dyspareunia. Incubation time: 2–4 wk. Syphilis **(1)** is characterized by chancres at the entry site; they have a red base with firm, rolled edges and are painless. Early infection is asymptomatic. Venereal warts **(2)** are caused by human papillomavirus; incubation period is 2–3 mo. Recurrent herpes **(4)** may be preceded by itching, a burning sensation in the genital area, tingling in the legs, or a slight increase in vaginal discharge. **AS, 1, HPM**

53. **(3)** Sitz baths would be the best method to promote the patient's comfort.

The actions in options **1, 2,** and **4** would not be the best measures to promote periurethral comfort. **IMP, 1, SECE**

54. **(3)** Ovulation occurs 14 days *before* the next menstrual period. 31 − 14 = day 17, her ovulation day; add 17 to March 15 to arrive at the answer, April 2. Options **1, 2,** and **4** do not reflect accurate calculations of her expected date of ovulation based on her LMP. **IMP, 5, HPM**

The Intrapartal Experience

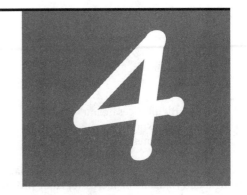

Chapter Outline

- Key Points
- Key Words
- Biophysical Foundations of Labor
  - Premonitory Signs
  - Etiology
  - Overview of Labor Process
  - Anatomic/Physiologic Determinants
    Maternal
    Fetal
    Assessment of Presentation and Position
    Mechanisms of Normal Labor
  - Warning Signs During Labor
- Pain Management During Labor and Birth
  - Neurologic Origins of Pain
  - Psychoprophylaxis—Lamaze Method
  - Warm-Water Immersion/Hydrotherapy
  - Pharmacologic Management of Pain
- Nursing Actions During First Stage of Labor
- Nursing Actions During Second Stage of Labor
- Nursing Actions During Third Stage of Labor

- Nursing Actions During Fourth Stage of Labor
- Nursing Management of the Newborn
  Immediately After Birth
- Nurse-Attended Emergency Birth
- Alterations Affecting Protective Function
  - Induction of Labor
    Assessment *Before* Induction
    Assessment *During* Induction and Labor
  - Operative Obstetrics—*Episiotomy*
  - Operative Obstetrics—*Forceps-Assisted Birth*
  - Operative Obstetrics—*Vacuum Cap and Pump-Assisted Birth*
  - Operative Obstetrics—*Cesarean Birth*
  - Vaginal Birth After Cesarean (VBAC): Trial of
    Labor
- Summary
- Study and Memory Aids
- Questions
- Answers/Rationale

☞ KEY POINTS

- The nurse assumes much of the responsibility of monitoring labor and keeping the physician/nurse midwife informed of normal findings and possible deviations from normal findings.
- Coaching, support, and comfort measures assist the woman (and her family) in using her energy constructively to relax and work with her contractions.
- During the *second stage* of labor, each woman must have someone in constant attendance to provide continuous monitoring, support, and coaching.
- The *fourth stage* of labor (the first 1–2 hr postbirth) is a critical period for mother and newborn; the primary concern is *hemorrhage*. Other important concerns are *bladder distention, safety, comfort,* and *nutrition* (including fluids).

Key Words

Apgar scoring system
Cardinal movements of labor
Dilatation
Effacement
Fetal
   Attitude
   Lie
   Presentation
   Position
Hyperventilation
Leopold's maneuvers
Lightening
Pain
   Somatic
   Visceral
Pelvis
   False
   True

Presentation
    Cephalic-vertex
    Breech
REEDA
Vaginal birth after cesarean (VBAC)
Valsalva maneuver
Warm water immersion/hydrotherapy

General overview: This review of the anatomic and physiologic determinants of successful labor provides baseline data against which the nurse compares findings of an ongoing assessment of the woman in labor. Nursing actions are planned and implemented to meet the present and emerging needs of the woman (and her family) in labor.

Biophysical Foundations of Labor

I. Premonitory signs
    A. *Lightening*—process in which the fetus "drops" into the pelvic inlet.
        1. *Characteristics*
            a. Nullipara—usually occurs 2–3 wk before onset of labor.
            b. Multipara—commonly occurs with onset of labor.
        2. *Effects*
            a. Relieves pressure on diaphragm—breathing is easier.
            b. Increases pelvic pressure
                (1) Urinary frequency returns.
                (2) Increased pressure on thighs.
                (3) Increased tendency to vulvar, vaginal, perianal, and leg varicosities.
    B. *Braxton-Hicks contractions*—may become more uncomfortable.
II. **Etiology:** unknown. *Theories* include:
    A. Uterine overdistention.
    B. Placental aging—declining estrogen/progesterone levels.
    C. Rising prostaglandin level.
    D. Fetal cortisol secretion.
    E. Maternal-fetal oxytocin secretion.
III. **Overview of labor process**—forces of labor (involuntary uterine contractions) overcome cervical resistance; cervix thins (*effacement*) and opens (0–10 cm *dilatation*) (Table 4.1 and Figure 4.1). Voluntary contraction of secondary abdominal muscles during the second stage (e.g., pushing, bearing-down) forces fetal descent. Changing pelvic dimensions force fetal head to accommodate to the birth canal by molding (cranial bones overlap to decrease head size).

Stages of labor
    A. *First*—begins with establishment of regular, rhythmic contractions; ends with complete effacement and dilatation (10 cm); divided into three phases:
        1. Latent and early active.
        2. Active.
        3. Transitional.
    B. *Second*—begins after complete dilatation and ends with birth of infant.
    C. *Third*—begins after birth of infant and ends with expulsion of placenta.
    D. *Fourth*—begins after expulsion of placenta; ends when maternal status is stable (usually 1–2 hr postpartum).

IV. **Anatomic/physiologic determinants**
    A. *Maternal*
        1. *Uterine contractions*—involuntary; birth, begin process of involution.
            a. *Characteristics:* rhythmic; increasing tone (*increment*), peak (*acme*), relaxation (*decrement*).
            b. *Effects*
                (1) Decreases blood flow to uterus and placenta.
                (2) Dilates cervix during first stage of labor.
                (3) Raises maternal blood pressure during contractions.
                (4) With bearing-down efforts (abdominal muscles, voluntary), expels fetus (second stage) and placenta (third stage).
                (5) Begins involution.
            c. **Assessment**
                (1) *Frequency*—time from beginning of one contraction to beginning of the next.
                (2) *Duration*—time from beginning of contraction to its relaxation.
                (3) *Strength (intensity)*—resistance to indentation.
                (4) False/true labor—differentiation (Table 4.2).
                (5) Signs of dystocia (dysfunctional labor) See p. 125.
        2. *Pelvic structures and configuration*
            a. *False pelvis*—above linea terminalis (line travels across top of symphysis pubis around to sacral promontory); supports gravid uterus during pregnancy.
            b. *True pelvis*—lies below linea terminalis; divided into
                (1) Inlet—"brim," demarcated by linea terminalis
                    (a) Widest diameter: transverse.
                    (b) Narrowest diameter: anterior-posterior (true conjugate).
                (2) Midplane—pelvic cavity.
                (3) Outlet
                    (a) Widest diameter: anterior-posterior (requires internal rotation of fetal head for entry).
                    (b) Narrowest diameter: transverse (intertuberous); facilitates birth in occiput anterior (OA) position.
            c. *Classifications*
                (1) Gynecoid—normal female pelvis; rounded oval.

TABLE 4.1 FIRST STAGE OF LABOR

Phases of First Stage	◄ Assessment: Expected Maternal Behaviors	◄ Nursing Care Plan/Implementation
0–4 cm—Latent Phase and Early Active Phase		
1. *Time*—nullipara 8–10 hr, average; multipara 5–6 hr	1. Usually comfortable, euphoric, excited, talkative, and energetic, but may be fearful and withdrawn	1. Provide encouragement, feedback for relaxation, companionship
2. *Contractions*—regular, mild 5–10 min apart, 20–30 sec duration	2. Relieved or apprehensive that labor has begun	2. *Coach* during contractions: signal beginning of contraction, mark the seconds, signal end of contraction; "Follow my breathing," "Watch my lips," etc.
3. Low-back pain and abdominal discomfort with contractions	3. Alert, usually receptive to teaching, coaching, diversion, and anticipatory guidance	3. *Comfort measures:* position for comfort; praise; keep aware of progress
4. Cervix thins; some bloody show		
5. *Station*—multipara −2 to +1; nullipara 0		
4–8 cm—Midactive Phase, Phase of Most Rapid Dilatation		
1. *Average time*—nullipara 1–2 hr; multipara 1½–2 hr	1. Tired, less talkative, and less energetic	1. *Coach* during contractions; husband (coach) may need some relief
2. *Contractions*—2–5 min apart, 30–40 sec duration, intensity increasing	2. More serious, malar flush between 5 and 6 cm, tendency to hyperventilate, may need analgesia, needs constant coaching	☞ 2. *Comfort measures* (to husband, too—as needed): position for comfort while preventing hypotensive syndrome; encourage relaxation, focusing her on areas of tension; provide counterpressure to sacrococcygeal area, prn; praise; keep aware of progress; minimize distractions from surrounding environment (loud talking, other noises); ▬ offer analgesics and anesthetics, as appropriate; provide hygiene: mouth care, ice chips, clean perineum; warmth, as needed
3. Membranes may rupture now		3. Monitor progress of labor and maternal-fetal response
4. Increased bloody show		☞ 4. If monitors are in use, attention on mother; periodically check accuracy of monitor readouts
5. *Station:* −1 to 0		

(continued)

(2) Android—normal male pelvis; funnel-shaped.
(3) Anthropoid—oval.
(4) Platypelloid—flattened, transverse oval.
  B. *Fetal*
    1. *Fetal head* (Figure 4.2)
      a. Bones—one occipital, two frontal, two parietals, two temporals.
      b. Suture—line of junction or closure between bones; sagittal (longitudinal), coronal (anterior), and lambdoidal (posterior); permit molding to accommodate head to birth canal.
  c. Fontanels—membranous space between cranial bones during fetal life and infancy
    (1) *Anterior* "soft spot"—diamond-shaped; junction of coronal and sagittal sutures; closes (ossifies) in *12–18 mo.*
    (2) *Posterior*—triangular; junction of sagittal and lambdoidal sutures; closes by *2 mo* of age.

TABLE 4.1   FIRST STAGE OF LABOR (Continued)

Phases of First Stage	▶ Assessment: Expected Maternal Behaviors	▶ Nursing Care Plan/Implementation
8–10 cm—Transition, Deceleration Period of Active Phase		
1. *Average time;* nullipara—40 min–1 hr; multipara—20 min	1. If not under regional anesthesia, more introverted; may be amnesic between contractions	1. Stay with woman (couple) and provide constant support
2. *Contractions*—1½–2 min, 60–90 sec duration, strong intensity	2. Feeling she cannot make it; increased irritability, crying, nausea, vomiting, and belching; increased perspiration over upper lip and between breasts; leg tremors; and shaking	☞ 2. Continue to *coach* with contractions: may need to remind, reassure, and encourage her to reestablish breathing techniques and concentration with each contraction; coach panting or "he-he" respirations to prevent pushing
3. Increased vaginal show; rectal pressure with beginning urge to bear down	3. May have uncontrollable urge to push at this time	3. *Comfort measures:* remind her and partner her behavior is normal and "OK"; coach breathing to quell nausea
4. *Station:* +3 to +4.		4. Assist with countertension techniques woman requested: *effleurage.*
		5. Monitor contractions, fetal heart rate (after each contraction), vaginal discharge, perineal bulging, maternal vital signs; record every 15 min.
		6. Assess for bladder filling
		7. Keep mother (couple) aware of progress
		8. Prepare husband/partner for birth (scrub, gown, etc.)

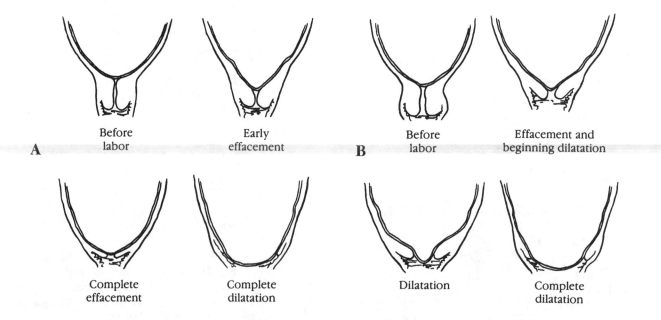

FIGURE 4.1   *Comparison of nullipara* (A) and **multipara (B) dilatation and effacement. (From Clinical Education Aid No. 13. Columbus, OH: Ross Laboratories.)

TABLE 4.2 ✉ ASSESSMENT: DIFFERENTIATION OF FALSE/TRUE LABOR

False Labor	True Labor
Contractions: Braxton-Hicks intensify (more noticeable at night); short, irregular, little change	Contractions: begin in lower back, radiate to abdomen ("girdling"); become regular, rhythmic; frequency, duration, intensity increase
Relieved by change of position or activity (e.g., walking)	Unaffected by change of position, activity, drinking 2 glasses of water, or moderate analgesia
Cervical changes—none; no effacement or dilatation progress	Cervical changes—progressive effacement and dilatation

2. *Fetal lie*—relationship of fetal long axis to maternal long axis (spine)
    a. *Transverse*—shoulder presents.
    b. *Longitudinal*—vertex or breech presents.
3. *Presentation*—fetal part entering inlet first (Figure 4.3)
    a. *Cephalic*—vertex (most common); face, brow.
    b. *Breech*
        (1) *Complete*—feet and legs flexed on thighs; buttocks and feet presenting.
        (2) *Frank*—legs extended on torso, feet up by shoulders; buttocks presenting.
        (3) *Footling*—single (one foot), double (both feet) presenting.
4. *Attitude*—relationship of fetal parts to one another (e.g., head flexed on chest).
5. *Position*—relationship of presenting fetal part to quadrants of maternal pelvis; vertex most common, occiput anterior on maternal left side (LOA). See Figure 4.3,a.

✉ **C. Assessment:** determine *presentation* and *position*

☞ 1. *Leopold's maneuvers*—abdominal palpation
    a. *First*—palms over fundus, breech feels softer, not as round as head would be.
    b. *Second*—palms on either side of abdomen, locates fetal back and small parts.
    c. *Third*—fingers just above pubic symphysis, grasp lower abdomen; if unengaged, presenting part is mobile.
    d. *Fourth*—facing mother's feet, run palms down sides of abdomen to symphysis; check for cephalic prominence (usually on right side), and if head is floating or engaged.

☞ 2. *Location of fetal heart tones* (FHTs)—heard best through fetal back or chest
    a. *Breech* presentation—usually most audible *above* maternal umbilicus.
    b. *Vertex* presentation—usually most audible *below* maternal umbilicus.
    c. Changing location of most audible FHTs—useful indicator of fetal descent.
    d. Factors affecting audibility:
        (1) Obesity.
        (2) Maternal position.
        (3) Hydramnios.
        (4) Maternal gastrointestinal activity.
        (5) Loud uterine souffle or bruit—origin: hissing of blood through maternal uterine arteries; synchronous with maternal pulse.
        (6) Loud funic souffle or bruit—origin: hissing of blood through umbilical arteries; synchronous with fetal heart rate (FHR).
        (7) External noise, faulty equipment.
3. *Vaginal examination:* palpable sutures, fontanels (triangular-shaped superior, diamond-shaped inferior = vertex presentation, OA position).

D. *Cardinal movements of the mechanisms of normal labor*—vertex presentation, positional changes of fetal head accommodate to changing diameters of maternal pelvis. (Figure 4.4)
1. *Descent*—head engages and proceeds down birth canal.
2. *Flexion*—head bent to chest; presents smallest diameter of vertex (suboccipital-bregmatic, 9.5 cm).
3. *Internal rotation*—during second stage of labor, transverse diameter of fetal head enters pelvis; occiput rotates 90° to bring back of neck (the nape) under symphysis (e.g., LOT to LOA to OA); presents smallest diameter (biparietal) to smallest diameter of outlet (intertuberous).
4. *Extension*—back of neck pivots under symphysis, allows head to be born by extension.
5. *Restitution*—head returns to normal alignment with shoulders (with LOA, results in head facing right thigh), presents smallest diameter of shoulders to outlet.
6. *Expulsion*—birth of neonate completed.
7. **Assessment:** relationship of fetal head to ischial spines (**degree of descent**)
    a. *Engagement*—widest diameter of presenting part has passed through pelvic inlet (e.g., biparietal diameter of fetal head).
    b. *Station*—relationship of presenting part to ischial spines (IS)
        (1) *Floating*—presenting part above inlet, in false pelvis.
        (2) Station——5 is at inlet (presenting part well above IS).
        (3) Station 0—presenting part at IS (engaged).

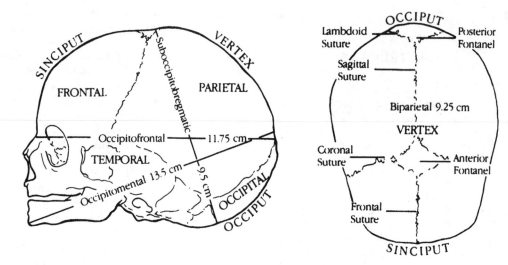

FIGURE 4.2   **THE FETAL HEAD. Bones:** two frontal, two temporal, one occipital.
Sutures: sagittal, frontal, coronal, lambdoid. **Fontanels:** anterior, posterior.
(From Clinical Education Aid No. 13. Columbus, OH: Ross Laboratories.)

(4) Station +4—presenting part at the outlet.

V. Warning signs during labor

> **A.** *Contraction*—hypertonic, poor relaxation, or tetanic (>90 sec long and ≤2 min apart).
> **B.** *Abdominal pain*—sharp, rigid abdomen.
> **C.** *Vaginal bleeding*—profuse.
> **D.** *FHR*—late decelerations, prolonged variable decelerations, bradycardia, tachycardia (Figure 4.5).
> **E.** *Maternal hypertension.*
> **F.** *Meconium-stained amniotic fluid (MSAF).*
> **G.** *Prolonged rupture of membrane (ROM)*

Pain Management During Labor and Birth

I. Neurologic origins of pain
  A. *First stage* of labor: Pain is *visceral,* caused by dilatation of the cervix and uterine ischemia; referred to the lower abdominal wall, the area over the lumbar region, and the sacrum.
  B. *Second stage* of labor: Pain is *somatic,* caused by hypoxia of the uterus, distention of the vagina and perineum, and pressure on adjacent tissues. Pain is felt in the lower back or suprapubic area, or referred to the flank and thighs.
  C. *Third stage* of labor: Pain is similar in origin to that of the first stage.
II. **Psychoprophylaxis—Lamaze method** (also, see discussion, Chapter 2, p. 42)
  A. Premise—conditioned responses to stimuli occupy nerve pathways, reducing perception of pain. Emphasis is on childbirth as a natural event, with an informed woman as the active participant. The ability to relax effectively reduces the perception

of pain, and the involvement of the coach fosters the family concept.
  B. Childbirth partners are taught
    1. Anatomy and physiology of labor.
    2. Psychology of man and woman.
    3. What to expect in the hospital setting.
    4. Conditioned responses to labor stimuli
      a. Concentration on focal point.
      b. Breathing techniques.
      c. Need for active coaching to enable woman to:
        (1) Use techniques appropriate to stage of labor.
        (2) *Avoid* hyperventilation.
    5. Specific stage—appropriate techniques
      a. *First stage of labor—early:* slow, deep chest-breathing.
      b. *Transition (8–10 cm)*—rapid, shallow breathing pattern, to prevent pushing prematurely
        (1) Panting.
        (2) Pant-blow.
        (3) "He-he" pattern.
      c. *Second stage of labor*
        (1) Pushing (or bearing-down)—aids fetal descent through birth canal.
        (2) Panting—aids relaxation between contractions; prevents explosive birth of head.
    6. Effects on labor behaviors/coping
      a. Help mother cope with and assist contractions.
      b. Prevent premature bearing-down; reduce possibility of cervical edema due to pushing on incompletely dilated cervix.
      c. When appropriate, improve efficiency of bearing-down efforts.

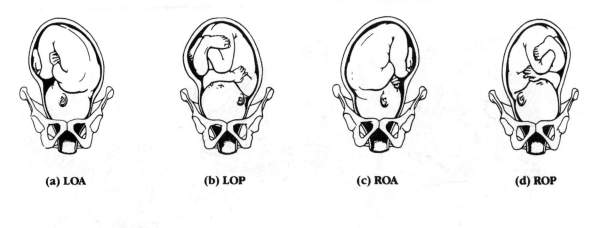

(a) LOA   **(b) LOP**   **(c) ROA**   **(d) ROP**

(e) LSP
(Frank Breech)   **(f) Shoulder presentation**   **(g) Prolapse of cord**

FIGURE 4.3   **CATEGORIES OF FETAL PRESENTATION.** (a) **LOA:** Fetal occiput is in left anterior quadrant of maternal pelvis. (b) **LOP:** Fetal occiput is in left posterior quadrant of maternal pelvis. (c) **ROA:** Fetal occiput is in right anterior quadrant of maternal pelvis. (d) **ROP:** Fetal occiput is in right posterior quadrant of maternal pelvis. (e) **LSP** (*frank breech*): Fetal sacrum is in left posterior quadrant of maternal pelvis. (f) **Shoulder** presentation with fetus in transverse lie. (g) **Prolapse of umbilical cord** with fetus in LOA position. (From Clinical Education Aid No. 18. Columbus, OH: Ross Laboratories.)

C. Other methods—include parent classes, classes for siblings, multiparas, and those who plan cesarean birth.
III. Warm-water immersion/hydrotherapy
   A. Proponents view labor as a normal biologic process; however, even with this type, an episiotomy may be needed.
   B. Bath temperature should be maintained at 32–37°C (89.6–98.6°F), which is most therapeutic for both the mother and fetus.
   C. **Assessment** before immersion
     1. Maternal and fetal vital signs—within normal limits.
     2. Cervical dilatation—4–5 cm; active phase of first stage.
     3. Membranes intact, or, if ruptured, fluid must be clear or only lightly stained with meconium.
     4. IV or an IV heparin lock may be in place.

   5. Following cervical priming with *prostaglandin* (*PGE₂*) gel: after fetus has been assessed for 2 hr.
   6. Stimulation with oxytocin is a contraindication.
   D. *Expected effects:* positive effect on labor pattern and cervical dilatation.
     1. Relief from discomfort and general body relaxation reduce a woman's anxiety, which decreases adrenalin production; an increase in oxytocin (to stimulate labor) and endorphins (to reduce pain perception) occurs.
     2. A 30-min whirlpool bath is expected to increase cervical dilatation an additional 2–3 cm.
     3. Increases *serum level of dopamine,* which increases renal blood flow: reduces blood pressure, encourages diuresis. Blood pressure drops within 2 min of immersion.

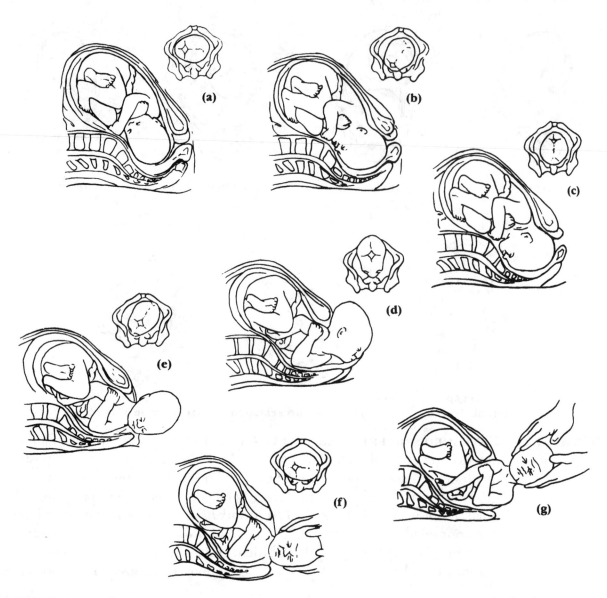

FIGURE 4.4 **CARDINAL MOVEMENTS IN THE MECHANISM OF LABOR** with the fetus in vertex presentation. (a) Engagement, descent, flexion. (b) Internal rotation. (c) Extension beginning (rotation complete). (d) Extension complete. (e) External rotation (restitution). (f) External rotation (shoulder rotation). (g) Expulsion. (From Clinical Education Aid No. 13. Columbus, OH: Ross Laboratories.)

E. Nursing interventions
  1. Continuous monitoring of labor: contractions, FHRs, BP, pulse, pain perception, signs of imminent birth, temperature.
  2. Keep woman well hydrated since dehydration may occur; can use sips of water, ice chips, IV fluids.
  F. Keep tub meticulously clean.
IV. Pharmacologic management of pain. See Table 4.3 for a discussion of categories of pain control, desired effects, nursing assessment and comments, and planning implementation.

Nursing Actions During First Stage of Labor

  I. Assessment—careful evaluation of:
    A. *Antepartal history*
      1. Expected date of birth (EDB)
      2. Genetic and familial problems.
      3. Pre- and coexisting medical disorders, allergies.
      4. Pregnancy-related health problems (hyperemesis, bleeding, etc.).

Pattern	Description	

A

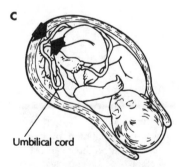

Head compression
(HC)

Early Decelerations

No intervention required.
Continue observation.

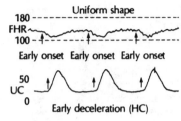

1. FHR begins to slow with the onset of the uterine contraction (UC) and returns to baseline when contraction is over.
2. Fetal head compression occurs.
3. Vagal nerve stimulation.
4. Transient slowing of FHR.

B

Compression
of vessels

Uteroplacental insufficiency
(UPI)

Late Decelerations

Change maternal position.
Turn off Pitocin; increase rate of maintenance IV.
Begin oxygen by face mask
Notify physician.
Check blood pressure and pulse rate.
Possible candidate for cesarean birth.

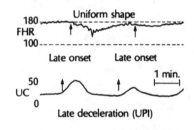

1. FHR begins to fall at height of the UC and returns to baseline after contraction has ceased.
2. FHR usually remains within normal range.
3. Indicates some degree of uteroplacental insufficiency.

C

Umbilical cord

Umbilical cord compression
(CC)

Variable Decelerations

Change maternal position to alleviate cord pressure.
Turn off Pitocin; increase rate of maintenance IV.
Begin oxygen by face mask.
Notify physician.
Check blood pressure and pulse rate.
Possible candidate for cesarean birth.
Possible candidate for amnio infusion.

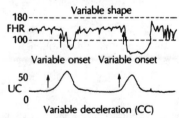

1. Slowing of FHR either with a contraction or in between contractions. Unrelated pattern of FHR and uterine contraction.
2. Pattern may be U shaped or V shaped. Transitory acceleration precedes or follows the deceleration.
3. FHR may fall below 100 beats/min; then returns immediately to baseline.
4. Usually indicates cord compression.

FIGURE 4.5   FHR DECELERATIONS AND NURSING INTERVENTIONS.

TABLE 4.3   PAIN MANAGEMENT DURING LABOR AND BIRTH

Category and Desired Effect	▷ *Assessment and Comments*	▷ *Planning and Implementation*
Systemic Medication		

Examples: sedatives
   Short duration (1 hr): *secobarbital*
     (Seconal)
   Intermediate (2 hr): *pentobarbital*
     (Nembutal)
   Long duration (3 hr): *phenobarbital*
     (Luminal sodium)*
 Desired effect: relieve anxiety and induce sleep only in prodromal or early latent labor:
 Route: oral or IM
	Before administration of medication note
	   Prenatal history of allergies or medical disorders
	   Prodromal labor
	   Degree of apprehension
	     Woman states she is anxious
	     Woman is clenching fists, restless, seems tense
	   Absence of pain
	 After administration of medication, note:
	   Strength and frequency of uterine contractions should *not* decrease appreciably
	   Little change in maternal vital signs; with decreased anxiety, pulse, respirations, and blood pressure do decrease but should not fall below woman's normal baseline in her prenatal record
	 Assess woman's response to medication
	 Assess FHR
	 Assess for pain
		Alert physician if chart reveals history of drug allergy, other disorders
		 Administer if
		   Woman is apprehensive, tense
		   Woman is in early latent phase of first stage of labor
		 Do not give without an analgesic if woman has pain
		 Continue with comfort measures and general hygiene given to any woman in labor
		 If changes occur in contractions or in maternal or fetal vital signs, record and notify physician
		 If woman becomes uncomfortable, confer with physician regarding need for analgesic relief

Examples: narcotic analgesics
   Morphine
   Meperidine hydrochloride (Demerol)
   Pentazocine (Talwin)
   Fentanyl
 Desired effect: relief of severe, persistent, or recurrent pain, without nausea and vomiting or respiratory depression of mother or fetus
 Route: IM or IV
	Before administration of medication note
	   Prenatal information regarding:
	     Drug allergies
	     Liver and kidney damage
	     Substance (drug) abuse
	     History of asthma
	   Stage of labor; progress in labor
	     Nullipara: before full dilatation
	     Multipara: before 7 cm dilatation
	   Degree of discomfort
	     Mother states she is having pain; cries out with pain; clenches teeth, fists
	   Maternal and fetal vital signs
	 After administration of medication, note:
	   Time between administration of narcotic and time of baby's birth
	   Maximum effect (IM) in 15 min, duration of 2 hr
	   Drug may slow labor, or it may accelerate labor as woman relaxes
	   Adverse, side effects assessed every 5–30 min—respiratory depression:
	     FHR deceleration and loss of short-term variability noted by electronic fetal monitor
	     Nausea, vomiting, dizziness, sweating, dysphoria
	     Bronchospasm in women who suffer from asthma
		Do *not* administer if birth is expected within 2 hr
		 Explain expected effect
		 Overdose management: oxygen, IV fluids, and vasopressors
		
		 If baby is born when drug reaches maximum effect, baby may be depressed and require resuscitation; prepare *Narcan* (0.01/kg) to be given IM into baby's thigh

(continued)

TABLE 4.3   PAIN MANAGEMENT DURING LABOR AND BIRTH (*Continued*)

Category and Desired Effect	▶ *Assessment and Comments*	▶ *Planning and Implementation*
Systemic Medication—cont'd		
Examples: narcotic antagonists Naloxone hydrochloride (Narcan) *Desired effect:* Reversal of narcotic depression of mother and/or baby *Route:* IV	Note which drug was given, time, amount, route; respiratory depression from any drug other than a narcotic *cannot* be reversed with these drugs	Do *not* give Narcan to mother addicted to narcotics because this causes instant withdrawal symptoms; Narcan given to mother reverses pain relief instantly, so that she must be prepared for return of pain or a second form of pain relief is given (e.g., epidural)
Examples: analgesic-potentiating drugs (ataractics, tranquilizers) *Promethazine hydrochloride (Phenergan)* *Propiomazine hydrochloride (Largon)* *Hydroxyzine pamoate (Vistaril)* *Promazine hydrochloride (Sparine)* *Desired effects:* increase desirable effects of analgesics without increasing dose of analgesics (i.e., ataractic potentiates effects of analgesic that is given with it and acts as antiemetic) *Route:* IV, IM	Same as for narcotic analgesics	Same as for narcotic analgesics
Inhalation Analgesia		
Mother breathes subanesthetic concentrations of inhalation anesthetic; if given properly, woman remains conscious but has profound pain relief		
Example: methoxyflurane (Penthrane)	Monitor vital signs closely (be alert for cardiac arrhythmias) q30 min and FHR q15 min	Stay with woman; *never* administer drug for woman because overdose is a risk
Desired effect: profound analgesia while remaining conscious; some amnesia for painful events		Alert physician and remove from mother's hand if: Mother has cardiac arrhythmia Mother loses consciousness; FHR abnormalities occur
Route: self-administered (usually) from a capsule and mask strapped to wrist; physician sets desired concentration; mother inhales drug during contractions	Assess mother's level of consciousness (LOC) and responsiveness; mother should remain conscious and not become delirious or excited	
Example: nitrous oxide (N_2O_2) *Desired effect:* analgesia *Route:* administered by trained personnel, during contractions, or continuously via face mask	☞ Monitor maternal-fetal vital signs q15 min	Trained personnel must remain with woman

(continued)

TABLE 4.3   PAIN MANAGEMENT DURING LABOR AND BIRTH (*Continued*)

Category and Desired Effect	✍ *Assessment and Comments*	✍ *Planning and Implementation*
General Anesthesia		
Rarely indicated for uncomplicated vaginal birth; woman is not awake; danger of aspiration and respiratory depression; safer than regional anesthesia for hypovolemic patients; does not depress neonate unless mother is anesthetized deeply *Examples: thiopental (Pentothal) sodium IV* produces rapid induction of anesthesia; depresses neonate; useful in controlling convulsions *Halothane (Fluothane) (inhalation)*—relaxes uterus quickly, facilitates intrauterine manipulation, version, and extraction *Desired effect:* produces general loss of sensitivity to touch, pain, and other stimulations	Anesthetist assesses woman continuously (intubation is necessary) ☞ Monitor fetal response continuously ☞ Provide *postanesthesia recovery care:* assess q15 min until vital signs are stable and woman is alert and reactive If woman had cesarean birth, do routine postsurgery assessment—wound assessment, intake and output, etc. *Routine postpartum assessment* Assess readiness to see baby Assess her response to anesthesia and event that necessitated birth under general anesthesia (e.g., giving birth by cesarean when vaginal birth was anticipated)	If general anesthesia is being considered: Keep woman NPO ☞ See that an IV infusion is established Premedicate with *cimetidine* to neutralize acid contents of stomach Assist with **cricoid pressure** before intubation ☞ *Recovery room care:* Maintain open airway Maintain cardiopulmonary functions Prevent postpartal hemorrhage *Routine postpartum care:* Facilitate parent-child attachment as soon as possible Answer mother's questions
Regional (Conduction) Anesthesia		

Local anesthetics injected to block primary neuropathways that result in temporary interruption of conduction of nerve impulses, notably pain; mother remains awake
Examples: common agents in 0.5–1.0% solution
  Lidocaine (Xylocaine) hydrochloride
  Bupivacaine (Marcaine) hydrochloride
Chloroprocaine
Tetracaine (Pontocaine) hydrochloride
Mepivacaine hydrochloride (Carbocaine)
	Used with epinephrine (or other vasoconstrictor drug) to delay absorption, prolong anesthetic effect, and decrease chance of hypotension	**Note any history of allergy:** note response: allergic reaction, hypotension, and lack of wearing off of anesthetic effect; observe for *hypertensive crisis* if agent combined with epinephrine and oxytocin (Pitocin) is also being given

Types of Nerve Blocks		
Peripheral nerve block *Pudendal* (5–10 mL on each side): anesthetizes lower two-thirds of vagina and perineum; of short duration (30 min)—given for birth and repair; local anesthesia, may be done by physician or anesthetist; simple and safe, does not depress neonate; may *inhibit bearing-down reflex*	☞ Monitor fetal response continuously Assist physician or anesthetist as necessary	See general nursing actions, below Provide explanation during procedure
Local infiltration: useful for perineal repairs	Assist physician or anesthetist as necessary	See general nursing actions, below Nurse informs physician of medication in syringe

(continued)

TABLE 4.3   PAIN MANAGEMENT DURING LABOR AND BIRTH (*Continued*)

Category and Desired Effect	✉ *Assessment and Comments*	✉ *Planning and Implementation*
Types of Nerve Blocks—cont'd		

Regional nerve block: Requires trained anesthesiologist; with proper administration, relieves pain completely, may prolong labor if given too early; *hypotension* from vasodilation (below anesthesia level) is likely; *fetal bradycardia* may occur as a result of maternal hypotension; *bearing-down reflex* partially or completely *eliminated,* necessitating *outlet forceps* at birth: mother remains awake; absence of pain may facilitate maternal-child attachment; can be used for women with metabolic, lung, and heart diseases	General assessment: note degree of hydration, history of allergy, skin infection over back, previous neural or spinal injury or disease, and attitude toward anesthesia
	Prebirth, monitor:
	☞ Maternal vital signs and FHR
	  Assess for return of pain
	  Monitor labor if anesthesia is established during late first stage
	☞ Rate of IV fluid infusion
	  Perineum to see if birth is imminent (or monitor progress by vaginal examination)
		General nursing actions:
		☞ Hydrate by IV infusion
		  Explain to woman expected feelings as anesthesia begins (warm toes) and as it wears off (tingling); help position her, offering reassurance and support; it is very frightening not to be able to see the procedure and to deal with only sensations and sounds; do not make promises of complete pain relief; each woman may have a differing perception of pain, or block may not provide complete relief
		☞ Treat hypotension: maintain *lateral position or elevate legs;* administer humidified oxygen by mask at 10–12 L/min; increase rate of IV maintenance fluids

Epidural: Useful during first and second stages; can be given as "one shot" or over a period of time; given on top of (or over) dura through third, fourth, or fifth lumbar interspace; risk of dural puncture
During labor, analgesic doses are given
For birth, anesthetic dose is given
Bearing-down reflex usually preserved
	Postbirth, monitor:
	  Uterine tone
	  Bladder tone
	  Return of sensation
		If contractions become *less* frequent, of *less* intensity, or of *shorter* duration, report to physician *immediately;* physician may need to augment labor; assist as necessary
		Add forceps to birth table
		Provide assistance to move from birth table to bed; maintain good uterine tone; prevent bladder distention; prevent injury by keeping side rails up and assisting her when she ambulates

Subarachnoid (low spinal, saddle nerve block): Usually given as "one shot" when fetal head is on perineum; medication is mixed with cerebrospinal fluid in subarachnoid space; injected through third, fourth, or fifth lumbar interspace Bearing-down reflex is *lost*	After subarachnoid block, observe for headache If indwelling catheter is threaded and woman feels a momentary twinge down her leg, hip, or back, anesthetist or nurse assures her it is *not* a sign of injury	For introduction of epidural anesthesia, position woman as for subarachnoid block or in *modified Sims' position:* place woman on her side, shoulders parallel, legs slightly flexed, and back arched An *alternative position* may be preferred by the anesthetist: position woman in a *sitting* position with her buttocks near edge of birth table, feet supported on a footstool; ask woman to place her arms between her knees, flex her head, and arch her back "like a rainbow"; after medication is injected, ask her to remain sitting up for 20–30 sec; then place her *supine* with a pillow under her head and a pelvic wedge to displace uterus to left *Postbirth:* encourage oral *fluids* (if permitted) or monitor IV fluids; ask her to report headache; keep bladder empty; maintain uterine tone

(continued)

TABLE 4.3	PAIN MANAGEMENT DURING LABOR AND BIRTH (*Continued*)	
Category and Desired Effect	⋈ *Assessment and Comments*	⋈ *Planning and Implementation*
Types of Nerve Blocks—cont'd		
Intrathecal (spinal) morphine	0.5 mg MS produces marked analgesia for 12–24 hr; onset in 20–30 min	Side effects: respiratory depression, pruritus, nausea, vomiting, sleepiness, urinary retention; keep *Naloxone*, 0.4 mg, at bedside and respiratory support equipment readily available

Modified from IM Bobak, M Jensen. *Essentials of Maternity Nursing—The Nurse and the Childbearing Family* (2nd ed). St. Louis: Mosby, 1987. P 415.

    5. Infectious diseases (past and present herpes, etc.).
    6. Past obstetric history, if any.
    7. Pelvic measurements.
    8. Height.
    9. Weight gain.
〰10. Laboratory results
      a. Blood type and Rh factor.
      b. Serology.
      c. Urinalysis.
   11. Prenatal care history.
   💊**12.** Use of medications.
  B. *Admission findings*
    1. Emotional status.
    2. Vital signs.
    3. Present weight.
    4. Fundal height.
    5. Present fetal size.
    6. Edema.
〰 **7.** Urinalysis (for protein and sugar).
☞ **C.** *Fetal heart rate (FHR)*—normal, 120–160/min (see Figure 4.5).
    1. Check and record every 30 min—to monitor fetal response to physiologic stress of labor.
    2. *Bradycardia* (mild, 100–119/min, or 30/min lower than baseline reading).
    3. *Tachycardia* (moderate, 160–179/min, or 30/min above baseline reading).
☞ **D.** *Contractions*—every 15–30 min.
    1. Place fingertips over fundus, use gentle pressure; contraction felt as hardening or tensing.
    2. *Time:* frequency and duration.
    3. *Intensity/strength* at acme
      a. *Weak*—easily indent fundus with fingers.
      b. *Moderate*—some tension felt, fundus indents slightly with finger pressure.
      c. *Strong*—unable to indent fundus.
⋈ **E.** *Maternal response to labor*—assess for effective coping, cooperation, and utilizing effective breathing techniques.
☞ **F.** *Maternal vital signs*—between contractions
    1. Response to pain or use of special breathing techniques alters pulse and respirations.
    2. B/P, P, RR—if *normotensive:* on admission,

and then every hour and prn; *after regional anesthesia:* every 30 min (every 5 min first 20 min).
    3. Temperature—if within normal range: on admission, and then every 4 hr and prn. Every 2 hr after rupture of membranes.
    4. Before and after analgesia/anesthesia.
    5. After rupture of membranes (see *Amniotic fluid embolism*, p. 127).
  G. Character and amount of *bloody show*
  H. *Bladder* status: encourage voiding every 1–2 hr, monitor output
☞ **1.** Determine bladder distention—palpate just above symphysis (full bladder may impede labor progress or result in trauma to bladder).
〰 **2.** Admission urinalysis—check for protein and sugar.
  I. Signs of deviations from normal patterns
  J. Status of membranes
    1. Intact.
〰 **2.** Ruptured (nitrazine [pH] paper turns blue on contact with alkaline amniotic fluid). Assess, record, and report
      a. Time—danger of infection if ruptured more than 24 hr.
☞   **b.** FHR stat and 10 min later—to check for prolapsed cord.
      c. Character and color of fluid (see below).
〰 **K.** Amniotic fluid
    1. Amount—hydramnios (>2000 mL)—associated with *congenital anomalies*.
    2. Character—thick consistency and/or odor associated with *infection*.
    3. Color—normally clear with white specks
      a. Yellow—indicates *fetal distress* about 35 hr previous; Rh or ABO incompatibility.
      b. Green or meconium stained; if fetus in vertex position, indicates recent fetal hypoxia secondary to *respiratory distress* in fetus.
      c. Port wine—may indicate *abruptio placentae*.
  L. Labor progress
    1. Effacement.

2. Dilatation.
3. Station.
4. Bulging membranes.
5. Molding of fetal head.
M. Perineum—observe for bulging.

✠ **II. Analysis/nursing diagnosis**

A. *Anxiety, fear* related to uncertain outcome, pain.
B. *Ineffective individual coping* related to lack of preparation for childbirth and/or poor support from coach.
C. *Altered nutrition: less than body requirements* related to physiologic stress of labor.
D. *Altered urinary elimination* related to pressure of presenting part.
E. *Altered thought processes* related to sleep deprivation, transition, analgesia.
F. *Fluid volume deficit* related to anemia, excessive blood loss.
G. *Impaired (fetal) gas exchange* related to impaired placental perfusion.

✠ **III. Nursing care plan/implementation**

A. Goal: *comfort measures*
1. Maintain hydration of oral mucosa. Encourage sucking on cool washcloth, ice chips, lollipops.
2. Reduce dryness of lips. Apply lip balm (Chapstick, petrolatum jelly).
☞ 3. Relieve backache. Apply sacral counterpressure (particularly with occiput posterior [OP] presentation).
4. Encourage significant other to participate.
5. Encourage ambulation when presenting part engaged.

B. Goal: *management of physical needs*
1. Encourage frequent voiding—to prevent full bladder from impeding oncoming head.
2. Encourage ambulation throughout labor; *lateral Sims' position* with head elevated to:
a. Encourage relaxation.
b. Allow gravity to assist in anterior rotation of fetal head.
c. Prevent compression of inferior vena cava and descending aorta (supine hypotensive syndrome); lateral Sims' with head elevated.
d. Promote placental perfusion.
☞ 3. Perineal prep, if ordered—to promote cleanliness.
! ☞ 4. Fleet's enema, if ordered—to stimulate peristalsis, evacuate lower bowel. **NOTE: contraindicated** if:
a. Cervical dilatation (4 cm or more) with unengaged head—because of possibility of cord prolapse.
b. Fetal malpresentation/malposition—because of possible fetal distress.
c. Preterm labor—may stimulate contractions.
d. Painless vaginal bleeding—because of possible placenta previa.
5. Provide *clear fluids* (tea, apple juice) with sugar (if ordered)—to provide energy and to maintain hydration.

C. Goal: *management of psychosocial needs. Emotional support*
1. Encourage verbalization of feelings, fears, concerns.
2. Explain all procedures.
3. Reinforce self-concept ("You're doing well!").

D. Goal: *management of discomfort*
⊕ 1. Analgesia and/or anesthesia—may be required or desired—to facilitate safe, comfortable birth.
☞ 2. Support/enhance/teach childbirth techniques
a. Reinforce appropriate *breathing techniques* for current labor status
(1) If **hyperventilating,** to increase PaCO$_2$, minimize fetal acidosis, and relieve symptoms of vertigo and syncope, suggest:
(a) Breathe into paper bag.
(b) Breathe into cupped hands.
(2) Demonstrate appropriate breathing for several contractions—to reestablish rate and rhythm.

E. Goal: *sustain motivation*
1. Offer support, encouragement, and praise, as appropriate.
2. Keep informed of status and progress.
3. Reassure that irritability is normal.
4. Serve as surrogate coach when necessary (if no partner, before arrival of partner, while partner is changing clothes, during needed breaks); assist with effleurage, breathing, focusing.
5. Discourage bearing-down efforts by pant-blow until complete (10 cm) dilatation—to avoid cervical edema.
6. Facilitate informed decision making regarding medication for relaxation or pain relief.
7. Keep woman and family informed of her progress.
8. Minimize distractions: quiet, relaxed environment; privacy.

✠ **IV. Evaluation/outcome criteria**

1. Woman manages own labor discomfort effectively.
2. Woman maintains control over own behavior.
3. Woman successfully completes first stage of labor without incident.

Nursing Actions During Second Stage of Labor

✠ **I. Assessment**

A. Maternal (or couple's) response to labor.
☞ B. FHR—continuous electronic monitoring, or after each contraction with fetoscope, Doppler.
C. Vital signs.
D. Time elapsed—average: 2 min–1 hr; prolonged second stage increases risk of fetal distress, maternal exhaustion, psychological stress, intrauterine infection.

E. Contraction pattern—average every 1½–3 min, lasting 60–90 sec.

F. Vaginal discharge—increases.

G. Nausea, vomiting, disorientation, tremors, amnesia between contractions, panic.

H. Response to regional anesthesia, if administered
   1. Signs of hypotension—reduces placental perfusion, increases risk of fetal hypoxia.
   2. Effect on contractions—note and report any slowing of labor.

I. Efforts to bear down—increases expulsive effects of uterine contractions.

J. Perineal bulging with contractions—fetal head distends perineum, crowns; head born by extension.

II. Analysis/nursing diagnosis
   A. *Pain* related to strong uterine contractions, pressure of fetal descent, stretching of perineum.
   B. *High risk for injury:*
      1. Infection related to ruptured membranes, repeated vaginal examinations.
      2. Laceration related to pressure of fetal head exceeding perineal elasticity and uterine rupture related to fundal pressure.
   C. *Impaired skin integrity* related to laceration, episiotomy.
   D. *Fluid volume deficit* related to hypotension secondary to regional anesthesia.
   E. *Anxiety* related to imminent birth of fetus.
   F. *Ineffective individual coping* related to prolonged sensory stimulation (contractions) and anxiety.
   G. *Altered urinary elimination* related to anesthesia and contractions.
   H. *Sleep pattern disturbance.*

III. Nursing care plan/implementation
   A. Goal: *emotional support*
      1. To sustain motivation/control
         a. Never leave mother and significant other alone now.
         b. Keep informed of progress.
         c. Direct bearing-down efforts (pushing) without holding breath° while pushing. Encourage pushing "out through vagina" and encourage mother to touch coming head; position mirror so woman can see perineal bulging with effective efforts; minimize distractions.
      2. To allay significant other's anxiety: reassure regarding mother's behavior if she is not anesthetized.
      3. Support family choices.
   B. Goal: *safeguard status*
      1. Precautions when putting legs in stirrups
         a. If varicosities, **do not put legs in stirrups.**

° The woman must be discouraged from using the **Valsalva maneuver** (holding one's breath and tightening abdominal muscles) for pushing during the *second* stage. This activity increases intrathoracic pressure, reduces venous return, and increases venous pressure. The cardiac output and blood pressure increase and pulse slows temporarily. During the Valsalva maneuver, fetal hypoxia may occur. The process is reversed when the woman takes a breath.

---

         b. *Avoid* pressure to popliteal veins; pad stirrups.
         c. Ensure proper, even alignment by adjusting stirrups.
         d. Move legs simultaneously into or out of stirrups—to *avoid* nerve, ligament, and muscle strain.
         e. Provide proper support to woman not using stirrups.
      2. Support woman in whatever position selected for birth, e.g., side-lying.
      3. Cleanse perineum, thighs, and lower abdomen, maintaining sterile technique.
   C. Goal: *maintain a comfortable environment*
      1. Free of unnecessary noise, light, conversation.
      2. Comfortable temperature (warm).
   D. *Medical management*
      1. Episiotomy may be performed to facilitate birth.
      2. Forceps may be applied to exert traction and expedite birth.
      3. Vacuum extraction also used.
   E. Birthing room birth with alternative positions.

IV. Evaluation/outcome criteria
   A. Woman is cooperative, actively participates in birth; maintains control over own behavior.
   B. Successful, uncomplicated birth of viable infant.
   C. All assessment findings within normal limits (vital signs, emotional status, response to birth).
   D. Presence of significant other.

Nursing Actions During Third Stage of Labor

I. Assessment
   A. Time elapsed—average: 5 min; prolonged third stage (>25 min) may indicate complications.

   ┌─────────────────────────────────────┐
   B. Signs of placental separation
      1. Increase in bleeding from vagina.
      2. Cord lengthens.
      3. Uterus rises in abdomen, assumes globular shape.
   └─────────────────────────────────────┘

   C. Assess mother's level of consciousness (LOC).
   D. Examine placenta for intactness and number of vessels in umbilical cord (*normal:* three. *NOTE:* two vessels only—associated with increased incidence of congenital anomalies); condition of placenta for calcification, infarcts, etc.

II. Analysis/nursing diagnosis
   A. *Family coping: potential for growth* related to bonding, beginning achievement of developmental tasks.
   B. *Fluid volume deficit* related to blood loss during third stage.

III. Nursing care plan/implementation
   A. Goal: *prevent uterine atony.* Administer *oxytocin,* as ordered (see Pharmacology Box 6.1).
   B. Goal: *facilitate parent-child bonding*

1. While protecting neonate from cold stress, encourage parents to see, hold, touch neonate.
2. Comment about neonate's individuality, characteristics, and behaviors.
3. After neonate is assessed for congenital anomalies (cleft palate, esophageal atresia), encourage breastfeeding, if desired.

C. Goal: *health teaching*
   1. Describe, discuss common neonatal behavior in transitional period (periods of reactivity, sleep, hyperactivity).
   ☞ 2. Demonstrate removal of mucus by aspiration with bulb syringe.
   ☞ 3. Demonstrate ways of facilitating breastfeeding.

⋈ **IV. Evaluation/outcome criteria**
   A. Woman has a successful, uneventful completion of labor
      1. Minimal blood loss.
      2. Vital signs within normal limits.
      3. Fundus well contracted at level of umbilicus.
   B. Parents express satisfaction with outcome, demonstrate infant attachment.

Nursing Actions During Fourth Stage of Labor— 1–2 hr postpartum

⋈ **I. Assessment**—every 15 min 4 times; then, every 30 min 2 times—or until stable—to monitor response to physiologic stress of labor/birth
   A. Vital signs
      1. *Temperature* taken once; if elevated, requires follow-up—may indicate infection, dehydration, excessive blood loss. Note, record, report temperature of 100.4°F (38°C) or more.
      2. *Blood pressure*—every 15 min × 4.
         a. Returns to prelabor level—due to loss of placental circulation and increased circulating blood volume.
         b. Elevation may be in response to use of oxytocic drugs or preeclampsia (first 48 hr).
         c. Lowered blood pressure—may reflect significant blood loss during labor/birth, or occult bleeding.
      3. *Pulse* and *respirations*—every 15 min × 4
         a. Physiologic bradycardia—due to normal vagal response.
         b. Tachycardia—may indicate excessive blood loss during labor/birth, dehydration, exhaustion, or occult bleeding.
   ☞ B. Location and tone of fundus—every 15 min × 4, to assure continuing contraction; prevent blood loss due to uterine relaxation
      1. Fundus—firm; at or slightly lower than the umbilicus; in midline.
      2. May be displaced by distended bladder—due to normal diuresis; common cause of bleeding in immediate postpartum, uterine atony.

C. Character and amount of *vaginal flow* every 15 min × 4
   1. Moderate lochia rubra.
   2. Perineal pad saturated in 15 min, or blood pools under buttocks, may indicate excessive loss.
   3. Bright-red bleeding may indicate cervical or vaginal laceration.
D. *Perineum* every 15 min × 4
   1. Edema.
   2. Bruising—due to trauma.
   3. Distention/hematoma, rectal pain.
E. *Bladder* fullness/voiding every 15 min × 4—to prevent distention.
F. Rate of IV, if present; response to added medication, if any.
G. Intake and output—to evaluate hydration.
H. Recovery from analgesia/anesthesia.
I. Energy level.
J. Verbal, nonverbal interaction between woman and significant other
   1. Dialogue.
   2. Posture.
   3. Facial expressions.
   4. Touching.
K. Interactions between parent(s) and newborn; signs of bonding
   1. Eye contact with newborn.
   2. Calls by name.
   3. Explores with fingertips, strokes, cuddles.
L. Signs of *postpartal emergencies*
   a. Uterine atony, hemorrhage.
   b. Vaginal hematoma.

II. Analysis/nursing diagnosis
   A. *Fluid volume deficit* related to excessive intrapartal blood loss, dehydration.
   B. *Altered urinary elimination* related to intrapartal bladder trauma, dehydration, blood loss.
   C. *Impaired skin integrity* related to episiotomy, lacerations, cesarean birth.
   D. *Altered family processes* related to role change.
   E. *Altered parenting* related to interruption in bonding secondary to:
      1. Compromised maternal status.
      2. Compromised neonatal status.
   F. *Knowledge deficit* related to self-care procedures.
   G. *Fatigue* related to sleep disturbances and anxiety.
   H. *Anxiety* related to status of self and infant.
   I. *Altered nutrition, less than body requirements,* related to decreased food and fluid intake during labor.

⋈ **III. Nursing care plan/implementation**
   ☞ A. Goal: *comfort measures*
      1. Maternal position.
      2. Pad change.
      3. Perineal care—to promote healing; to reduce possibility of infection.
      4. Ice pack to perineum, as ordered—to reduce edema, discomfort, and pain related to hemorrhoids.

B. Goal: *nutrition/hydration.* Offer fluids, foods as tolerated.

C. Goal: *urinary elimination*
  1. Encourage voiding—to avoid bladder distention.
  2. Record: time, amount, character.
  3. Anticipatory guidance related to nocturnal diuresis and increased output.

D. Goal: *promote bonding*
  1. Provide privacy, quiet; encourage sustained contact with newborn.
  2. Encourage: touching, holding baby; breast-feeding (also promotes involution).

E. Goal: *health teaching*
  1. Perineal care—front to back, labia closed (after *each* void/bowel movement).
  2. Handwashing—before and after each pad change; after voiding, defecating; before and after baby care.
  3. Signs to report
     a. Uterine cramping.
     b. Increased vaginal bleeding, passage of large clots.
     c. Nausea, dizziness.

IV. Evaluation/outcome criteria
  A. Woman expresses comfort, satisfaction in fourth stage.
  B. Vital signs stable, fundus contracted, moderate lochia rubra, perineum undistended.
  C. Woman tolerates food and fluids well.
  D. Woman voids in adequate amount.
  E. Woman demonstrates eye contact with infant, cuddles.
  F. Woman verbalizes abnormal signs to report to physician.
  G. Woman returns demonstration of appropriate perineal care.
  H. Woman ambulates without pain, dizziness, numbness of legs.

Nursing Management of the Newborn Immediately After Birth

I. Assessment
  A. Mucus in nasopharynx, oropharynx.
  B. *Apgar score:* note and record—at 1 and 5 min of age.

Apgar Scoring System			
	Points Given According to Status		
Clinical Sign	0 Points	1 Point	2 Points
Appearance (color)	Blue, pale	Body pink, extremities blue	Completely pink
Pulse (HR)	Absent	Below 100	Over 100
Grimace (reflex irritability to a gentle slap)	No response	Grimaces	Cries
Activity (muscle tone)	Limp	Some flexion of extremities	Active motion, general flexion
Respiratory effort	Absent	Slow, irregular	Good, strong cry

  1. *Score of 7–10:* good condition.
  2. *Score of 4–6:* fair condition; assess for CNS depression; resuscitate as necessary.
  3. *Score of 0–3:* poor condition; requires immediate resuscitative measures. **Asphyxia neonatorum**—fails to breathe spontaneously within 30–60 sec after birth.

  C. Number of vessels in umbilical stump.
  D. Passage of meconium stool, urine.
  E. General physical appearance/status
    1. Signs of *respiratory distress* (nasal flaring, grunting, sternal retraction, cyanosis, tachypnea).
    2. *Skin* condition (meconium-stained, cyanosis, jaundice, lesions).
    3. *Cry*—presence, pitch, quality.
    4. Signs of *birth trauma* (lacerations, dislocations, fractures).
    5. *Symmetry* (absent parts, extra digits, gross malformations, ears, palm creases, sacral dimples).
    6. Head: molding, caput succedaneum, cephalohematoma.
    7. Assess *gestational age.*
  F. Identify high-risk infant.

II. Analysis/nursing diagnosis
  A. *Ineffective airway clearance* related to excessive nasopharyngeal mucus.
  B. *Ineffective breathing pattern* related to CNS depression secondary to intrauterine hypoxia narcosis, prematurity, and lack of pulmonary surfactant.
  C. *Impaired gas exchange* related to respiratory distress.
  D. *Fluid volume deficit* related to birth trauma; hemolytic jaundice.
  E. *Impaired skin integrity* related to cord stump.
  F. *High risk for injury* (biochemical, metabolic) related to impaired thermoregulation.
  G. *Ineffective thermoregulation* related to environmental conditions.

III. Nursing care plan/implementation
  A. Goal: *ensure patent airway*
    1. Suction mouth first, then nose; when stimulated, sensitive receptors around entrance to nares initiate gasp, causing aspiration of mucus present in mouth.
    2. Suction with bulb syringe
       a. If deeper suctioning necessary, use DeLee mucus trap attached to suction. Oral use of DeLee is discouraged due to risk of con-

tact with baby's secretions (new Delee now available has no such risk).
  b. *Avoid* prolonged, vigorous suctioning
    (1) Reduces oxygenation.
    (2) May traumatize tissue, cause edema, bleeding, laryngospasm, and cardiac arrhythmia.
  3. Assist gravity drainage of fluids; *position:* head-dependent (Trendelenburg), and side-lying.
B. Goal: *maintain body temperature*—to conserve energy, preserve store of brown fat, decrease oxygen needs; prevent acidosis. Prevent chilling:
  1. Minimize exposure; dry quickly.
  2. Warm; apply hat.
  3. Take temperature hourly until stable.
C. Goal: *identify infant*
  1. Apply Identiband or name beads.
  2. Take infant's footprints and maternal fingerprints.
D. Goal: *prevent eye infection* (gonorrheal and chlamydial *ophthalmia neonatorum*). Within 2 hrs of birth, apply ophthalmic antibiotic drops (2 drops in each eye) or ointment (1 line in each eye).
E. Goal: *facilitate prompt identification/vigilance for potential neonatal complications*
  1. Record significant data from mother's chart
    a. History of pregnancy, diabetes, hypertension, current drug abuse, excessive caffeine, medications, alcohol, malnutrition.
    b. Course of labor, evidence of fetal distress, medications received in labor.
    c. Birth history of anesthesia.
    d. Apgar; resuscitative efforts.
F. Goal: *facilitate prompt identification/intervention in hemolytic problems of the newborn*
  1. Collect and send cord blood for appropriate tests
    a. Blood type and Rh factor.
    b. Coombs test.
  2. Give vitamin K to facilitate clotting.
IV. Evaluation/outcome criteria: successful transition to extrauterine life
  A. Status satisfactory; all assessment findings within normal limits.
  B. Responsive in bonding process with parents.

Nurse-Attended Emergency Birth (precipitate birth)

When woman presents without prenatal care to ER, may represent drug abuse.

Imminent Birth

I. Assessment: identify signs of **imminent birth**
  A. Strong contractions.

  B. Bearing-down efforts.
  C. Perineal bulging; crowning.
  D. Mother states, "It's coming."
II. Analysis/nursing diagnosis
  A. *Pain* related to:
    1. Strong, sustained contractions.
    2. Descent of fetal head.
    3. Stretching of perineum.
  B. *Anxiety/fear* related to imminent birth.
  C. *Ineffective individual coping* related to circumstances surrounding birth; anxiety, fear for self and infant.
  D. *Injury* (mother) related to
    1. Lacerations (vaginal, perineal).
    2. Infection secondary to unsterile birth.
  E. *Fluid volume deficit* related to
    1. Lacerations.
    2. Uterine atony.
    3. Retained placental fragments.
  F. *Impaired gas exchange* (infant) related to intact membranes during birth.
  G. *Risk for injury* (infant) related to
    1. Precipitate birth.
    2. Trauma.
    3. Hypoxia.
III. Nursing care plan/implementation
  A. Goal: *reduce anxiety/fear*—reassure mother.
  B. Goal: *delay birth,* as possible
    1. Discourage bearing-down.
    2. Encourage panting.
    3. *Side-lying position* to slow descent and allow for more controlled birth.
  C. Goal: *prevent infection*
    1. Provide sterile (or clean) field for birth.
    2. *Avoid* touching birth canal without gloved hands.
    3. Support perineum (and advancing head) with sterile (or clean) towel.
  D. Goal: *facilitate/assist birth* (Figure 4.6)
    1. If membranes intact as head emerges, tear them at neck to facilitate first breath.
    2. Support head in both hands.
    3. Feel for cord around neck (if present, and if possible, slip cord over head; if tight, *and* sterile equipment at hand, clamp cord in 2 places, cut between clamps, unwrap cord). If *unsterile* environment, keep fetus and placenta attached—*do not* cut cord.
    4. After restitution, apply gentle downward pressure to bring anterior shoulder under pubic symphysis.
    5. Gently lift head to ease birth of posterior shoulder.
    6. Support infant as body slips free of mother's body.
  E. Goal: *facilitate drainage of mucus and fluid* → patent airway.
    1. Hold infant in *head-dependent position* (see Figure 4.6, E).
    2. Clear mucus with bulb syringe (if available), or use fingertip, wipe with towel.

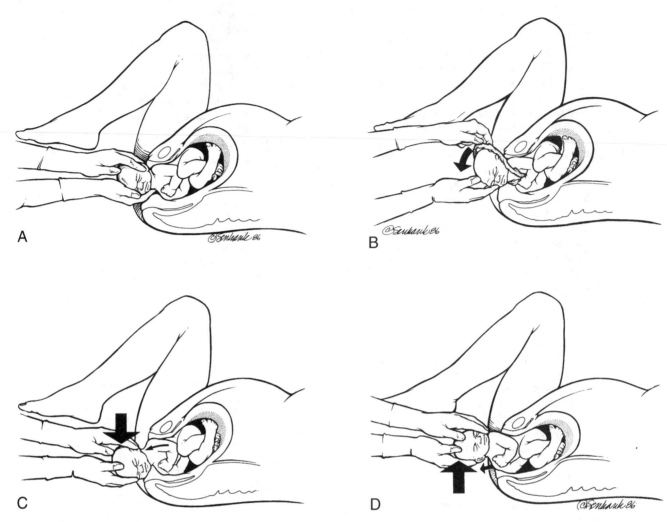

FIGURE 4.6   **EMERGENCY BIRTH.** See caption on facing page.

☞ **F.** Goal: *prevent placental transfusion*—hold infant level with placenta until cord stops pulsating. If sterile supplies are available, cut cord (Figure 4.7).

☞ **G.** Goal: *prevent chilling*
   1. Wrap infant in towel or other clean material.
   2. Place infant on *side, head-dependent,* on mother's abdomen.
   3. Dry head, cover with cap or material.

Placental Separation

◄ **I. Assessment**—*third stage:* identify signs of **placental separation** (review p. 106).

II. Nursing care plan/implementation—*third stage*
   A. Goal: *avoid/minimize potential for complications* (everted uterus, tearing of placenta with fragments remaining, separation of cord from placenta)
      1. *Avoid* traction (pulling) on cord.
      2. *Avoid* vigorous fundal massage.
      3. *Discourage* maternal bearing-down efforts unless placenta visible at introitus.
      4. With fundus well contracted, and placenta visible at introitus, encourage mother to bear down to expel placenta.

☞ **B.** Goal: *stimulate respiration.* If neonate *fails to breathe spontaneously*
   1. Maintain body temperature—dry and cover.
   2. Clear airway: Position head downs, turn head to side.
      a. Position: head down.
      b. Turn head to side.
   3. Stimulate.
      a. Rub back gently.
      b. Flick soles of feet.
   4. If no response to stimulation:
      a. Slightly extend neck to "sniffing" position (head tilt-chin lift method).
      b. Place mouth over newborn's nose and mouth and exhale air in cheeks, saying "ho" (prevents excessive pressure).

C. Goal: begin *cardiopulmonary resuscitation (CPR)* if no heart rate.
      a. Place infant on firm, flat surface.
      b. With two–three fingers on sternum, depress ½–¾ in. 100 times/min.

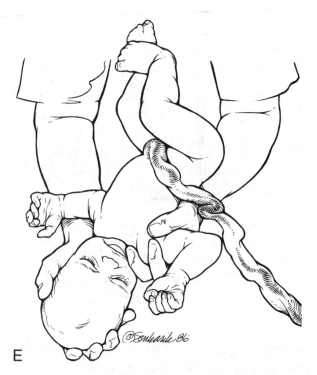

E

FIGURE 4.6   **EMERGENCY BIRTH.** (A) **Support infant's head** as it delivers. (B) **Loosen cord** from around neck. (C) Gently guide head downward to **help upper shoulder deliver.** (D) Guide head upward to **help lower shoulder deliver.** (E) Babies are slippery! **Hold the baby firmly,** with the head dependent to, facilitate drainage of secretions. (From N. Caroline. *Emergency Care in the Streets* (5th ed). Boston: Little, Brown, 1995. Pp 863–864.)

    c. Assist ventilation on upstroke of every fifth compression (5:1 ratio).
    d. Go immediately to emergency room.
    e. See *Teaching parents CPR, Chapter 8,* p. 170.

D. Goal: *maintain infant's body temperature*
    1. Wrap placenta with baby, if cord intact.
    2. Place infant in mother's arms.
E. Goal: *prevent maternal hemorrhage* (uterine atony)
    1. Encourage breastfeeding, or stimulate nipple.
☞ **2.** Gently massage fundus, support lower part of uterus and express clots when uterus is contracted.
    3. Encourage voiding if bladder is full.
    4. Get to a medical facility.
F. Goal: *encourage bonding/stimulate uterine contractions.* Encourage breastfeeding.
G. Goal: *legal accountability* as birth attendant. Record date, time, birth events, maternal and fetal status.
⋈ **III. Evaluation/outcome criteria**
  A. Woman experiences normal spontaneous birth of viable infant over intact perineum.

  B. Uncomplicated fourth stage—status satisfactory for both mother and infant.
  C. Woman expresses satisfaction with management and result.

Alterations Affecting Protective Function

I. Induction of labor—deliberate initiation of uterine contractions
  A. Indications for
    1. History of rapid or silent labors, precipitate birth.
    2. Woman resides some distance from hospital (controversial).
    3. Coexisting medical disorders:
      a. Uncontrolled diabetes.
      b. Progressive preeclampsia.
      c. Severe renal disease.
    4. Premature rupture of membranes (PROM)—spontaneous rupture of membranes before onset of labor and less than 37 wk from last menstrual period. **Hazards:**

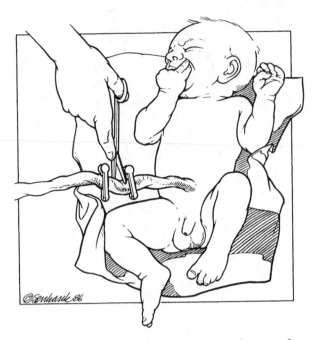

FIGURE 4.7   **CUTTING THE UMBILICAL CORD.** Place clamps about 2 in. apart along the cord after it has stopped pulsating, and cut between them. (From N. Caroline. *Emergency Care in the Streets* (5th ed). Boston: Little, Brown, 1995. P 866.)

a. *Maternal*—intrauterine infection (amnionitis, endometritis).

   b. *Fetal*—sepsis; prolapsed cord.

5. Rh or ABO incompatibility, fetal hemolytic disease.

6. Congenital anomaly (e.g., anencephaly).

7. Postterm pregnancy with nonreactive (nonstress test) (NST).

8. Intrauterine fetal death.

B. *Criteria for induction*

   1. Absence of cephalopelvic disproportion (CPD), malpresentation, or malposition.

   2. Engaged vertex of single gestation.

   3. Nearing, or at, term.

   4. Fetal lung maturity

      a. Survival rate—better at 32 wk or more.

      b. Lecithin-sphingomyelin (L/S) ratio greater than $2:1$.

      c. Diabetic mother—*phosphatidylglycerol* is present in amniotic fluid.

   5. "Ripe" cervix—softening, partially effaced, or ready for effacement/dilatation (if not already present). NOTE: Intravaginal or paracervical application of prostaglandin gel, or laminaria, may be used to prepare cervix for labor.

C. *Methods*

   1. *Amniotomy*—artificial rupture of membranes (AROM) with fetal head engaged.

   2. Intravenous *oxytocin infusion.*

D. *Potential complications*

   1. *Amniotomy*—irrevocably committed to birth

      a. Prolapsed cord.

      b. Infection.

   2. *IV oxytocin infusion:*

      a. Overstimulation of uterus.

      b. Decreased placental perfusion/fetal distress.

      c. Precipitate labor and birth.

      d. Cervical/perineal lacerations.

      e. Uterine rupture.

      f. Water intoxication—if large doses given in dextrose in water (D/W) over prolonged period (antidiuretic effect increases water reabsorption).

      g. Hypertensive crisis.

Before Induction

A. Assessment—*before induction*

   1. Estimate of gestation (EDB, fundal height, cervical status).

   2. *Bishop Score:* evaluation of cervical inducibility.

   3. General health status:

      a. Weight, vital signs, FHR, edema.

      b. Status of membranes.

      c. Vaginal bleeding.

      d. Coexisting disorders.

   4. History of previous labors, if any.

5. Emotional status.
6. Knowledge/understanding of anticipated procedures:
   a. Amniotomy (artificial rupture of membranes).
   ☞ b. IV oxytocin infusion.
   c. Fetal monitoring.
7. Preparation for childbirth (Lamaze, etc.); coping strategies. Identify support person.

B. Analysis/nursing diagnosis
1. *Knowledge deficit* related to process of induction.
2. *Anxiety/fear* related to need for induction of labor.
3. *Ineffective individual coping* related to psychological stress.
4. *Pain* related to uterine contractions.

C. Nursing care plan/implementation
1. Goal: *health teaching*
   a. Explain rationale for procedures
      (1) Amniotomy
         (a) Induces labor.
         (b) Relieves uterine overdistention.
         (c) Increases efficiency of contractions, shortening labor.
      (2) Oxytocin infusion
         (a) Induces labor.
         (b) Stimulates uterine contractions.
      (3) Internal fetal monitor
         (a) Provides continuous assessment of uterine response to oxytocin stimulation.
         (b) Provides continuous assessment of fetal response to physiologic stress of labor.
   b. *Describe procedure*—to reduce anxiety and increase cooperation.
   c. *Explain advantages/disadvantages*—to ensure "informed consent."
2. Goal: *emotional support*—encourage verbalization of concerns, reassure, as possible.

D. Evaluation/outcome criterion: Woman verbalizes understanding of process, rationale, procedures, and alternatives.

During Induction

A. Assessment—*during induction and labor*
1. *Amniotomy*—same as for spontaneous rupture of membranes (SROM)
   a. Observe fluid—note color, amount.
   ☞ b. Monitor FHR; assess for fetal distress.
   c. Observe for signs of prolapsed cord.
   d. Assess fetal activity
      (1) Excessive activity may indicate distress.
      (2) Absence of activity may indicate distress or demise.
2. *IV oxytocin infusion*
   ☞ a. Continually assess response to oxytocin stimulation/flow rate; always given via controlled infusion.

(1) Uterine contractions.
(2) Maternal vital signs, FHR.
b. Identify signs of:
   (1) *Deviation* from normal patterns:
      (a) Lack of response to increasing flow rate.
      (b) Uterine hyperirritability (contractions—<2 min apart).
      (c) Lack of adequate uterine relaxation between contractions.
   (2) *Side effects* of oxytocin: diminished output—potential water intoxication.
   (3) **Hazards** to mother or fetus:
      (a) Sustained (>90 sec duration) or tetanic (strong, spasmlike) contractions—potential abruptio placentae, uterine rupture, fetal hypoxia/anoxia/death.
      (b) *Fetal* arrhythmias, decelerations.
      (c) *Maternal* hypertension—potential for hypertensive crisis, cerebral hemorrhage.

B. Nursing care plan/implementation
1. Same as for other women in labor.
2. Treatment for indications of deviations from normal patterns (see Figure 4.5)
   a. Change maternal position.
   b. Stop oxytocin infusion, maintain IV with 5% D/W or other (Ringer's lactate, etc.).
   ☞ c. Begin oxygen per mask; up to 8–10 L/min.
   d. Notify physician promptly.
   e. Check maternal blood pressure and pulse rate.
3. Anticipatory guidance: may have strong contractions soon after induction starts.

C. Evaluation/outcome criteria
1. Woman demonstrates response to oxytocin stimulation.
   a. Establishes desired contraction pattern, not hyperstimulated.
   b. Progresses through labor—within normal limits
      (1) Normotensive.
      (2) Voids in adequate amounts.
      (3) No evidence of deviation from normal contraction patterns.
2. Fetus shows no evidence of distress.
3. Woman experiences normal vaginal birth of viable infant.

II. Operative obstetrics—*episiotomy*
   A. Definition—incision of perineum to facilitate infant's birth.
   B. Rationale
   1. Surgical incision reduces possibility of laceration.
   2. Heals more easily than a laceration.
   3. Protects infant's head from pressure exerted by resistant perineum.
   4. Shortens second stage of labor.
   C. Types

1. *Midline*—chance of extension into anal sphincter greater than with mediolateral.
2. *Mediolateral*—healing is more painful than midline.

✉ **D. Assessment**
   1. "REEDA"
      a. Color: (**r**edness).
      b. Swelling: (**e**dema).
      c. Bruising: (**e**cchymosis).
      d. Drainage: (**d**ischarge).
      e. Suture line intact, or separated (**a**pproximation).
   2. Healing.
   3. Hematoma.
   4. Tenderness; pain. NOTE: evaluate complaints of pain carefully. If intense, and unrelieved by usual measures, report promptly. May indicate vulvar, paravaginal, or ischiorectal abscess or hematoma.

✉ **E. Analysis/nursing diagnosis**
   1. *Pain* related to labor process.
   2. *Impaired skin integrity* related to surgical incision.
   3. *Fluid volume deficit* related to hematoma.
   4. *Sexual dysfunction* related to discomfort.

✉ **F. Nursing care plan/implementation**
   1. Goal: *prevent/reduce edema, promote comfort and healing*
      👉 **a.** Place covered ice pack during immediate postpartum.
      💊 **b.** Administer analgesics, topical sprays, ointments, witch hazel pads.
      c. Encourage use of sitz bath or rubber ring.
      👉 **d.** Encourage *Kegel's* exercises.
      e. Do *health teaching*
         (1) Instruct in tightening gluteal muscles before sitting.
         (2) Instruct to *avoid* sitting on one hip.
   2. Goal: *minimize potential for infection*
      👉 **a.** Teach/provide perineal care during fourth stage of labor.
      b. *Health teaching*: instruct in self-perineal care after voiding, defecation, and with each pad change.

✉ **G. Evaluation/outcome criteria**
   1. Woman's incision heals by primary intention.
   2. Woman demonstrates appropriate self-perineal care.
   3. Woman evidences no signs of hematoma, infection, or separation of suture line.
   4. Woman experiences minimal discomfort.

III. Operative obstetrics—*forceps-assisted birth*
  A. *Indications*
   1. Fetal distress.
   2. Maternal need
      a. Exhaustion.
      b. Coexisting disease, such as cardiac disorder.
      c. Poor progress in second stage.
      d. Persistent fetal occiput transverse (OT) or occiput posterior (OP) position.

  B. *Criteria* for forceps application:
   1. Engaged fetal head.
   2. Ruptured membranes.
   3. Full dilatation.
   4. Absence of cephalopelvic disproportion.
   5. Some anesthesia has been given; usually, episiotomy has been performed.
   6. Empty bladder.
  C. *Types:*
   1. Low—outlet forceps.
   2. Pipers—applied to after-coming head in selected breech births.
⚡ **D.** Potential *complications:*
   1. *Maternal:*
      a. Lacerations of birth canal, rectum, bladder.
      b. Uterine rupture/hemorrhage.
   2. *Neonatal:*
      a. Cephalohematoma.
      b. Skull fracture.
      c. Intracranial hemorrhage, brain damage.
      d. Facial paralysis.
      e. Direct tissue trauma (abrasions, ecchymosis).
      f. Umbilical cord compression.

✉ **E. Assessment**
   👉 **1.** FHR immediately before—and after—forceps application (forceps blade may compress umbilical cord).
   ✉ **2.** Observe mother/newborn for injury or signs of complications.

✉ **F. Analysis/nursing diagnosis**
   1. *Self-esteem disturbance* related to inability to give birth without surgical assistance.
   2. *Anxiety/fear* related to infant's appearance (forceps marks) or awareness of potential complications.

✉ **G. Nursing care plan/implementation**
   1. Goal: *minimize feelings of failure due to inability to give birth "naturally"*
      a. Explain, discuss reasons/indications for forceps-assisted birth.
      b. Emphasize no maternal control over circumstances.
   2. Goal: *reduce parental anxiety, maternal guilt over infant bruising/forceps marks.* Explain condition is temporary and has no lasting effects on child's appearance.

✉ **H. Evaluation/outcome criteria**
   1. Woman verbalizes understanding of reasons for forceps-assisted birth.
   2. Woman evidences no interruption in bonding with infant.
   3. Woman experiences uncomplicated recovery.

IV. Operative obstetrics—*vacuum cap and pump-assisted birth*

V. Operative obstetrics—*cesarean birth:* incision through abdominal wall and uterus to give birth
  A. *Indications* for elective cesarean birth
   1. Known CPD.
   2. Previous uterine surgery (e.g., myomectomy), repeated cesarean births (depends on type of incision done).

3. Active maternal genital herpes II infection.
4. Breech presentation (*NOTE:* to reduce infant morbidity/mortality, elective cesarean birth is common method of choice).
5. Neoplasms of cervix, uterus, or birth canal.
6. Maternal diabetes with placental aging; fetal macrosomia (cephalopelvic disproportion).

B. *Criteria* for elective cesarean birth: L/S ratio greater than 2:1—indicates presence of pulmonary surfactant; less risk of respiratory distress syndrome.

C. *Indications for emergency cesarean birth*
1. *Fetal*
   a. *Fetal distress:* prolapsed cord.
   b. *Fetal jeopardy:* Rh or ABO incompatibility.
   c. *Fetal malposition*/malpresentation.
   d. *Medical evaluation:* fetal blood sampling—low O_2, elevated CO_2, pH below 7.20 (indicates fetal hypoxia, acidosis).

2. *Maternal*
   a. Uterine dysfunction.
   b. Placental disorders:
   (1) Placenta previa.
   (2) Abruptio placentae, with Couvelaire uterus.
   c. Severe maternal preeclampsia/eclampsia.
   d. Fetopelvic disproportion.
   e. Sudden maternal death.
   f. Carcinoma.
   g. Failed induction.

D. Types
1. *Low segment*—method of choice
   a. Transverse incision through abdominal wall and lower uterine segment.
   b. Transverse incision through abdominal wall, with vertical incision of lower uterine segment.
   c. Advantages—fewer complications:
   (1) Less blood loss.
   (2) More comfortable convalescence.
   (3) Less adhesion formation.
   (4) Lower risk of uterine rupture in subsequent pregnancy/labor and birth.
   (5) Cosmetically more acceptable.
2. *Classic*—vertical incision through abdominal wall and uterus. Necessary for anterior placenta previa and transverse lie.
3. *Porro's*—hysterotomy followed by hysterectomy. Necessary in presence of:
   a. Hemorrhage from uterine atony.
   b. Placenta previa, accreta.
   c. Large uterine myomas.
   d. Ruptured uterus.
   e. Cancer of uterus or ovary.

E. Assessment
1. *Maternal* physical status
   a. Vital signs.
   b. Labor status, if any.
   c. Contractions (if any).
   d. Membranes (intact; ruptured).

   e. Signs of complications.
2. *Fetal* status
   a. FHR pattern.
   b. Color and amount of amniotic fluid.
   c. Biophysical profile (BPP).
3. Maternal emotional status.
4. Understanding of procedure, indications for, implications.
5. Other—as for any abdominal surgery.

F. Analysis/nursing diagnosis
1. *Self-esteem disturbance* related to perceived failure to give birth vaginally.
2. *Anxiety/fear* related to impending surgery and/or reasons for cesarean birth.
3. *Ineffective individual coping* related to anxiety and fear for self, infant.
4. *Fluid volume deficit* related to abdominal surgery and/or reason for cesarean birth.
5. *Pain* related to abdominal surgery.
6. *Constipation* related to decreased bowel activity.
7. *Altered urinary elimination* related to fluid volume deficit.

G. Nursing care plan/implementation
1. *Preoperative*
   a. Goal: *safeguard fetal status*
   (1) Monitor fetal heart rate continually.
   (2) Notify neonatology and NICU of scheduled surgical birth.
   b. Goal: *health teaching*
   (1) Describe, discuss anticipated anesthesia.
   (2) Explain rationale for preoperative antacids: cimetidine, a histamine blocker, to decrease production of gastric acid; *metoclopramide (Reglan)* to hasten gastric emptying.
   (3) Describe, explain anticipated procedures—abdominal shave, indwelling catheter, intravenous fluids—to woman and support person.
   c. Other—as for any abdominal surgery.
   d. Prepare for cesarean birth.
2. *Postoperative*
   a. Same as for other abdominal surgical patients.
   b. Same as for other postpartum women.

H. Evaluation/outcome criteria
1. Woman verbalizes understanding of reasons for cesarean birth.
2. Successful birth of viable infant.
3. Evidence of no surgical/birth complications.
4. Woman evidences no interference with bonding.
5. Woman expresses satisfaction with procedure and result.

VI. Vaginal birth after cesarean (VBAC): *trial of labor*
   A. Candidates:
   1. Previous low-transverse cesarean birth.
   2. Fetal head well engaged in pelvis; *no* evidence of CPD or feto-pelvic disproportion (FPD).
   3. Woman in active labor, including adequate

contractions, engagement and descent of presenting part, effacement and dilatation in progress; soft anterior cervix.
  4. Preexisting reason for cesarean birth *not* apparent.
  5. *No* history of sepsis with previous cesarean
birth that may hinder new incision from healing properly.
  6. *No* herpetic infection.
▶ **B. Assessment**
  ☞ **1.** Monitor FHR carefully.
  ☞ **2.** Monitor uterus for adequacy of contractions
and for progress of labor.
    3. Observe mother for signs of complications.
▶ **C. Analysis/nursing diagnosis**
    1. *Knowledge deficit* related to trial of labor.
    2. *Fear* related to outcome for fetus.
    3. *Ineffective individual coping* related to labor
progress and outcome.
▶ **D. Nursing care plan/implementation**
    1. *Latent* phase of labor: encourage normal ac-
tivities for any woman in this phase of labor.
    2. *Active* phase of labor
      a. Monitor uterine activity and FHR elec-
tronically.
    ☞ **b.** Establish IV access (e.g., heparin lock).
      c. Attend to woman's and family's anxiety, as
well as her physical needs.
▶ **E. Evaluation/outcome criteria**
    1. Woman gives birth vaginally to a healthy in-
fant; or,
    2. If a repeat cesarean birth is necessary,
woman/family are supported and encouraged
to verbalize feelings about outcome.
    3. Whether birth is vaginal or abdominal, woman
verbalizes positive feelings about herself.

Summary

The perinatal nurse requires very special skills of assessment,
analysis, planning, implementation, and evaluation to provide
safe, quality nursing care during the intrapartal phase of the
childbearing process. Nursing care is based on knowledge of
the *biologic foundations of labor, pain management,* nursing
care of the *mother-fetus/newborn and family* during the *four
stages* of labor and birth, *nurse-attended emergency birth, induction of labor, operative obstetrics,* and *VBAC.* From admission to the hospital (or birth center) through the fourth
stage of labor, the nurse considers all members of the childbearing family, encouraging and promoting early family participation and attachment.

💡 Study and Memory Aids

FHT—Assessment of Sound

Funis: hissing sound of blood through umbilical
arteries

Cardinal Movements of Labor

Descent
Flexion
Internal rotation
Extension
Restitution
Expulsion/birth

Length of Labor

Stage	Nullipara	Multipara
First	8–12 hr	6–8 hr
Second	1–2 hr	30 min
Third	5–60 min	5–60 min

Labor: Breathing Techniques— Hyperventilation Treatment

Breathe into paper bag or cupped hands.

Alert: Labor

Avoid Valsalva maneuver when bearing down

Examine Placenta for Blood Vessels in Cord: "AVA"

Artery
Vein
Artery

"APGAR"—Newborn Assessment

Appearance
Pulse
Grimace
Activity
Respiratory effort

APGAR Scores—Points for Status

Good	7–10
Fair	4–6
Resuscitate	0–3

Alert: Newborn
_____

Suction **mouth** first!

Fourth Stage of Labor—Postpartum
Assessments Taken q15 Min × 4
_____

P, R, BP
Fundus
Lochia
Perineum
Bladder
Mother's recovery

"REEDA"—Episiotomy
_____

Redness—color
Edema—swelling
Ecchymosis—bruising
Discharge—drainage
Approximation—suture line

Questions

1. The nurse informs the pregnant woman that, with lightening, the primigravida may experience
   1. Urinary frequency, dyspnea, and leg pains.
   2. Dyspnea, constipation, and dysuria.
   3. Constipation, dysuria, and abdominal pain.
   4. Leg cramps, urinary frequency, and easier breathing.
2. The nurse knows that a woman is experiencing false labor when she reports that
   1. She has been having bloody show.
   2. Lightening occurred 10 days ago.
   3. She is feeling her contractions beginning in the lower back.
   4. She has experienced diarrhea in the past few hours.
3. A woman in labor, sitting in a rocking chair, becomes nauseated and beads of perspiration appear over her upper lip. What is the nurse's first action?
   1. Notify the obstetrician because she is going into shock.
   2. Examine her to see if she is fully dilated.
   3. Quickly assess her blood pressure for hypotension.
   4. Move her to the birth bed for immediate birth.
4. The nurse should discourage the use of the Valsalva maneuver during pregnancy (in exercise programs) or bearing-down during the second stage of labor because it causes:
   1. A marked increase in venous return to the heart.
   2. A transient hypotension followed by hypertension.
   3. An increased cardiac output blood flow to the brain.
   4. A decrease in fetal pH and PO_2 and an increase in fetal PCO_2.
5. A pregnant woman expresses concern because the doctor told her that her "spines are blunt and somewhat widely separated." The nurse's reassurance is based on knowledge that the ischial spines of the female pelvis are important in labor and birth because:
   1. They form the inlet of the true pelvis.
   2. The distance between them is the narrowest diameter of the pelvis.
   3. They are landmarks of the widest measurement of the pelvis.
   4. They bear the weight of the body when sitting.
6. Which statement by a nurse to a laboring woman shows understanding of the physiology of maternal positioning as related to labor progress?
   1. "When you begin pushing, you'll have your legs comfortably supported in stirrups and a pillow under your head."
   2. "Sit in the rocking chair and rest while we do a 15-min monitor strip, then we'll walk again."
   3. "You can raise the head of your bed a little and we'll support your knees with pillows."
   4. "Just stay on your left side here in bed; that will help keep your baby's heart as strong as it is now."
7. While assisting a woman to give birth, the nurse knows not to pull on the umbilical cord, because the placenta is still attached, when which finding is noted?
   1. Cord lengthens.
   2. Silver-colored tissue appears at vaginal opening.
   3. A gush of blood is seen.
   4. Uterus is discoid-shaped.
8. The labor nurse knows that maternal visceral pain is characteristic of which phase/stage of labor and birth?
   1. Latent phase of first stage.
   2. First stage.
   3. Second stage, until presenting part is on perineum.
   4. Second stage, during expulsion of baby.
9. The labor nurse knows that maternal somatic pain is characteristic of which phase/stage of labor and birth?
   1. Latent phase of first stage.
   2. First stage.
   3. Second stage.
   4. Third stage.
10. The labor nurse knows that systemic medication is best given to a nullipara when her cervix is dilated to:
    1. 3–4 cm.
    2. 5–6 cm.
    3. 8 cm.
    4. 10 cm.
11. During a vaginal examination on a woman in active labor, the nurse palpates a triangular-shaped fontanel. These data suggest:
    1. Excessive molding of fetal skull bones.
    2. The biparietal diameter is presenting.
    3. The occipitomental diameter is presenting.
    4. The suboccipitobregmatic diameter is presenting.
12. A multipara is 7–8 cm dilated. She is working, using breathing to keep in control during her frequent and strong contractions. She tells the nurse that she feels lightheaded and her fingers tingle. What is the nurse's first action?
    1. Prepare her for imminent birth.
    2. Change her position.

3. Ask her to breathe into a paper bag.

4. Give her oxygen by face mask.

13. During oxytocin induction of labor, the nurse must be alert for a potential complication of oxytocin, such as:
    1. Pregnancy-induced hypertension (PIH).
    2. Water intoxication.
    3. Amniotic fluid embolism.
    4. Urinary retention.

14. Assessment of a woman in labor reveals an active labor pattern and cervix dilated 4–5 cm. A 30-min whirlpool bath at this time can be expected to:
    1. Slow her labor pattern.
    2. Increase her cervical dilatation an additional 2–3 cm.
    3. Result in a precipitous birth.
    4. Have no effect on labor pattern or cervical dilatation.

15. At which time will a nullipara probably be taken to the birth room?
    1. When the vertex is seen at the introitus with contractions.
    2. When full cervical dilation occurs.
    3. At approximately 8 cm dilation.
    4. When her contractions last 50–60 sec.

16. To plan for and provide nursing care that supports a woman's self-concept and feelings of self-worth, as well as meeting her physical care needs, the nurse knows that the best description of a woman's emotional changes during labor is:
    1. She becomes increasingly dependent and needs to be handled like a child.
    2. She becomes more demanding as labor becomes more painful.
    3. She becomes more irritable as labor progresses and should be left alone.
    4. She becomes more and more introspective as labor progresses.

17. To meet the standard for care, the nurse should know that for a primigravida who is 2 cm dilated:
    1. Her blood pressure will be assessed every half hour.
    2. Vaginal examination will be done every 2 hr.
    3. The FHR will be assessed every 30 min.
    4. Her temperature will be assessed every hour.

18. The physician's examination of a woman in labor reveals the following data: Cervix is 6 cm dilated and 100% effaced; the presenting part is at +1 station. Suddenly, the woman is out of emotional control, crying hysterically. The best way for the coach to assist the Lamaze-prepared woman is to:
    1. Leave the room until she is composed.
    2. Suggest that she take pain medications.
    3. Tell her it will soon be over.
    4. Talk to her, using direct eye contact, and demonstrate breathing for her.

19. The nurse is confident in judging that a pregnant woman's membranes have probably ruptured if the nitrazine (pH) paper turns to the color:
    1. Dark blue.
    2. Yellow.
    3. Olive.
    4. White.

20. What nursing action should be implemented when a woman in labor in the lithotomy position experiences supine hypotension?
    1. Have the woman sit up quickly.
    2. Give oxygen by face mask.
    3. Turn the woman to her side.
    4. Have the woman stand up.

21. Immediately following the administration of epidural anesthesia, the nurse's first assessment should be the:
    1. Fetal heart rate.
    2. Maternal heart rate.
    3. Maternal blood pressure.
    4. Length of contractions.

22. The nurse's plan of care is based on knowledge that the pregnant woman who would likely be given a "trial of labor" for vaginal birth after cesarean (VBAC) is one who previously had a:
    1. Cesarean through a classic uterine incision because of severe fetal distress.
    2. Low transverse cesarean for breech presentation; this pregnancy, fetus is in vertex presentation.
    3. Cesarean for fetopelvic disproportion.
    4. Low transverse cesarean for active vaginal/perineal herpes infection; culture at 39 wk in this pregnancy was positive for herpes.

23. A woman is in the transition phase of labor. The fetal monitor shows a baseline FHR of 140–150 beats/min, with accelerations noted to 160 beats/min with fetal movement and occasionally with contractions. During a particularly long contraction, the nurse notes that the fetal heart slowed to 115 beats/min at the onset of the contraction and returned to baseline by the end of the contraction. What is the priority nursing action?
    1. Turn the woman to her side.
    2. Start an intravenous infusion of D/5/RL.
    3. Start oxygen by face mask.
    4. Document and continue to observe.

24. If the fetal position is right occiput anterior (ROA), the nurse would locate the point of maximum impulse (PMI) of fetal heart tones (FHTs) in the mother's:
    1. Left upper quadrant (LUQ).
    2. Right upper quadrant (RUQ).
    3. Left lower quadrant (LLQ).
    4. Right lower quadrant (RLQ).

25. The nurse applies an ice pack to a new mother's episiotomy area immediately following vaginal childbirth, to reduce discomfort by:
    1. Freezing the area, thus preventing pain.
    2. Minimizing the amount of edema.
    3. Helping her focus on the cold rather than on the pain.
    4. Increasing circulation to the area for more rapid healing.

26. Which nursing assessment is appropriate during the fourth stage of labor (the 2 hr following birth)?
    1. Fundus, every 30 min × 4.
    2. Blood pressure, once at 1 hr, than per hospital protocol.
    3. Temperature, every 15 min × 4.
    4. Bladder, every 15 min × 4, then every 30 min × 2.

27. What is the nurse's first action immediately following rupture of the membranes of a woman in labor?

1. Note the color and consistency of the fluid.
2. Assess the fetal heart rate.
3. Look for presence of the umbilical cord at the vaginal orifice.
4. Keep her in bed until the MD is contacted.

28. The labor nurse determines that the woman is experiencing false labor when:
    1. Contractions occur at regular intervals.
    2. Intensity of contractions is lessened by walking.
    3. Intervals of contractions gradually shorten.
    4. Duration of contractions increase.

29. A woman in the second stage of labor is preparing to push. The nurse must intervene immediately when the coach is heard to say:
    1. "Try to relax completely between contractions."
    2. "Your semirecumbent position is very good."
    3. "Push in short bursts as you feel the urge to bear down."
    4. "Push with your mouth closed and no noise!"

30. A spiral electrode and an intrauterine catheter are inserted for direct monitoring of a woman in labor. The nurse observes the following data on the monitor strip: contractions every 3 min lasting 80 sec, fetal heart rate (FHR) baseline of 135–145 beats/min, fall in FHR to 110 beats/min that begins when contraction begins and ends when contraction ends, variability 6–10 beats/min. Which nursing action is most appropriate?
    1. Implement measures for fetal distress; this is an ominous pattern.
    2. Continue monitoring per standard; this is a benign pattern.
    3. Troubleshoot the monitor; this pattern contains artifact.
    4. Notify the physician; this situation requires fetal scalp pH assessment.

31. As part of the admission procedure, the nurse performs and evaluates findings from Leopold's maneuvers as a basis for individualizing the plan of care. Leopold's maneuvers reveal the breech in the fundus and nodulations noted in the mother's left flank. This fetus is:
    1. Left sacrum posterior (LSP).
    2. Right sacrum anterior (RSA).
    3. Left occiput posterior (LOP).
    4. Right occiput anterior (ROA).

Answers/Rationale

1. **(4)** Leg cramps, urinary frequency, and easier breathing often occur with lightening. Lightening refers to the sensation of decreased abdominal distention produced by uterine descent into the pelvic cavity, as the fetal presenting part settles into the pelvis; it occurs about 2 wk before the onset of labor in nulliparas. Lightening does *not* cause *dyspnea* (**1** and **2**) or *dysuria* (**2** and **3**), both of which would require further assessment and possible intervention (dysuria is a symptom of urinary tract infection). Lightening also does *not* result in *abdominal pain* (**3**); abdominal pain may be the result of abruptio placentae or other complications. **IMP, 5, HPM**

2. **(4)** Although diarrhea is often a prodromal symptom of labor, it may to due to a variety of other causes. The signs/symptoms in options **1, 2,** and **3** *are* commonly experienced by women beginning *true* labor. **AN, 5, HPM**

3. **(2)** The signs and symptoms described suggest that she is fully dilated (10 cm); the nurse should examine her to confirm this. These are signs/symptoms of full dilatation, not *shock* (**1**) or *hypotension* (**3**). They signify the end of the first stage and *only* the beginning of the second stage; birth (**4**) may still be *some time away*. NOTE: Other symptoms/signs include belching and shaking of the legs. **IMP, 5, HPM**

4. **(4)** The Valsalva maneuver (closed glottis) does result in a decrease in fetal pH and PO_2, and an increase in fetal PCO_2. There is a marked *decrease,* not increase (**1**), in venous return to the heart. There is a transient *hypertension*, followed by a *decrease* in maternal blood pressure, rather than the reverse (**2**). There is a decrease in cardiac output blood flow to the brain, *not an increase* (**3**), that may cause orthostatic hypotension (aortocaval syndrome). **PL, 6, HPM**

5. **(2)** The ischial spines are the landmarks for *station* of the presenting part; the distance between them is the narrowest diameter of the pelvis. (The description given is that of an adequate, gynecoid pelvis.) The *brim* forms the inlet of the true pelvis (**1**); linea terminalis, sacral promontory, and symphysis pubis form the brim. The distance between the ischial spines is the narrowest, *not* the widest (**3**), measurement of the pelvis. The body's weight is borne by the ischial *tuberosities* when the person is sitting (**4**). **IMP, 5, HPM**

6. **(2)** The upright position (sitting in a rocking chair, walking) is the position of preference to let gravity assist in the cervical effacement and dilatation equally around the cervix (lying in bed leads to complete effacement/dilatation "except for an anterior lip"). *Squatting* is the most efficient position for pushing with the fetus in vertex position (but not posterior); lying down (**1**) does not put the woman in best anatomic/physiologic position for pushing. Knees are *never* supported with pillows while in bed (**3**); if lying down, the woman should be side lying. Side lying (**4**) does enhance renal and uteroplacental perfusion, but, because it does not allow gravity to work for the woman in labor, it is not the *best* choice. **EV, 3, HPM**

7. **(4)** Before the placenta separates, the uterus is discoid-shaped; after separation, the uterus is globular in shape. The other options are the signs that the placenta

Key to Codes

Nursing process: AS, assessment; **AN,** analysis; **PL,** planning; **IMP,** implementation; **EV,** evaluation. (See Appendix I for explanation of nursing process steps.)

Category of human function: 1, protective; **2,** sensory-perceptual; **3,** comfort, rest, activity, and mobility; **4,** nutrition; **5,** growth and development; **6,** fluid-gas transport; **7,** psychosocial-cultural; **8,** elimination. (See Appendix K for explanation.)

Client need: SECE, safe, effective care environment; **PhI,** physiologic integrity; **PsI,** psychosocial integrity; **HPM,** health promotion/maintenance. (See Appendix L for explanation.)

has separated: The cord lengthens (1), amniotic membranes are seen at the vaginal introitus (2), and a gush of blood is seen (3). **EV, 5, HPM**

8. (2)   During the first stage of labor, pain is visceral, caused by dilatation of the cervix and uterine ischemia. This pain is referred to the lower abdominal wall, the area over the lumbar region, and the sacrum. Visceral pain characterizes the *entire* first stage, not just the latent phase (1). *Somatic* pain characterizes the second stage (3 and 4). **AN, 3, HPM**

9. (3)   Pain of somatic origin characterizes the second stage. It is caused by hypoxia of the uterus, distention of the vagina and perineum, and pressure on adjacent tissues. Pain may be felt in the lower back or suprapubic area, or referred to the flank and thighs. Throughout the first stage (1 and 2), and in the third stage (4), pain is *visceral* in origin. **AN, 3, HPM**

10. (2)   Ideally, there is less effect on the labor of the nullipara if systemic medication is given when she is in active labor, about 5–6 cm. It is *too early* to give systemic medication to a nullipara at cervical dilatation of 3–4 cm (1). It is *unnecessary to wait* until dilatation is 8 cm (3) before administering pain medication to the nullipara, and 10 cm dilatation (4) is *too late* to give systemic medication to a nullipara. **EV, 1, PhI**

11. (4)   When the suboccipitobregmatic diameter is presenting, the posterior triangular-shaped fontanel is presenting; the fetus is in an attitude of general flexion and is presenting the smallest head diameter for birth. With excessive molding (1), it may be difficult to feel the fontanel. (Excessive molding refers to the overlapping of cranial bones or shaping of the fetal head to accommodate and conform to the bony and soft parts of the mother's birth canal during labor.) If the fetus was presenting with the biparietal diameter (2), the nurse would have felt the sagittal suture. If the fetus was presenting with the largest diameter of the fetal head, the occipitomental diameter (3), the nurse would have felt the fetal brow or the anterior, diamond-shaped fontanel. **AN, 5, HPM**

12. (3)   Since these are the symptoms of hyperventilation, the nurse should ask her to breathe into a paper bag. These symptoms are not those of imminent birth (1). For hyperventilation, the first action is to ask her to breathe into a paper bag, *not* to change the position (2). She needs to rebreathe her carbon dioxide and does *not need oxygen* (4) at this time. **IMP, 6, PhI**

13. (2)   Water intoxication is a complication associated with oxytocin induction/augmentation of labor. Neither PIH (1) nor urinary retention (4) is associated with induction. Amniotic fluid embolism (3) is associated with rupture of membranes, *not* with oxytocin induction. **EV, 6, PhI**

14. (2)   A 30-min whirlpool bath is expected to increase this woman's cervical dilatation an additional 2–3 cm. Relief from discomfort and general body relaxation reduce the woman's anxiety, which decreases adrenaline production. An increase in oxytocin and endorphins occurs. Labor is facilitated, *not* slowed (1), unless she is in the latent phase of the first stage. The woman's labor is monitored continuously; if birth is imminent (3), she

is removed from the bath. The whirlpool bath has a *positive* effect on the labor pattern and cervical dilatation (4). **IMP, 3, HPM**

15. (1)   Is correct: The woman will probably be taken to the birth room when the vertex is seen at the introitus with contractions; at this point, there is usually still time to move a nullipara. Options 2, 3, and 4 are incorrect since birth may still be hours away. **IMP, 5, HPM**

16. (4)   She turns inward into herself. Only conversation directed at her should be initiated now; she perceives all she hears as pertaining to her. She does become more dependent (1), but she is an *adult* and should be treated as such. No woman is "demanding" in labor (2)—there is only the woman whose needs have not been met. She may become more irritable (3), but should *never be left alone.* To leave her alone would be abandonment (legally speaking). **PL, 7, HPM**

17. (3)   During the early first stage of labor (2 cm dilatation), in most cases, the FHR is assessed every 30 min, if labor is progressing to the active phase and when membranes rupture. Blood pressure (1) is assessed every *hour.* Vaginal examination (2) is performed *as necessary* to identify progress of labor. Temperature (4) is usually assessed every *4 hr;* it may be assessed every 2 hr if membranes are ruptured. **IMP, 5, HPM**

18. (4)   The woman needs to know that someone is in control and requires firm, direct coaching with demonstration of breathing techniques. Leaving the room (1) is abandonment, and can be seen by the woman as punishment for her "inappropriate" behavior. Suggesting pain medication (2) may be interpreted by the woman that the coach has no confidence in her; it also does not acknowledge the woman's perception of discomfort. Saying that "it will soon be over" (3) may be false reassurance; it is always difficult to predict the time of birth ("soon" can be interpreted as 5 min!). This response also fails to acknowledge the woman's perception of discomfort. **IMP, 7, PsI**

19. (1)   The litmus (pH) paper turns dark blue when exposed to an alkaline fluid such as amniotic fluid. The paper does *not* turn yellow (2), olive (3), or white (4) in the presence of amniotic fluid. **EV, 5, HPM**

20. (3)   The side-lying position relieves supine hypotension by reducing compression of the vena cava and aorta. The woman may faint if she rises quickly (1 and 4). Oxygen (2) is not needed, and would be of little value as long as the major vessels remain compressed. **IMP, 3, PhI**

21. (3)   A side effect of epidural anesthesia is maternal hypotension, and therefore the nurse should check the BP *immediately* after administration of the drug. FHR deceleration (1) would be *caused* by a drop in maternal BP, putting the fetus at risk for hypoxia; therefore, the maternal BP is the *priority.* The maternal heart rate (2) is *not* affected. Although contraction strength and frequency (4) *may* decrease, the effect of maternal BP on *fetal oxygenation* is the *main concern.* **AS, 6, PhI**

22. (2)   The reason for the previous cesarean in this case was breech presentation, which is not present now. The women described in the other options would not be good candidates for VBAC. In **1**, the vertical incision

through the uterus, and subsequent scar, is considered to weaken the uterus and compromise its ability to withstand stretching and contracting. In **3**, original cause for the previous cesarean (fetopelvic disproportion) may remain. In **4**, the infant may acquire herpes during passage through an infected birth canal. **PL, 5, HPM**

23. **(4)** The situation describes an *early deceleration,* one that "mirrors" the contraction by falling as the contraction increases and returning to the baseline as the contraction decreases. Early decelerations are caused by the baby's vagal response to fetal head compression. These decelerations are thought to be *benign* with good fetal outcome and show little or no response to interventions geared to increase fetal oxygen. The nurse should simply document these baseline changes and continue to observe the fetal heart pattern. The measures in options **1, 2,** and **3** are taken in times of *fetal distress* and are therefore *inappropriate* and *ineffective* in this case. **IMP, 5, HPM**

24. **(4)** The FHR is best heard through the fetus' back; with vertex presentation and with the fetal occiput to the mother's right, the fetal back is also on the mother's right side and in the lower quadrant. The fetus would have to be left sacrum anterior (LSA) for the FHR to be in the mother's LUQ **(1)**. The fetus would have to be right sacrum anterior (RSA) for the FHR to be in the mother's RUQ **(2)**. The fetus would have to be left occiput anterior (LOA) for the FHR to be in the mother's LLQ **(3)**. **AS, 5, HPM**

25. **(2)** Minimizing the amount of edema at this time (*immediately* after birth) will reduce discomfort later. Freezing **(1)** *destroys* tissues. The purpose of applying cold is *not to distract* **(3)**; distraction does little to decrease discomfort. Ice packs (covered) *decrease, not in-crease* **(4)**, circulation to the area. **PL, 1, SECE**

26. **(4)** During the first hour, every 15 min × 4, the nurse assesses BP, heart rate, respiration, lochia, fundal tone and position, *bladder filling,* perineum, recovery from medications, and reaction to birth experience; temperature is assessed at 1 hr. If complications occur, the frequency and number of assessments are adjusted, prn. The fundus **(1)** and BP **(2)** are checked every *15 min × 4;* then every 30 min × 2; then per hospital protocol if the assessments reveal no complications. The temperature **(3)** is checked *once* at the end of the

first hour and then per hospital protocol if the values remain within normal limits. **AS, 5, HPM**

27. **(2)** This assessment is the only one that could diagnose prolapse of the umbilical cord that may not be visible in the vagina or at the vaginal orifice or palpable with vaginal examination. If the cord is prolapsed out of the vagina, keep it warm and moist with continuous applications of warm, sterile saline compresses. Option **1** is incorrect because the fluid needs to be assessed, but that is done *following* assessment of the FHR. Option **3** is incorrect because the FHR is the *only* way to diagnose whether the fetus is being well oxygenated; a prolapsed cord may not be visible. Option **4** is incorrect because this may be indicated, but is not the *priority* action. **IMP, 5, PhI**

28. **(2)** With false labor, the intensity of contractions lessens with walking. The other options all describe the contractions of *true* labor: intervals are regular **(1)** and shorten gradually **(3)**, and duration increases **(4)**. **AN, 5, HPM**

29. **(4)** The nurse needs to intervene immediately when a coach is heard to say, "Push with your mouth closed and no noise!" because this pushing method encourages the Valsalva maneuver with cardiovascular risks and other sequelae. Encouraging relaxation between contractions **(1)** and semi-Fowler's (or side-lying) position **(2)** *is appropriate* at this time. Short bursts of pushing when the woman feels the urge to push **(3)** are effective for the second stage of labor. **EV, 5, HPM**

30. **(2)** The fetal monitor readings are consistent with early (head compression) deceleration; continue to monitor per standard. Options **1, 3,** and **4** are incorrect because this is *not* an ominous pattern. **EV, 5, PhI**

31. **(4)** With the breech in the fundus, the fetus must be vertex; nodulations (elbows, hands, knees, feet) on the mother's left mean that the fetal back must be in the mother's right flank. LSP **(1)** means that the fetus is breech (the head is in the fundus) and the nodulations would be felt over the entire maternal abdomen since the fetal back would be to the mother's back. RSA **(2)** means that the fetus is breech and the nodulations would not be easily felt; the fetal back would be in the anterior of the mother's abdomen. LOP **(3)** means that the vertex is presenting but the nodulations would be easily felt all over the maternal abdomen; the fetal back would be to the maternal back. **EV, 5, HPM**

Complications During the Intrapartal Period

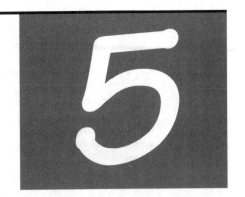

Chapter Outline

🔑 KEY POINTS

- Dystocia results from differences in the normal relationships among the *six* essential factors of labor.
- Uterine contractility is increased by oxytocin and prostaglandin, and decreased by tocolytic agents.
- *Medical emergencies* can occur secondary to dystocia: disseminated intravascular coagulopathy (DIC), adult respiratory distress syndrome (ARDS), thrombophlebitis, cardiac decompensation.
- *Management* of preterm labor includes prenatal education of signs and symptoms, home monitoring and therapy, tocolysis, and, in the event that tocolysis is not possible, stimulation of fetal lung maturity.

Key Words

Adult respiratory distress syndrome (ARDS)
Amniotic fluid (pulmonary) embolus
Dystocia
Prolapsed umbilical cord
Tocolysis
Uterine rupture

General Aspects

I. **Pathophysiology**—interference with normal processes and patterns of labor/birth result in maternal and/or fetal jeopardy (e.g., *preterm* labor, *dysfunctional* labor patterns; *prolonged* [>24 hr] labor; *hemorrhage: uterine rupture/inversion, amniotic fluid embolus*).

II. **Etiology**

A. *Preterm labor*—unknown.

B. *Dysfunctional labor* (**dystocia:** see p. 127)

1. Physiologic response to anxiety/fear/pain—results in release of catecholamines, increasing physical/psychological stress → myometrial dysfunction; painful and ineffectual labor.

2. *Iatrogenic factors:* premature or excessive analgesia, particularly during latent phase.

3. *Maternal factors*

a. Pelvic contractures.

b. Uterine tumors (e.g., myomas, carcinoma).

c. Congenital uterine anomalies (e.g., bicornate uterus).

d. Pathologic contraction ring (*Bandl's* ring).

e. Rigid cervix, cervical stenosis/stricture.

f. Hypertonic/hypotonic contractions.

g. Prolonged rupture of membranes. **NOTE:** Intrauterine infection may have caused rupture of membranes, or may follow rupture.

123

   h. Prolonged first or second stage.
   i. Medical conditions: diabetes, hypertension.
  4. *Fetal factors*
      a. Macrosomia (large for gestational age [LGA]).
      b. Malposition/malpresentation.
      c. Congenital anomaly (e.g., hydrocephalus, anencephaly).
      d. Multi-fetal gestation (e.g., interlocking twins).
      e. Prolapsed cord.
      f. Postterm.
  5. *Placental factors*
      a. Placenta previa.
      b. Inadequate placental function with contractions.
      c. Abruptio placentae.
      d. Placenta accreta.
  6. Physical restrictions: when confined to bed, *flat position,* etc.

III. Assessment
   A. Prenatal history, physical examination, laboratory and other diagnostic test results, e.g., ultrasound, nonstress test (NST).
   B. Emotional status.
   ☞ **C.** Vital signs, fetal heart rate (FHR).
   D. Labor assessment
      1. *Preadmission events:* contractions, membranes, etc.
      2. *Physical examination:* lung status, edema, rashes, respiratory conditions, etc.
      ☞ **3.** *Contraction pattern:* frequency, duration, intensity.
      ☞ **4.** *Leopold's* maneuvers (abdominal palpation): presentation, position (identification of presenting part, the fetal lie, and attitude), degree of descent into the pelvis, and location of point of maximal impulse (PMI) of FHR in relation to maternal abdomen.
      5. *Vaginal examination:* presentation, position, station; cervical effacement, dilatation; status of membranes; fullness of rectum.
   E. Collection of specimens: urine, blood; assessment of amniotic fluid from vaginal vault (color, character, amount).
   F. Assessment for **risk factors:** warning signs
      1. *Contractions:* intrauterine pressure 75 mm Hg, or greater (by intrauterine pressure catheter [IUPC]), lasting 90 sec or longer, occurring at intervals of less than 2 min.
      2. *FHR:* bradycardia, tachycardia, or persistent decreased variability; irregular; absence of.
      3. *Vaginal discharge:* meconium stained or bloody; foul smelling; persistent bright or dark red.
      4. *Prolapsed umbilical cord.*
      5. Arrest in progress of *cervical dilatation/effacement* and/or descent of the fetus (see Length of Labor, Chapter 4, p. 115).
      6. *Maternal temperature* 100.4°F (38°C) or greater.

IV. Analysis/nursing diagnosis
   A. *Anxiety/fear* for self and infant related to implications of prolonged or complicated labor/birth.
   B. *Pain* related to hypertonic contractions/dysfunctional labor.
   C. *Ineffective individual coping* related to physical/ psychological stress of complicated labor/birth, lowered pain threshold secondary to fatigue.
   D. *High risk for injury* related to prolonged rupture of membranes, infection.
   E. *Fluid volume deficit* related to excessive blood loss secondary to placenta previa, abruptio placentae, Couvelaire uterus, disseminated intravascular coagulopathy (DIC).

V. Nursing care plan/implementation
   A. Goal: *minimize physical/psychological stress during labor/birth.* Assist woman in coping effectively
      1. Reinforce relaxation techniques.
      2. Support couple's effective coping techniques/ mechanisms.
      3. Utilize warm-water immersion/hydrotherapy, prn.
      4. Meet woman's comfort needs.
   B. Goal: *emotional support*
      1. Encourage verbalization of anxiety/fear/concerns.
      2. Explain all procedures—to minimize anxiety/ fear, encourage cooperation/participation in care.
      3. Provide quiet environment conducive to rest.
   ☞ **C.** Goal: *continuous monitoring of maternal-fetal status and progress through labor*—to identify early signs of dysfunctional labor, fetal distress; facilitate prompt, effective treatment of emerging complications.
   D. Goal: *minimize effects of complicated labor on mother, fetus*
      1. *Position* change: lateral Sims'—to reduce compression of inferior vena cava and descending aorta.
      ☞ **2.** Oxygen per mask, as indicated.
      3. Institute interventions appropriate to emerging problems (see specific disorder).

VI. Evaluation/outcome criteria
   A. Woman has successful birth of viable infant.
   B. Maternal/infant status stable, satisfactory.

Disorders Affecting Protective Functions: *Preterm Labor*

Preterm labor occurs after 20 wk gestation and before beginning of week 38.

   I. Pathophysiology—physiologic events of labor (i.e., contractions, spontaneous rupture of membranes, cervical effacement/dilatation) occur before completion of normal, term gestation.

II. Etiology—unknown. Theory: may be due to fetal factors released when placental function begins to diminish and intrauterine environment is hostile to continuing fetal well-being.

III. *Coexisting disorders*

   A. Infections that may cause premature rupture of membranes (PROM).

   B. PROM of unknown etiology.

   C. Hypertension (preeclampsia/eclampsia).

   D. Uterine overdistention

      1. Hydramnios.

      2. Large baby.

      3. Multi-fetal gestation.

   E. Maternal diabetes, renal or cardiovascular disorder.

   F. Severe maternal illness (e.g., pneumonia, acute pyelonephritis, urinary tract infection [UTI]).

   G. Abnormal placentation

      1. Placenta previa.

      2. Abruptio placentae.

   H. Iatrogenic: miscalculated estimated date of birth (EDB) for repeat cesarean birth.

   I. Fetal death.

   J. Incompetent cervical os (small percentage).

   K. Uterine anomalies (rare)

      1. Intrauterine septum.

      2. Bicornate uterus.

   L. Uterine fibroids.

IV. *Prevention*

   A. *Primary*—close obstetric supervision; education in warning signs/symptoms of preterm labor.

> **1.** Dull lower backache that radiates like a wave to the front of the abdomen (characteristic of a true labor contraction).
>
> **2.** Contractions every 10 min for 2 hr even after position changes and drinking some glasses of water; low back pain and light bloody discharge (*"bloody show"*).
>
> **3.** Constant menstrual-like cramping low in the abdomen.
>
> **4.** Pelvic pressure extending to the back and thighs.

   B. *Secondary*—prompt, effective treatment of associated disorders (see *III* above).

   C. *Tertiary*—suppression of preterm labor.

      1. Bedrest.

      2. *Position:* side lying—to promote placental perfusion.

      3. Hydration.

      4. Pharmacologic (may require "informed consent"; follow hospital protocol). Beta-adrenergic agents (*take ECG first*) to reduce sensitivity of uterine myometrium to oxytocic and prostaglandin stimulation; increase blood flow to uterus.

      5. May be maintained at home with adequate follow-up and health teaching.

V. Contraindications for suppression—labor is *not* suppressed in presence of:

   A. Placenta previa or abruptio placentae.

   B. Chorioamnionitis.

   C. Erythroblastosis fetalis.

   D. Severe preeclampsia.

   E. Severe diabetes (e.g., "brittle").

   F. Increasing placental insufficiency.

   G. Cervical dilatation of 4 cm or more.

   H. Ruptured membranes (depends on cause and if sepsis).

VI. Assessment

   A. Maternal vital signs. Response to medication:

      1. Hypotension.

      2. Tachycardia, arrhythmia.

      3. Dyspnea, chest pain.

      4. Nausea and vomiting.

   B. Signs of infection:

      1. Increased temperature.

      2. Tachycardia.

      3. Diaphoresis.

      4. Malaise.

      5. Increased baseline fetal heart rate.

   C. Contractions: frequency, duration, strength.

   D. Emotional status—signs of denial, guilt, anxiety, exhaustion.

   E. Signs of continuing and progressing labor. NOTE: vaginal examination *only* if indicated by other signs of continuing labor progress.

      1. Effacement.

      2. Dilatation.

      3. Station.

   F. Status of membranes.

   G. Fetal heart rate, activity (continuous monitoring).

VII. Analysis/nursing diagnosis

   A. *Anxiety/fear* related to possible outcome.

   B. *Self-esteem disturbance* related to feelings of guilt, failure.

   C. *Impaired physical mobility* related to imposed bedrest.

   D. *Knowledge deficit* related to medication side effects.

   E. *Ineffective individual coping* related to possible outcome.

   F. *Impaired gas exchange* related to side effects of medication (circulatory overload; pulmonary edema).

   G. *Diversional activity deficit* related to imposed bedrest, decreased environmental stimuli.

   H. *Altered urinary elimination* related to bedrest.

   I. *Constipation* related to bedrest.

VIII. Nursing care plan/implementation

   A. Goal: *tocolysis* (inhibition) of uterine activity.

      a. Administer tocolytic medications as ordered—*ritodrine (Yutopar), terbutaline,* or *magnesium sulfate.*

   B. Goal: *safeguard status*

      1. Continuous maternal-fetal monitoring.

      2. Maternal *position:* side lying to increase placental perfusion, prevent supine hypotension.

      3. I&O—to identify early signs of possible circulatory overload.

> **4.** Report **warning signs/symptoms** promptly to physician
>
>   **a.** Maternal pulse of 110 or more.
>
>   **b.** Diastolic pressure of 60 mm Hg or less.

c. Respirations of 25 or more; crackles (rales).
d. Complaint of shortness of breath and chest tightness.°
e. Contractions: increasing frequency, strength, or duration or cessation of contractions.
f. Intermittent back and thigh pain.
g. Rupture of membranes.
h. Vaginal bleeding.
i. Fetal distress, e.g., tachycardia, 180 beats/min or more.
j. Laboratory results: hyperglycemia, hyperkalemia.

5. Give *antidote*, per order: *propranolol,* 1 mg, for beta-mimetic drugs (e.g., *ritodrine, terbutaline*); toxicity, or *calcium gluconate* or *calcium chloride,* 1 g for IV injection given over 3-min period for magnesium sulfate toxicity.

6. *Home care:* preterm labor
   a. Teaching about medications: dosage ordered, etc.
   b. Teaching about *signs/symptoms of toxicity* to report stat: severe dizziness, drowsiness, headache, nervousness, restlessness; severe muscle cramps and weakness; continuous nausea and vomiting; dyspnea; pulmonary edema, respirations of 25/min or more; continuous palpitations, chest pain.
   c. Teaching about side-lying *position* for resting.
   d. Teach/practice stress reduction/relaxation techniques.
   e. Make appropriate referrals, if assistance is needed in the home, e.g., child care.

C. Goal: *comfort measures*
   1. Basic hygienic care—bath, mouth care, cold washcloth to face, perineal care.
   2. Backrub, linen change—to promote relaxation.

D. Goal: *emotional support*
   1. Encourage verbalization of guilt feelings, anxiety, fear, concerns; provide factual information.
   2. Support positive self-concept.
   3. Keep informed of progress.

E. Goal: *provide quiet diversion.* Television, reading materials, handcrafts.

F. Goal: *health teaching*
   1. Explain, discuss proposed management to suppress preterm labor.
   2. Describe, discuss side effects of medication.
   3. Explain rationale for bedrest, position.

If Labor Continues to Progress

A. Goal: *facilitate infant survival*

°Alert: If a steroid, such as beta-*methasone (Celestone, Solup),* is used (to stimulate fetal lung maturity) in conjunction with beta-mimetic drugs (e.g., *ritodrine, terbutaline*), **risk for cardiac decompensation is greatly increased.** (Maternal HR: ≥140 beats/min; continuous palpitations, chest pain.)

1. Administer *betamethasone,* as ordered, 24 hr before birth—to increase/stimulate production of pulmonary surfactant.
2. Notify perinatal team—to increase chances for fetal survival, ensure prompt, expert management of neonate and provide information and support to parents.
3. Monitor progress of labor to identify signs of impending birth. NOTE: May give birth before complete (10 cm) dilatation.
4. Consider transfer to high-risk facility.
5. Prepare for birth or cesarean birth if infant less than 34–36 wk gestation.

B. Goal: *emotional support*
   1. Do *not* leave woman (or couple) alone.
   2. Encourage verbalization of anxiety, fear, concern.
   3. Explain all procedures.

C. Goal: *comfort measures.* NOTE: Analgesics may be *contraindicated*—to prevent depression of fetus/neonate.

D. Goal: *support effective coping techniques.* Encourage/support Lamaze (or other) techniques—coach, as necessary; discourage hyperventilation.

E. Goal: *health teaching*—for *preterm birth*
   1. Discuss need for episiotomy, possibility of outlet forceps-assisted birth—to reduce stress on fetal head, *or*
   2. Prepare for cesarean birth—to reduce possibility of fetal intraventricular hemorrhage.
   3. Rationale for avoiding use of medications to reduce contraction pain.

Immediate Care of Neonate

A. Goal: *safeguard status*
   1. Stabilize environmental temperature—to prevent chilling (isolette or other controlled-temperature bed).
   2. Suction, oxygen, as needed; may need intubation.
   3. Parenteral fluids, as ordered—to support normal acid-base balance, pH; administer antibiotics, as necessary.
   4. Arrange transport to high-risk facility, as necessary.

B. Goal: *continuous monitoring of status*
   1. Electronic monitors—to observe respiratory and cardiac functions.
   2. Blood samples—to monitor blood gases, pH, hypoglycemia.

Postpartum Care

A. Goal: *emotional support*
   1. Facilitate attachment.
   2. If couple, foster sense of mutual experience and closeness.
   3. Help her/them maintain a positive self-image.
   4. Encourage touching of infant before transport to nursery or high-risk facility; father/partner

may accompany infant and report back to
mother.
5. Encourage early contact—to facilitate
mother's need to ventilate her feelings.
6. Assist parent(s) with grieving process if necessary.
7. Refer to support group if necessary.
⋈ **IX. Evaluation/outcome criteria:** The woman:
A. Verbalizes understanding of medical/nursing recommendations and treatments.
B. Complies with medical/nursing regimen.
C. Experiences no discomfort from side effects of
therapy.
D. Experiences successful outcome—labor inhibited.
E. Carries pregnancy to successful termination.
F. If preterm birth occurs, copes effectively with outcome (physiologically compromised neonate, neo-
natal demise).

Grief and Childbearing Experience

The loss of a pregnancy or a newborn, or the birth of a physiologically compromised child (premature, congenital disorder), is a crisis situation. The unexpected outcome can cause
the parent(s) to suffer a sense of loss of self-esteem, self-
concept, positive body image, feelings of worth (see Table 3.4,
p. 72).

⋈ **I. Assessment**
A. Response to loss of the "fantasy child"/real child
1. *Behavioral*—anger, hostility, depression, dis-
interest in activities of daily living, withdrawal.
2. *Biophysical*—somatic complaints (stomach
pain, malaise, anorexia, nausea).
3. *Cognitive*—feelings of guilt.
B. Knowledge/understanding/perception of situation.
C. Coping abilities, mechanisms.
D. Support system.
⋈ **II. Analysis/nursing diagnosis**
A. *Ineffective family coping: compromised* related to
psychological stress associated with fear for infant,
guilt feelings, impact on self-image.
B. *Ineffective individual coping* related to anxiety,
stress.
C. *Ineffective family coping: disabling* related to disturbance in intrafamily relations secondary to individual coping deficits, recriminations.
D. *Altered parenting* related to lack of effective bonding secondary to emotional separation from infant,
feelings of guilt.
E. *Dysfunctional grieving* related to guilt feelings,
impact of loss on self-concept.
F. *Disturbance in body image, self-esteem, role performance* related to perceived failure to complete
gestational task and produce perfect, healthy infant; associated with sleep deprivation.
G. *Social isolation* related to severe coping deficit,
dysfunctional grieving, disturbance in self-esteem.
⋈ **III. Nursing care plan/implementation**

A. Goal: *emotional support*
1. Provide privacy; encourage open expression/
verbalization of feelings, fears, concerns, perceptions.
2. Crisis intervention techniques.
B. Goal: *facilitate bonding, effective coping, and/or
anticipatory grieving processes*
1. Encourage contact and participation in care of
premature or compromised infant.
2. Keep informed of infant's status.
3. Provide realistic data.
C. Goal: *health teaching*
1. Clarify misperceptions, as appropriate.
☞ 2. Discuss, demonstrate infant care techniques
(e.g., feeding infant who has cleft lip and/or
palate).
3. Refer to appropriate community resources.
⋈ **IV. Evaluation/outcome criteria:** The parent:
A. Verbalizes recognition and acceptance of diagnosis.
B. Verbalizes understanding of relevant information
regarding treatment, prognosis.
C. Makes informed decision regarding infant care.
D. Demonstrates comfort and increasing participation
in care of neonate.
E. Shows evidence of bonding (eye contact, cuddles,
calls infant by name).

Disorders Affecting Comfort, Rest, Mobility: *Dystocia*

I. *Definition:* difficult labor, birth.
II. *Etiology:* the six "Ps"
A. Position (*maternal*).
B. Psychological response (maternal).
C. Placenta—previa, abruptio (see Chapter 3, p. 78).
D. **Power:** forces of labor (uterine contractions, use
of abdominal muscles)
1. Premature analgesia/anesthesia.
2. Uterine overdistention (multifetal pregnancy,
fetal macrosomia).
3. Uterine myomas.
E. **Passageway:** resistance of cervix, pelvic structures
1. Rigid cervix.
2. Distended bladder.
3. Distended rectum.
4. Dimensions of the bony pelvis: pelvic contractures.
F. **Passenger:** accommodation of the presenting part
to pelvic diameters
1. Fetal malposition/malpresentation
a. Transverse lie.
b. Face, brow presentation.
c. Breech presentation.
d. Cephalopelvic disproportion (CPD) or feto-
pelvic disproportion (FPD).
2. Fetal anomalies

a. Hydrocephalus.
b. Conjoined ("Siamese") twins.
c. Myelomeningocele.
3. Fetal size

⚡ **III. Hazards**
  A. *Maternal*
    1. Fatigue, exhaustion, dehydration—due to prolonged labor.
    2. Lowered pain threshold, loss of control—due to prolonged labor, continued uterine contractions, anxiety, fatigue, lack of sleep.
    3. Intrauterine infection—due to prolonged rupture of membranes and frequent vaginal examinations.
    4. Uterine rupture—due to obstructed labor.
    5. Cervical, vaginal, perineal lacerations—due to obstetric interventions.
    6. Postpartum hemorrhage—due to uterine atony and/or trauma.
  B. *Fetal:*
    1. Hypoxia, anoxia, demise—due to decreased oxygen concentration in cord blood.
    2. Intracranial hemorrhage—due to changing intracranial pressure.

IV. Hypertonic dysfunction
  A. **Pathophysiology**—increased resting tone of uterine myometrium; diminished refractory period; prolonged latent phase
    1. *Nullipara*—more than 20 hr.
    2. *Multipara*—more than 14 hr.
  B. **Etiology**—unknown. Theory—ectopic initiation of incoordinate uterine contractions.
  ⬦ C. **Assessment**
    1. Onset—early labor (latent phase).
    2. Contractions
      a. Continuous fundal tension, incomplete relaxation.
      b. Painful.
      c. Ineffectual—no effacement or dilatation.
    3. Signs of fetal distress
      a. Meconium-stained amniotic fluid.
      ☞ b. Fetal heart rate irregularities.
    4. Maternal vital signs.
    5. Emotional status.
    ⟿ 6. *Medical* evaluation: vaginal examination, X-ray pelvimetry, ultrasonography—to rule out CPD.
  ⬦ D. **Analysis/nursing diagnosis**
    1. *Pain* related to hypertonic contractions, incomplete uterine relaxation.
    2. *Anxiety/fear* for self and infant related to strong, painful contractions without evidence of progress.
    3. *Ineffective individual coping* related to fatigue, exhaustion, anxiety, tension, fear.
    4. *Impaired gas exchange (fetal)* related to incomplete relaxation of uterus.
    5. *Sleep pattern disturbance* related to prolonged ineffectual labor.
  ⬦ E. **Nursing care plan/implementation**
    1. Medical management

⬬ a. Short-acting barbiturates (see Table 4.3)—to encourage rest, relaxation.
☞ b. Intravenous fluids—to restore/maintain hydration and fluid-electrolyte balance.
  c. If CPD, cesarean birth.
2. *Nursing management*
  a. Goal: *emotional support*—assist coping with fear, pain, discouragement
    (1) Encourage verbalization of anxiety, fear, concerns.
    (2) Explain all procedures.
    (3) Reassure. Keep couple informed of progress.
  b. Goal: *comfort measures*
    (1) *Position:* Side lying—to promote relaxation and placental perfusion.
    (2) Bath, backrub, linen change, clean environment.
    (3) Environment: quiet, darkened room—to minimize stimuli and encourage relaxation, warmth.
    ⟿ (4) Encourage voiding—to relieve bladder distention; to test urine for *ketones.*
  ☞ c. Goal: *prevent infection.* Strict aseptic technique.
  d. Goal: *prepare for cesarean birth* if necessary.
⬦ F. **Evaluation/outcome criteria:** The woman:
  1. Relaxes, sleeps, establishes normal labor pattern.
  2. Demonstrates no signs of fetal distress.
  3. Successfully completes uneventful labor.

V. Hypotonic dysfunction during labor
  A. **Pathophysiology**—after normal labor at onset, contractions diminish in frequency, duration, and strength; lowered uterine resting tone; cervical effacement and dilatation slows/ceases.
  B. **Etiology**
  ⬬ 1. Premature or excessive analgesia/anesthesia (caudal or epidural block).
    2. CPD.
    3. Overdistention (hydramnios, fetal macrosomia, multifetal pregnancy).
    4. Fetal malposition/malpresentation.
    5. Maternal fear/anxiety.
  ⬦ C. **Assessment**
    1. Onset—may occur in latent phase; most common during active phase.
    2. Contractions: normal previously, demonstrate:
      a. Decreased frequency.
      b. Shorter duration.
      c. Diminished intensity (mild to moderate).
      d. Less uncomfortable.
    3. Cervical changes—slow or cease.
    4. Signs of fetal distress—rare
      a. Usually occur late in labor due to infection secondary to prolonged rupture of membranes.
      b. Tachycardia.
    5. Maternal vital signs may indicate infection (↑ temperature).

MMM 6. Medical diagnosis—procedures: vaginal examination, X-ray pelvimetry, ultrasonography—to rule out CPD (most common cause).

☒ D. Analysis/nursing diagnosis
  1. *Knowledge deficit* related to limited exposure to information.
  2. *Anxiety/fear* related to failure to progress as anticipated; fear for fetus.
  3. *High risk for injury* (infection) related to prolonged labor and/or ruptured membranes.

☒ E. Nursing care plan/implementation
  1. Medical management
    a. Amniotomy—artificial rupture of membranes.
    ● b. Oxytocin augmentation of labor—intravenous infusion of *oxytocin* to increase frequency, duration, strength, and efficiency of uterine contractions (see *Induction of labor*, p. 110).
    c. If CPD, cesarean birth.
  2. *Nursing management*
    a. Goals: *emotional support, comfort measures, prevent infection*—as for *Hypertonic dysfunction* (see p. 128).
    b. Other—see *Induction of labor*, p. 110.
F. Evaluation/outcome criteria: The woman:
  1. Reestablishes normal labor pattern.
  2. Experiences successful birth of viable infant.

Disorders Affecting Fluid-Gas Transport: Maternal

I. Uterine rupture
  A. Pathophysiology—stress on uterine muscle exceeds its ability to stretch.
  B. Etiology
    1. Overdistention—due to large baby, multifetal gestation.
    2. Old scars—due to previous cesarean births or uterine surgery.
    3. Contractions against CPD, fetal malpresentation, pathologic retraction ring (*Bandl's*).
    4. Injudicious obstetrics—malapplication of forceps (or application without full effacement/dilatation).
    ● 5. Tetanic contraction—due to hypersensitivity to oxytocin (or excessive dosage) during induction/augmentation of labor.
  ☒ C. Assessment
    1. Identify predisposing factors early.
    ⚑ 2. *Complete rupture*
      a. Pain: sudden, sharp, abdominal; followed by cessation of contractions; tender abdomen.
      b. Signs of shock; vaginal bleeding.
      c. Fetal heart tones—absent.
      d. Presenting part—not palpable on vaginal examination.
    3. *Incomplete rupture*

    a. Contractions: continue, accompanied by abdominal pain and failure to dilate.
    b. Signs of shock.
    c. May demonstrate vaginal bleeding.
    d. Fetal heart tones—absent.
  D. *Prognosis*
    1. Maternal—guarded.
    2. Fetal—grave.
  ☒ E. Analysis/nursing diagnosis
    1. *Pain* related to rupture of uterine muscle.
    2. *Fluid volume deficit* related to massive blood loss secondary to uterine rupture.
    3. *Anxiety/fear* related to concern for self, fetus.
    4. *Altered tissue perfusion* related to blood loss secondary to uterine rupture.
    5. *Altered urinary elimination* related to necessary conservation of intravascular fluid secondary to blood loss.
    6. *Anticipatory grieving* related to expected loss of fetus; inability to have more children.
  ☒ F. Nursing care plan/implementation
    1. *Medical management*
      a. Surgical—laparotomy, hysterectomy.
      b. Replace blood loss—transfusion, packed cells.
      ● c. Reduce possibility of infection—antibiotics.
    2. *Nursing management*
      a. Goal: *safeguard status.*
        (1) Report *immediately;* mobilize staff.
        (2) Prepare for immediate laparotomy.
        ☞ (3) Oxygen per mask—to increase circulating oxygen level.
        MMM (4) Order stat type and cross-match for blood—to replace blood loss.
        ☞ (5) Establish intravenous line—to infuse fluids, blood, medications.
        ☞ (6) Insert indwelling catheter—to deflate bladder.
        ☞ (7) Abdominal prep—to remove hair, bacteria.
        (8) Surgical permit (informed consent) for hysterectomy.
      b. Goal: *emotional support*—to allay anxiety (woman and family)
        (1) Encourage verbalization of fears, anxiety, concerns.
        (2) Explain all procedures.
        (3) Keep family informed of progress.
  ☒ G. Evaluation/outcome criteria
    1. Woman experiences successful termination of emergency; minimal blood loss.
    2. Woman's postoperative status is stable.

II. Amniotic fluid (pulmonary) embolus
  A. Pathophysiology: *acute cor pulmonale* —due to embolus blocking vessels in pulmonary circulation; massive hemorrhage—due to DIC resulting from entrance of thromboplastinlike material into bloodstream.
  B. Etiology—amniotic fluid (with any meconium, lanugo, or vernix) enters maternal circulation

through open venous sinuses at placental site; travels to pulmonary arterioles

   1. Rare.

   2. Associated with tumultuous labor, abruptio placentae, rupture of membranes.

C. *Prognosis*—carries a high rate of maternal mortality.

D. Assessment

   1. May occur during labor, at time of rupture of membranes, or immediately postpartum.

   2. Sudden dyspnea, tachypnea, and cyanosis; apprehension.

   3. Chest pain; pleuritic pain.

   4. Hypotension, tachycardia.

   5. Frothy sputum.

   6. **Signs of DIC**

      a. Purpura—local hemorrhage.

      b. Increased vaginal bleeding—massive.

      c. Rapid onset of shock.

   7. Signs of **adult respiratory distress syndrome (ARDS)**

      a. Pale color; diaphoresis; dyspnea; cyanosis, nonresponsive to nasal oxygen or intermittent positive pressure breathing.

      b. Apprehension; disorientation

      c. Distended neck veins.

      d. Pulse rate increased.

      e. History of dystocia: labor with failure to progress, difficult forceps-assisted birth, amniotic fluid (pulmonary) embolus.

E. Analysis/nursing diagnosis

   1. *Impaired gas exchange* related to pulmonary edema.

   2. *Risk for fluid volume deficit* related to DIC.

   3. *Anxiety/fear* for self and fetus related to severity of symptoms, perception of jeopardy.

F. Nursing care plan/implementation

   1. Medical management

      a. IV heparin, whole blood.

      b. Birth: immediate, by forceps, if possible.

      c. Digitalize, as necessary.

   2. *Nursing management*

      a. Goal: *assist ventilation*

        (1) *Position:* semi-Fowler's for breathing comfort.

        (2) Oxygen under positive pressure and emergency equipment should be readily available.

        (3) Suction, prn.

      b. Goal: *facilitate/expedite administration of fluids, medications, blood*

        (1) Establish intravenous line with large-bore needle.

        (2) Administer heparin, fluids, as ordered.

      c. Goal: *restore cardiopulmonary function, if needed.* Cardiopulmonary resuscitation techniques.

      d. Goal: *emotional support* of woman, family.

        (1) Reassurance and coaching in relaxation techniques to lessen anxiety.

        (2) Explain all procedures.

        (3) Keep informed of status.

G. Evaluation/outcome criteria

   1. Dyspnea relieved.

   2. Bleeding controlled.

   3. Successful birth of viable infant.

   4. Uneventful postpartum course.

Disorders Affecting Fluid-Gas Transport: Fetal

I. Fetus in jeopardy—general aspects

  A. Pathophysiology—maternal hypoxemia, anemia, ketoacidosis, Rh isoimmunization, or decreased uteroplacental perfusion.

  B. Etiology—*maternal*

    1. Preeclampsia/eclampsia.

    2. Heart disease.

    3. Diabetes.

    4. Rh or ABO incompatibility.

    5. Insufficient uteroplacental/cord circulation due to

      a. Maternal hypotension/hypertension.

      b. Cord compression:

        (1) Prolapsed.

        (2) Knotted.

        (3) Nuchal.

      c. Hemorrhage; anemia.

      d. Placental problem:

        (1) Malformation of the placenta/cord.

        (2) Premature "aging" of placenta.

        (3) Placental infarcts.

        (4) Abruptio placentae.

        (5) Placenta previa.

    6. Postterm gestation.

    7. Maternal infection.

    8. Hydramnios.

    9. Hypertonic uterine contractions.

      a. PROM with chorioamnionitis.

      b. Dystocia (e.g., from CPD).

  C. Assessment—*intrapartal*

    1. Amniotic fluid examination—at/or after rupture of membranes. *Signs of fetal distress:* meconium-stained, vertex presentation—due to relaxation of fetal anal sphincter secondary to hypoxia/anoxia. NOTE: Fetus "gasps" in utero—may aspirate meconium and amniotic fluid.

    2. Fetal activity

      a. Hyperactivity—due to hypoxemia, elevated carbon dioxide.

      b. Cessation—possible fetal death.

    3. *Methods of monitoring* FHR

      a. Stethoscope or fetoscope.

      b. Phonocardiography with microphone application.

      c. Internal fetal electrode—attached directly to fetus through dilated cervix after membranes ruptured.

      d. Doppler probe using ultrasound flow.

      e. Cardiotocograph—transducer on maternal abdomen transmits sound.

☞ 4. *Abnormal FHR* patterns (see Figure 4.5).
  a. Persistent irregularity.
  b. Persistent tachycardia of 160 or more beats/min.
  c. Persistent bradycardia of 100 or fewer beats/min.
  d. *Early deceleration*—due to vagal response to head compression.
  e. *Late deceleration*—due to uteroplacental insufficiency.
  f. *Variable deceleration*—due to cord compression.
  g. Decreased or loss of variability in FHR pattern.
〰 5. *Medical* evaluation—procedures: fetal blood gases, pH
  a. Purpose—to identify fetal acid-base status.
  b. Requirements for
   (1) Ruptured membranes.
   (2) Cervical dilatation.
   (3) Engaged head.
  c. Procedure—under sterile condition, sample of fetal scalp blood obtained for analysis.
  d. Signs of fetal distress
   (1) pH below 7.20 (normal range is 7.3–7.4).
   (2) Increased carbon dioxide.
   (3) Decreased PO_2.
✖ D. **Analysis/nursing diagnosis**
  1. *Impaired gas exchange, fetal*, related to decreased placental perfusion/insufficient cord circulation.
  2. *Altered tissue perfusion* related to hemolytic anemia.
  3. *High risk for fetal injury* related to hypoxia.
II. **Prolapsed umbilical cord**
  A. **Pathophysiology**—cord descent in advance of presenting part; compression interrupts blood flow, exchange of fetal-maternal gases → fetal hypoxia, anoxia, death (if unrelieved).
  B. **Etiology**
   1. Spontaneous or artificial rupture of membranes before presenting part is engaged.
   2. Excessive force of escaping fluid, as in hydramnios.
   3. *Malposition*—breech, compound presentation, transverse lie.
   4. Preterm or small-for-gestational-age (SGA) fetus—allows space for cord descent.
✖ C. **Assessment**
  1. Visualization of cord outside (or inside) vagina.
  2. Palpation of pulsating mass on vaginal examination.
  3. Fetal distress—variable deceleration and persistent bradycardia.
✖ D. **Analysis/nursing diagnosis**
  1. *Impaired gas exchange (fetal)*, related to interruption of blood flow from placenta/fetus.

2. *Anxiety/fear (maternal)*, related to knowledge of fetal jeopardy.
✖ E. **Nursing care plan/implementation**
  1. Goal: *reduce pressure on cord*
   a. Position: knee to chest; lateral modified Sims' with hips elevated; modified Trendelenburg.
   b. With gloved hand, support fetal presenting part off cord.
☞ 2. Goal: *increase maternal-fetal oxygenation*: oxygen per mask (8–10 L/min).
☞ 3. Goal: *protect exposed cord*: cover cord with warm sterile wet saline dressing.
  4. Goal: *identify fetal response* to above measures, reduce threat to fetal survival: monitor FHR continuously.
☞ 5. Goal: *expedite termination of threat to fetus*: prepare for immediate vaginal/cesarean birth.
  6. Goal: *support mother and significant other* by staying with them and explaining.
✖ F. **Evaluation/outcome criteria**
  1. FHR returns to normal rate and pattern.
  2. Uncomplicated birth of viable infant.

Summary of Warning Signs During Labor

I. Contractions—strong, every 2 min or less, lasting 90 sec or more; poor relaxation between contractions.
II. Sudden sharp abdominal pain followed by boardlike abdomen and shock—abruptio placentae or uterine rupture.
III. Marked vaginal bleeding.
IV. FHR periodic pattern decelerations—late, variable, absent (see Figure 4.5).
V. Baseline
  A. Bradycardia (<100 beats/min).
  B. Tachycardia (>160 beats/min).
VI. Amniotic fluid
  A. Amount: excessive; diminished.
  B. Odor.
  C. Color: meconium stained; port-wine; yellow.
  D. 24 hr or more since rupture of membranes.
VII. Maternal hypotension.

Summary

Complications during the intrapartal period have both physical and emotional sequelae. The mother (family) faces life-threatening hazards. A long and difficult labor is both physically and emotionally draining. These difficulties and fatigue may negatively affect a new parent's initial response to the newborn. The family may face short-term or long-term grief reactions if the outcome is tragic. The nurse's care-taking skills are important: the ability to assist the mother (family) develop/maintain effective individual coping and a sense of self-worth.

Study and Memory Aids

Definition: Tocolysis—from Greek:

toco-, toko- = a combining form meaning childbirth, labor

lysis = to break down or dissolve

Definition: Dystocia—from Greek:

dys- = a prefix meaning abnormal, diseased; difficult, painful, faulty

toco-, toko- = a combining form meaning childbirth, labor

Dystocia Etiology—"Six Ps"

Position
Psychological response
Placenta
Power
Passageway
Passenger

Questions

1. Ritodrine (Yutopar) IV is chosen as the beta-adrenergic agent to treat a woman's preterm labor. The nurse can expect which common *Maternal* side effect?
   1. Hypoglycemia.
   2. Decreased reflexes.
   3. Tachycardia.
   4. Hyperkalemia.

2. A woman is hospitalized for preterm labor at 28 wk. She is given beta-methasone (Celestone, Solupan). She asks the nurse what the drug is for. The nurse's explanation should be based on the knowledge that the drug is used to:
   1. Treat fetal respiratory distress syndrome (RDS).
   2. Prevent chorioamnionitis.
   3. Promote fetal pulmonary maturity.
   4. Increase uteroplacental exchange.

3. A woman is in labor with a large fetus. She experiences sudden, sharp abdominal pain, which is followed by a cessation of contractions and a tender abdomen. The nurse notifies the physician stat because these signs and symptoms indicate
   1. Abruptio placentae.
   2. Placenta previa.
   3. Uterine rupture.
   4. Uterine inversion.

4. The nurse is legally obligated to recognize the types of fetal heart rate (FHR) tracings on electronic fetal monitor strips. The nurse recognizes a late FHR deceleration as:
   1. A transitory decrease of FHR below baseline, concurrent with uterine contractions.
   2. An abrupt transitory decrease in FHR that varies in duration, intensity, and timing related to onset of contractions.
   3. A transitory decrease in FHR below baseline rate, starting at peak of contraction and lasting beyond end of contraction.
   4. An FHR below 120 beats/min lasting longer than 10 min.

5. The nurse is legally obligated to recognize the types of fetal heart rate (FHR) tracings on electronic fetal monitor strips. The nurse recognizes a variable FHR deceleration as:
   1. A transitory decrease of FHR below baseline, concurrent with contractions.
   2. A transitory decrease in FHR below baseline rate, starting at peak of contraction and lasting beyond end of contraction.
   3. An FHR below 120 beats/min lasting longer than 10 min.
   4. An abrupt transitory decrease in FHR that varies in duration, intensity, and timing related to onset of contractions.

6. Heart failure (HF) is one cause of maternal mortality during labor. Under what condition must the maternity nurse be on the alert for development of HF in a healthy woman in labor?
   1. During a long second stage of labor with prolonged bearing down.
   2. If the woman becomes exhausted during a difficult (dystotic) labor.
   3. Secondary to other therapy, such as tocolysis and use of beta-methasone.
   4. Secondary to other therapy, such as use of prostaglandins to augment/induce labor.

7. A woman in preterm labor is undergoing tocolysis and has shown signs/symptoms of toxicity. The nurse prepares and administers the antidote for ritodrine hydrochloride (Yutopar) toxicity, which is:
   1. Terbutaline, 10 µg.
   2. Calcium gluconate, 10 mg.
   3. Propranolol, 1 mg.
   4. Naloxone hydrochloride (Narcan).

8. The nurse will discontinue ritodrine tocolysis for a woman in premature labor, and notify the physician in the presence of which clinical occurrence?
   1. Maternal pulse of 104 and regular.
   2. Maternal blood pressure of 140/68.
   3. The woman complains of shortness of breath and chest tightness.
   4. The woman complains of palpitations.

9. The nurse's plan of care must include an alert for possible complications that can arise from therapeutic interventions. The nurse bases care on the knowledge that a healthy primigravida in preterm labor is at increased risk for cardiac decompensation if she
   1. Receives betamethasone during tocolysis.

2. Has a prolonged second stage of labor.
3. Becomes fatigued during a 24-hr labor.
4. Receives IV fluids and sucks on ice chips.

10. Preterm labor/birth give rise to physical, emotional, and financial stress for the family and possible physical/intellectual/sensory impairment for the child; therefore, nurses assure that all pregnant women know and have a list of signs and symptoms that indicate preterm labor. Which symptoms reported to the nurse by a pregnant woman are likely due to preterm labor?
1. Irregular contractions during the day, groin pain, heavy discharge.
2. Abdominal pain, occasional contractions, mucousy discharge.
3. Pelvic pressure, contractions during position changes, watery discharge.
4. Contractions every 10 min for 2 hr, low back pain, light bloody discharge.

11. The labor and birth room nurse notes that moments after a woman's membranes rupture, she becomes dyspneic, tachypneic, and apprehensive, and she is experiencing pleuritic pain. The nurse suspects:
1. Placenta abruptio.
2. Placenta previa.
3. Imminent birth.
4. Amniotic fluid embolus.

12. A 17-year-old, para 0-0-0-0, is admitted at 38 wk gestation and diagnosed with mild preeclampsia. Her condition stabilizes and induction of labor is begun with Pitocin. Cervical dilation is 2 cm and effacement is 70%. Amniotomy is done and scalp electrode and intrauterine contraction monitors are inserted. Which nursing action would be inappropriate?
1. Promote rest by checking on her less frequently.
2. Position her in lateral decubitus position.
3. Monitor intake and output hourly.
4. Observe for blood pressure changes related to Pitocin.

13. The nurse knows that oxytocin stimulation of labor must be discontinued immediately if which danger sign occurs?
1. Contractions last 60 sec and occur every 3 min.
2. FHR is 182 beats/min for longer than 10 min.
3. FHR falls from 138 to 128 beats/min with contractions.
4. The woman complains of discomfort with contractions.

14. For 3 hr, a woman in labor has stayed at 6 cm dilated, −1 station (vertex) with molding extending to +2 station. The physician orders Pitocin augmentation of labor. The nurse's responsibility is to:
1. Assist in initiating induction.
2. "Piggy-back" IV fluid containing Pitocin.
3. Start an accurate record.
4. Challenge the order.

15. A woman is admitted to the hospital in early labor; her membranes ruptured before admission. The nurse anticipates that the physician will order "bedrest" if assessment shows
1. Cervical dilatation: 3 cm.
2. Effacement: 90%.

3. Station: −2.
4. Contractions every 3 min, lasting 30 sec.

16. Complications can occur at any time when a woman is in labor. All nurses must be ready to intervene for emergencies such as prolapsed umbilical cord. The nurse knows that the primary goal of emergency care given when prolapsed cord occurs during labor is to:
1. Prevent cold air from prematurely stimulating fetal respiration.
2. Apply water to the cord to prevent it from drying while it is still pulsating.
3. Stimulate and restore circulation in the cord by vasodilation.
4. Prevent or relieve pressure on the umbilical cord.

17. During a woman's labor, the nurse must be alert for life-threatening umbilical cord prolapse, especially
1. During the second stage of labor.
2. When the woman is ambulatory.
3. When the presenting part is not engaged in the pelvic brim.
4. If the amniotic sac is intact.

18. In addition to changing the mother's position, what other independent nursing intervention is indicated when the umbilical cord is prolapsed out of the vagina?
1. Wash the cord immediately with warm antiseptic solution and replace it into the vagina.
2. Cover the cord with a wet sterile sponge.
3. Keep the cord warm and moist with continuous applications of warm sterile saline compresses.
4. Apply a clamp to the exposed cord and cover with a sterile towel.

19. When a woman is admitted to the labor area with a questionable diagnosis of placenta previa or abruptio placentae, which admission procedure would the nurse omit?
1. Giving an enema.
2. Collecting a urine specimen.
3. Starting an IV infusion.
4. Leopold's maneuvers.

Answers/Rationale

1. **(3)** Tachycardia is a side effect of ritodrine. The findings in options **1, 2,** and **4** are *not* among the common side effects of this drug. **EV, 6, PhI**
2. **(3)** Corticosteroids have been found to hasten production of surfactant in fetal lungs. This drug is used to *prevent* RDS, not treat it **(1).**

Key to Codes

Nursing process: AS, assessment; **AN,** analysis; **PL,** planning; **IMP,** implementation; **EV,** evaluation. (See Appendix I for explanation of nursing process steps.)

Category of human function: 1, protective; **2,** sensory-perceptual; **3,** comfort, rest, activity, and mobility; **4,** nutrition; **5,** growth and development; **6,** fluid-gas transport; **7,** psychosocial-cultural; **8,** elimination. (See Appendix K for explanation.)

Client need: SECE, safe, effective care environment; **PhI,** physiologic integrity; **PsI,** psychosocial integrity; **HPM,** health promotion/maintenance. (See Appendix L for explanation.)

This drug does *not* prevent infection of the fetal membranes, or chorioamnionitis (2), and it does not affect uteroplacental exchange (4). **IMP, 5, PhI**

3. (3) These signs and symptoms describe uterine rupture, which occurs when the stress on the uterine muscle exceeds its ability to stretch, e.g., overdistention with a large fetus or fetuses, previous cesarean births, tetanic contractions (secondary to Pitocin induction/augmentation of labor).

    The uterus remains contracted (tone is increased) with abruptio (1), but rupture does *not* occur. Signs and symptoms of placenta previa (2) include painless bright-red bleeding; uterine tone is within *normal* limits. Inversion (4), turning inside out, does *not* occur during *labor;* it may occur after the baby's birth if the cord is pulled to try to remove the placenta before it is detached from the uterine wall. **IMP, 3, PhI**

4. (3) A late FHR deceleration is defined as a transitory decrease in FHR below baseline rate, starting at peak of contraction and lasting beyond end of contraction.

    The other options describe *early* FHR deceleration (1), *variable* FHR deceleration (2), and FHR *bradycardia* (4). **AN, 5, HPM**

5. (4) Variable FHR decelerations are abrupt transitory decelerations that vary in duration, intensity, and timing related to onset of contractions.

    The other options describe *early* FHR deceleration (1), *late* FHR deceleration (2), and FHR *bradycardia* (3). **AN, 5, HPM**

6. (3) Therapy such as use of a beta-mimetic (ritodrine, terbutaline) for tocolysis and the use of beta-methasone (Celestone, Solup) to stimulate fetal lung development (production of surfactant) increases a healthy woman's risk of heart failure.

    A healthy woman will become exhausted with a long labor (1), but heart failure will not develop because of it. Neither a difficult labor in itself (2) nor use of prostaglandins (4) predisposes the healthy woman to heart failure. **EV, 6, HPM**

7. (3) Propranolol, 1 mg, is the antidote for ritodrine hydrochloride (Yutopar) toxicity. Terbutaline (1) is similar in action to ritodrine. Calcium gluconate (2) is the antidote for magnesium sulfate toxicity. Narcan (4) is the antidote for narcosis and depressed respirations. **IMP, 1, PhI**

8. (3) Shortness of breath and chest tightness are symptoms of cardiac decompensation. In addition, be especially alert for heart failure if a steroid such as beta-methasone (Celestone, Solup) is used to stimulate fetal lung maturity. The antidote for ritodrine hydrochloride (Yutopar) is propranolol, 1 mg. A maternal pulse of 130 exceeds the therapeutic range.

    The findings in 1, 2, and 4 represent side effects of ritodrine therapy, but remain within acceptable normal limits. **IMP, 6, PhI**

9. (1) A corticosteroid such as beta-methasone (Celestone, Solup; used to stimulate fetal lung maturity) plus a beta-mimetic drug such as ritodrine or terbutaline (used for tocolysis, stopping preterm labor) increases risk of cardiac decompensation. Signs/symptoms: shortness of breath, chest tightness; $P \geq 140$; $R \geq 25$.

None of the situations in options 2, 3, and 4 leads to cardiac decompensation in the healthy pregnant woman. **IMP, 6, PhI**

10. (4) Contractions occurring every 10 min for 2 hr (even after position changes and drinking glasses of water), low back pain, and light bloody discharge (bloody show) are common signs of true labor. Other symptoms of preterm labor include constant menstrual-like cramping low in the abdomen, dull lower backache that radiates like a wave to the front of the abdomen, and pelvic pressure extending to the back and thighs.

    Option 1 is incorrect because irregular contractions throughout the day, pain in the groin, and heavy vaginal discharge (leukorrhea) are common in *normal* pregnancy. Option 2 is incorrect because abdominal pain is *not* a sign of preterm labor and needs to be further evaluated; occasional contractions and mucousy discharge are commonly seen in *normal* pregnancy. Option 3 is incorrect because pelvic pressure could result from a low-lying baby, and contractions can be stimulated by position changes; watery discharge could be due to ruptured membranes (amniotic fluid), and does need to be assessed more thoroughly. **EV, 5, HPM**

11. (4) These signs suggest amniotic fluid embolism. This can also follow placental separation after the birth of the baby. Immediate recognition of the condition is important for timely, prompt intervention. DIC and adult respiratory distress syndrome (ARDS) are possible sequelae. None of the conditions in options 1, 2, and 3 would cause this type of patient response. **EV, 6, PhI**

12. (1) This critically ill woman now has an additional medication with powerful side effects that must be monitored regularly; it would be inappropriate to monitor her *less* frequently. The actions in options 2, 3, and 4 *are all proper* nursing measures for a hypertensive woman undergoing induction of labor. **IMP, 3, SECE**

13. (2) Persistent tachycardia (acceleration) is one sign of fetal distress. The findings in options 1, 3, and 4 are all within *normal* range. **EV, 1, SECE**

14. (4) The data suggest that the labor may be complicated by cephalopelvic disproportion (CPD). Augmenting labor with exogenous oxytocin may serve to wedge the presenting part deeper into the maternal pelvis and severely compromise the fetus. Labor should not be augmented as ordered (1 and 2) under these conditions, since CPD may be present. While maintaining an accurate record (3) is important, the nurse needs to *challenge* this order, not just document it. **IMP, 1, SECE**

15. (3) Station at -2 means that the presenting part of the fetus is high enough to allow the umbilical cord to slip down in front of the presenting part. Cervical dilatation (1), effacement (2), and contractions (4) are *irrelevant* to umbilical cord prolapse.

    NOTE: When membranes rupture, the nurse's primary responsibility is to assess for FHRs, since the umbilical cord can be "washed down" at the time the membranes rupture. **EV, 1, PhI**

16. (4) Compression of the umbilical cord compromises fetal oxygenation and, therefore, fetal well-being. Cold air (1) does not enter the uterus via the vagina follow-

ing rupture of membranes. The cord should be kept moist with sterile warm *saline* compresses, *not water* (**2**), to prevent it from drying. (Maintenance of *pulsation* is a goal since it indicates that fetal circulation continues.) Vasodilation (**3**) does *not* occur during cord compression; if the cord is external to the vagina, *vasoconstriction* will occur if it is not kept warm and moist, secondary to the effect on Wharton's jelly, which surrounds the vessels in the cord (on exposure to cold, the jelly expands and constricts the vessels in the cord, since the covering of the cord is not elastic and cannot expand). **PL, 6, PhI**

17. (**3**)   The umbilical cord can slip past the presenting part *before* it engages snugly in the pelvic brim. There is no room for the cord to slip past the full-term fetus during the *second* stage (**1**). Women *can* be ambulatory (**2**) when membranes are intact or after the presenting part has engaged, when prolapse is *not* likely. Sufficient amniotic fluid in an intact sac (**4**) *cushions* the umbilical cord. **AS, 6, PhI**

18. (**3**)   This action maintains cord integrity; warmth prevents Wharton's jelly from expanding and closing off umbilical blood vessels. The actions in options **1** and **2**

do not protect the cord. Clamping the cord (**4**) cuts off any uteroplacental-fetal circulation, and the fetus will die. **IMP, 1, PhI**

19. (**1**)   Giving an enema may result in dislodging a low-lying placenta, and severe hemorrhage may follow. Touching the cervix through the rectal and vaginal mucosas causes reflex uterine contractions, which result in cervical changes. These changes (dilatation and effacement) pull up and away from the low-lying placenta, thus dislodging it from its implantation site.

A urine analysis (**2**) *is* appropriate for admission to a labor floor to rule out infection. Starting an intravenous infusion (**3**) on admission *is* appropriate for someone who is bleeding and when anesthesia and surgical intervention may be required. Leopold's maneuvers (**4**) *could* assist in diagnosing an abnormally high fetus (commonly seen when the placenta occupies the lower uterine segment) and the general tone of the uterus (muscle tone is unaffected by placenta previa; it is increased in the presence of abruptio placentae). In addition, a blood specimen is obtained to assess for low platelets, a sign of DIC, which can occur with abruptio placentae. **IMP, 6, SECE**

The Postpartal Period

6

Chapter Outline

- Key Points
- Key Words
- Biologic Foundations
  - Uterine Involution
  - Birth Canal
  - Abdominal Wall
  - Cardiovascular System
  - Urinary Tract
  - Integument (Skin)
  - Legs
  - Weight
- Menstruation and Ovarian Function
- Nursing Management
- Psychological/Behavioral Changes
- Breastfeeding and Lactation
- Formula Feeding
- Critical Path/Case Management
- Home Care Following Early Discharge
- Summary
- Study and Memory Aids
- Questions
- Answers/Rationale

🔑 KEY POINTS

- Following expulsion of the placenta, levels of estrogen and progesterone fall rapidly, resulting in many of the anatomic and physiologic changes in the postpartum period.
- "Motherliness" can be exhibited by either parent.
- The interactional structure of a family must be restructured with the addition of the new member.
- The biggest differences between Western and non-Western beliefs and practices in childbearing occur in the postpartal period and require sensitive and knowledgeable consideration in the nursing plan of care.
- Careful assessment is essential in order to detect any deviations from the norm, to provide comfort measures for the relief of discomfort or pain, and to guard against injury and/or infection in the care of the newborn and mother.

Colostrum
Critical path/case management
Engorgement (breast)
Homan's sign
Home care
Involution
Let-down reflex
Lochia
   Rubra
   Serosa
   Alba
Oxytocic medications
Puerperium ("fourth trimester")
Telephone follow-up
Warm lines/help lines

General overview: This review of the normal physiologic and psychological changes occurring during the postpartal period—the "fourth trimester" (birth to 6 wk after)—provides the database necessary for assessing the woman's progress through involution, planning and implementing care, anticipatory guidance, health teaching, and evaluating the results. Emerging problems are identified by comparing the woman's status against established standards.

Key Words

"After pains"
Autolysis
"Baby blues"

Biologic Foundations

I. **Uterine involution**—integrated processes by which the uterus returns to nonpregnant size, shape, and consistency.

▷ I. Assessment

A. *Contractions* ("after pains")—shorten muscles, close venous sinuses, restore normal tone
1. Frequency, intensity, and discomfort decrease after first 24 hr.
2. More common in multiparas, and after birth of a large baby; primiparous uterus remains contracted.
3. Increased by breastfeeding.

B. Autolysis—breakdown and excretion of muscle protein (decreasing size of myometrial cells). Lochia—sloughing of decidua (the upper 2 layers of the endometrium, leaving the basal layer to regenerate the endometrium) and blood.

C. Formation of *new endometrium*—4–6 wk until placental site healed; heals without scarring.

D. *Cervix*
1. Immediately following birth—bruised, small tears; admits one hand.
2. Eighteen hr after birth—becomes shorter, firmer; regains normal shape.
3. One wk postpartum—admits two fingers.
4. Never returns fully to prepregnant state
   a. Parous os is wider and not perfectly round.
   b. Lacerations heal as scars radiating out from the os.

E. *Fundal height and consistency*
1. After birth—at umbilicus; size and consistency of firm grapefruit.
2. Day 1 (first 12 hr)—one finger breadth (about 1 cm) above umbilicus.
3. Descends by one fingerbreadth (about 1 cm) daily until day 10.
4. Day 10—behind symphysis pubis, nonpalpable.

F. *Lochia*
1. Character
   a. *Rubra* (red): from birth to about day 3 or 4; consists of blood, endometrial decidua, bacteria, fetal lanugo, vernix, small shreds of placental tissue and membranes.
   b. *Serosa* (pink to brown): apparent about day 3 until about day 7. The amount of blood decreases; the placental site exudes serous material and lymph.
   c. *Alba* (creamy yellowish-white to gray-white): appears during *second* or *third* wk. As endometrial epithelialization progresses, the amount of lochia decreases markedly and takes on a seromucinous consistency. Cessation of flow occurs at about 6 wk. It contains numerous leukocytes and bacteria.
2. Amount: scant, light, moderate, or heavy
   a. Moderate: 4–8 pads/d (average 6 pads/d).
   b. Following cesarean birth: less lochia—due to manipulation during surgery.
3. Odor: normal lochia has characteristic "fleshy" odor; foul odor is characteristic of infection.
4. Clots: normal: a few small clots, most commonly on arising—due to pooling in vagina.

NOTE: Clots and *heavy* bleeding are associated with uterine atony, retained placental fragments.

II. Birth canal
A. *Vagina*—never returns fully to prepregnant state
1. First few weeks postpartum—thin-walled, due to lack of estrogen; few rugae.
2. Week 3: Rugae may reappear.
3. Hymen—if torn, may heal.

B. *Pelvic floor*
1. Immediately after birth—infiltrated with blood, stretched, torn.
2. Month 6: Considerable tone regained.

C. *Perineum* (see REEDA, p. 113)
1. Immediately following birth—edematous; may have episiotomy (or repaired lacerations); hemorrhoids.
2. Healing, incisional line clean; no separation.
3. Hematoma—blood in connective tissue beneath skin; complains of pain, unrelieved by mild analgesia or heat; perineal distention; painful, tense, fluctuant mass.

III. Abdominal wall
A. Overdistention during pregnancy may cause rupture of elastic fibers, persistent striae, and diastasis of the rectus muscles.
B. Usually takes 6–8 wk to retrogress, dependent on previous muscle tone, obesity, and amount of distention during pregnancy.
C. Strenuous exercises discouraged until 8 wk postpartum.

IV. Cardiovascular system—characteristic changes
A. Immediately after birth—*increased* cardiac load, due to:
1. Return of uterine blood flow to general circulation.
2. Diuresis of excess interstitial fluid.
B. Volume—returns to prepregnant state (4 L) in about 3 wk. Major reduction—during first week, due to diuresis and diaphoresis.
C. Blood values (see Table 2.2).
1. High WBC during labor (25,000/mL); drops to normal level in first few days.
2. Week 1—Hgb, RBC, Hct, elevated fibrinogen return to normal.
D. Blood coagulation
1. During *labor*: rapid consumption of clotting factors.
2. During *postpartum*: increased consumption of clotting factors. Hypercoagulability maintained during first few days postpartum; predisposes to thrombophlebitis, pulmonary embolism.
▷ E. Assessment: potential complications—vital signs:
1. *Temperature*—elevated in
   a. Excessive blood loss, dehydration, exhaustion, infection.
   b. Puerperal infection: 100.4°F (38°C) after first day postpartum.
2. *Pulse*—physiologic bradycardia (50–70) common through second day postpartum; may persist 7–10 days; etiology: unknown.

Tachycardia—associated with excessive blood loss, dehydration, exhaustion, infection.

3. *Blood pressure*—generally unchanged. *Elevation*—associated with: preeclampsia, essential hypertension.

V. Urinary tract—characteristic changes:

A. *Output*—increased due to diuresis (12 hr–5 days postpartum); daily output to 3000 mL.

B. *Urine constituents:*
1. Sugar—primarily lactose.
2. Acetonuria—after prolonged labor; dehydration.
3. Proteinuria—first 3 days in response to the catalytic process of involution.

C. Dilatation of ureters—subsides in first few weeks.

D. **Assessment: potential complications**—measure first few voidings, palpate bladder to determine emptying
1. Edema, trauma, and/or anesthesia may lead to retention with overflow.
2. Overdistended bladder—common cause of excessive uterine bleeding in immediate postpartum.

VI. Integument (skin)—characteristic changes:

A. Striae—persist as silvery or brownish lines.

B. Diastasis recti abdominis—some midline separation may persist.

C. Diaphoresis—excessive perspiration for first few (approximately 5) days.

D. Breast changes—see I. C. *Breasts,* below.

VII. Legs

A. Should have no redness, tenderness, local areas of increased skin temperature, or edema.

B. May have some soreness from birth position.

C. *Homans' sign* should be negative (no calf pain when knee is extended and gentle pressure applied to dorsiflex the foot).

VIII. Weight—characteristic changes:

A. Initial weight loss—fetus, placenta, amniotic fluid, excess tissue fluid.

B. Weighs more than in prepregnant state (weight maintained in breasts).

C. Week 6—weight loss is individualized.

IX. Menstruation and ovarian function—first menstrual cycle may be anovulatory

A. *Nonnursing*—ovulation at 4–6 wk; menstruation at 6–8 wk.

B. *Nursing*—anovulatory period varies (39 days–6 mo or more); some for duration of lactation; contraceptive value: *very unreliable.*

Nursing Management

I. Assessment—minimum of twice daily

A. Vital signs.

B. Emotional status, response to baby.

C. *Breasts*
1. Observe: size, symmetry, placement and condition of nipples, leakage of colostrum. Normal: Although one breast is usually larger than

the other, breasts are essentially symmetrical in shape; nipples: in breast midline, erectile, intact (no signs of fissure); bilateral leakage of colostrum is common.
2. Note: reddened areas, elevations, supernumerary nipples, inverted nipples, cracks.
3. Observe for signs of (normal) *engorgement* (i.e., tenderness, distention, prominent veins). Transient; normally occurs shortly before lactation is established—due to venous and lymphatic stasis.
4. Palpate for local heat, edema, tenderness, swelling (signs of localized infection).

D. Fundus, lochia, perineum.

E. Voiding and bowel function.

F. Legs (see point VII above).

G. Signs of complications (see p. 142).

II. Analysis/nursing diagnosis: (See *Analysis/nursing diagnosis during the fourth stage of labor,* p. 107.)

III. Nursing care plan/implementation

A. Goal: *safety* (prevent hemorrhage)
1. Review prenatal and labor/birth history to identify predisposing factors: previous history of bleeding after birth, large baby (or twins, triplets, etc.), hydramnios, saddle-block anesthesia, long difficult labor (dystocia), intrauterine infection.
2. Take precautionary measures: remind woman to keep bladder empty so that "living ligature" can contract; keep uterus empty of clots, provide gentle massage, prn, to allow uterus maximum capacity to contract well.
3. Administer oxytocic medications, prn. See Pharmacology Box 6.1.

B. Goal: *comfort measures*
1. Perineal care—to promote healing, prevent infection.
2. Sitz baths—to promote healing.
3. Apply topical anesthetics, witch hazel to episiotomy area, hemorrhoids.
4. Administer mild analgesia, as ordered.
5. Instruct in tensing buttocks on position change—to reduce stress on suture line, discomfort.
6. Breast care: *bottle-feeding* mother
   a. Wash daily with clear water and mild soap.
   b. Support with well-fitting brassiere.
   c. For engorgement
      (1) Prevent with tight binder.
      (2) Treat with ice pack and mild analgesic.
      (3) *Avoid* nipple stimulation.
   d. See also *Breastfeeding and lactation,* p. 143.

C. Goal: *encourage normal bowel function* (normal to take 1–3 days for function to resume)
1. Administer stool softeners, as ordered.
2. Encourage ambulation.
3. Increase *dietary fiber* (salads, fresh fruit, vegetables, bran cereals).
4. Provide adequate *fluid* intake.

Pharmacology Box 6.1   MEDICATIONS TO STIMULATE UTERINE TONE

Drug/Dosage	Indication/Action	▶ Assessment: Side Effects	▶ Nursing Management
Oxytocin Injection			
USP (*Pitocin, Syntocinon, Uteracon*); oxytocic, synthetic posterior pituitary hormone IV injection, 10 U/mL; onset in 1 min IV infusion, 10–40 U/1000 mL 5% dextrose or physiologic electrolyte solution IM injection, 3–10 U; onset in 3–7 min; duration 30–60 min	Treat uterine atony: stimulate phasic uterine muscle contraction Assist breastfeeding: promote milk-ejection (letdown) reflex, facilitate flow of milk during engorgement	Hypertension, if patient is concurrently receiving *ephedrine, methoxamine,* or other vasopressors Hypersensitivity	Monitor for return of atony when effect wears off Store in cool place
Ergonovine			
USP, NF (*Ergotrate maleate*); oxytocic, ergot alkaloid Oral: 0.2–0.4 mg q6–12 h for 48 hr; onset in 6–15 min IM injection, 0.2 mg (1 mL) if nausea precludes oral preparation, onset "in a few minutes" Initial response: firm, tetanic contraction Subsequent response: alternating minor relaxations and contractions for 1½ hr; then vigorous rhythmic contractions for 3–4 hr after injection	Treat uterine atony: stimulate prolonged nonphasic uterine contractions	*Hypertension* Severe hypertensive episodes may occur if woman is hypertensive, or receiving vasoconstrictors. *Hypersensitivity* Nausea, vomiting Sudden change in BP, pulse	*Assess for hypertension before administering!* Monitor for changes in BP, pulse Store in cool place Note: keep record of count of ampules on unit; ampules "disappear," presumably taken for those wishing for induce abortion in early stages of pregnancy

(continued)

D. Goal: *health teaching and discharge planning*
1. Reinforce appropriate perineal self-care.
2. Reinforce handwashing (see Nursing actions during the fourth stage of labor, p. 107).
3. *Infant care*
   a. Bathing, cord care, circumcision care, diapering.
   b. Feeding, burping, scheduling.
   c. Assessment—temperature, skin color, newborn rash, jaundice.
   d. Normal stool cycle and voiding pattern.
   e. Common sleep/activity patterns.
   f. Newborn warning signs to report **immediately**
      (1) Diarrhea, constipation.
      (2) Colic, vomiting.
      (3) Fever.
      (4) Signs of inflammation and/or infection at cord stump.
      (5) Bleeding at circumcision site.
      (6) Rash, jaundice.
      (7) Deviation from normal patterns.
4. *Self-care*
   a. Adequate rest, nutrition, hydration.
   b. Breast self-examination (see Fig. 1.4, p. 5); wear bra to support breasts, and promote comfort.
   c. Normal process of involution; lochial patterns.
5. Resumption of *sexual intercourse*
   a. Sexual intercourse can be resumed by end of third or fourth postbirth week if bleeding has stopped and the episiotomy is healed.
   b. Physiologic reactions to sexual stimulation for the first three postbirth months are reduced in both rapidity and intensity of response.

Pharmacology Box 6.1	**MEDICATIONS TO STIMULATE UTERINE TONE (*Continued*)**		
Drug/Dosage	*Indication/Action*	◄ *Assessment: Side Effects*	◄ *Nursing Management*
Methylergonovine			
NF (*Methergine*); *oxytocic, ergot alkaloid* and conge- ner of lysergic acid (LSD) Oral: 0.2 mg tab, q6–8 h for maximum of 1 wk; onset in 5–10 min IM injection, 0.2 mg (1 mL) q2–4 h; onset in 2–5 min IV infusion (*emergency only*); 0.2 mg (1 mL) *slowly over 60 sec*; onset immediate	Treat uterine atony: stimu- late rapid, sustained te- tanic uterine contractions Treat subinvolution of uterus	Nausea, vomiting Transient hypertension (has only minimum vasocon- strictive effect) CNS effects: dizziness, headache, tinnitus Diaphoresis Palpitations Temporary chest pains	*Avoid* administering about the time woman re- ceives analgesic such as *oxycodone* and *aspirin* (Percodan)—may result in hallucinations Monitor BP Store in cool place away from light
Carboprost			
(*Prostin/*M15); *oxytocic, prostaglandin* IM injection, 1 ampule (250 µg), onset within minutes; intramyometrial injection (by physician only), ½–2 ampules (125–500 µg) di- luted with 10 mL saline (injected transabdominally into anterior wall of uterus); onset within min- utes	Treat uterine atony and uterine inversion: stimu- late rapid, sustained uter- ine contractions	Severe hypertension (sys- tolic > 170 mm Hg or di- astolic > 100 mm Hg) Diarrhea commonly seen with dosage above 1 am- pule Possible bronchoconstriction and wheezing	Review patient history: *avoid* use in patients with severe symptomatic asthma Observe for adverse reac- tions Monitor BP Store in refrigerator

c. For first 6 weeks to 6 months, vagina does not lubricate well because steroid hormone depletion following birth inhibits the vaso- congestive response to sexual tension.

d. Use of a water-soluble gel (K-Y), cocoa butter, or a contraceptive cream or jelly is recommended for lubrication.

e. Vaginal tenderness may be present.

  (1) To relax vagina and identify possible areas of discomfort, partner can be in- structed to insert one or more clean, lubricated fingers into vagina and ro- tate them.

  (2) Coital position of comfort is chosen in which woman can control depth of penile penetration, e.g., side-by-side or female-superior.

f. Presence of baby influences postbirth love- making

  (1) A common concern is that baby will hear them.

  (2) Sexual response cycle may be inter- rupted by hearing the baby cry or move, leaving both partners frustrated and unsatisfied.

  (3) Fatigue from child care affects desire.

6. Postbirth *contraception*

  a. Explain that time interval varies as to first postpartal ovulation.

  b. Family planning options may resume if de- sired (see Table 1.2)

  (1) If not breastfeeding, oral contracep- tives after first menstrual period (low dose given to breastfeeding mothers).

  (2) Use of IUD or diaphragm decided at postpartal check-up.

  (3) Emphasize need to recheck size and fit of diaphragm.

  (4) Other options: condom plus spermi- cides.

7. *Exercises*—to restore muscle tone, relieve tension

  a. Mild exercise during first few weeks

  (1) Deep abdominal breathing.

  (2) Supine head-raising.

  (3) Stretching from head to toe.

  (4) Pelvic tilt.

  (5) Kegel's—to regain perineal muscle tone (see p. 42).

  b. Strenuous exercises (sit-ups, leg lifts)—de- ferred until later in postpartum.

8. Maternal warning signs to report stat
  a. *Vaginal discharge:* prolonged lochia rubra, excessive lochia or vaginal discharge, foul-smelling lochia or vaginal discharge, recurrence of bright-red vaginal bleeding after lochia has changed to rust color.
  b. Pelvic or perineal *pain*.
  c. *Fever*, with or without chills.
  d. Burning sensation during urination (*dysuria*); inability to urinate.
  e. Swollen area on leg that is painful, red, or hot to the touch.
  f. Localized swelling or a painful, hot area on the breast.
  g. See also *Home care following early discharge*, p. 145.

  E. Goal: *anticipatory guidance*—discharge planning: Mothers are discharged earlier in their postpartum recovery today—(6–24 hr after birth if asymptomatic). See discussion at end of this chapter, *Critical path/case management* (p. 144), and *Home care following early discharge* (p. 145).
    1. Discuss, assist in organizing time schedule. Nap, when possible, when infant asleep—to minimize fatigue.
    2. Common maternal emotional/behavior changes, feelings:
      a. Jealous of infant; guilt feelings.
      b. "Baby blues"—due to hormonal fluctuations, fatigue, change of life-style.
      c. Feelings of inadequacy.
    3. Discuss support groups, aid in identifying supportive people.

⋈ **IV. Evaluation/outcome criteria**
  A. Woman experiences normal, uncomplicated postpartal period. All assessment findings within normal limits.
  B. Woman returns demonstrations of appropriate self-care measures/techniques
    1. Perineal care, pad change, handwashing.
    2. Breast care, breast self-examination.
  C. Woman verbalizes understanding of
    1. Need for adequate rest and diversion.
    2. Appropriate time for resumption of intercourse and exercise.
    3. Appropriate nutritional intake to meet needs (own and, if breastfeeding, infant).
    4. Signs to be reported immediately.
    5. Returns demonstration of appropriate infant care measures.
    6. Evidences beginning comfort and increasing confidence in parenting role.

⋈ **V. Postpartal assessment**—6 wk or less after birth:
  A. Weight, vital signs, urine for protein, complete blood count.
  B. Breast examination—lactating or not.
  C. Pelvic examination—involution and position of uterus; perineal healing; tone of pelvic floor.
  D. Desire for selection of method of contraception.

Psychological/Behavioral Changes

Achievement of developmental tasks—progress in assumption of maternal role

⋈ **I. Assessment**
  A. *Taking-in* phase°—1–3 days following birth
    1. Talkative; verbally relives labor/birth experience.
    2. Passive, dependent, concerned with own needs (eating, sleeping, elimination).
  B. *Taking-hold phase*°—day 3–2 wk
    1. Impatient to control own bodily functions, care for self.
    2. Expresses interest/concern in learning how to care for baby (desire to assume "mothering" role).
    3. Responds to positive reinforcement.
  C. *Letting-go phase*°—mother "lets go" of former self-concept, role, life-style; begins to integrate new role and self-concept as "mother."
    1. Feelings of insecurity, inadequacy.
    2. Hesitancy in approaching infant-care tasks.
  D. "*Baby blues*"—may appear on day 4 or 5. (NOTE: Often, father/partner experiences same feelings.)
    1. Thought to result from fatigue (sleep deprivation), realization of need for role change, recognition of new responsibilities.
    2. Mild depression, cries without provocation.
    3. Frightened—intimidated by own perceptions of responsibilities.
  E. Lag in experiencing "maternal feelings"—usually resolved within 6 wk.
    1. May contribute to "baby blues."
    2. Guilt regarding lack of "maternal feelings."
    3. Diminished by prompt bonding experience.
  F. *Attachment:* a feeling of affection or loyalty that binds one person to another. Occurs at critical periods, e.g., birth or adoption; it is unique, specific, and enduring.
  G. *Bonding:* describes the initial mutual attraction between people, such as between parent and child, at first meeting.

⋈ **II. Analysis/nursing diagnosis**
  A. *Ineffective family coping: compromised,* related to achieving developmental tasks.
  B. *Situational low self-esteem* related to perceived inadequacy in acceptance of maternal role.
  C. *Ineffective individual coping* related to "baby blues," lag in experiencing maternal feelings.

⋈ **III. Nursing care plan/implementation**
  A. *Taking-in.* Goal: *emotional support*
    1. Encourage verbalization of labor/birth experiences; compliment parents on "how well" they did.
    2. Explore feelings of disappointment, if any.

°This section is based on a study written by Reva Rubin.

3. Meet dependency needs; comment on appearance, hair, personal gowns.
4. Encourage rooming in.
- **B.** *Taking-hold.* Goal: *health teaching*
  1. Discuss self-care, postpartal physiologic/psychological changes.
  ☞ 2. Demonstrate infant care; mother returns demonstration.
- **IV. Evaluation/outcome criteria**
  - **A.** Woman demonstrates beginning comfort in maternal role.
  - **B.** Woman develops confidence and competence in infant care.
  - **C.** Woman expresses satisfaction with self, infant; eager to return home.
  - **D.** Woman is successful in breastfeeding. (Tension inhibits let-down reflex; baby nurses poorly.)

Breastfeeding and Lactation

I. Biologic foundations
- **A.** *Antepartal* alterations:
  1. High estrogen/progesterone levels—stimulate proliferation and development of breast ducts.
  2. High progesterone levels—also → development of mammary lobules and alveoli.
- **B.** *Postpartum* alterations:
  1. Rapid drop in estrogen/progesterone levels.
  2. Increased secretion of **prolactin**—stimulates alveolar cells → milk.
  3. Suckling—stimulates release of **oxytocin** → contraction of ducts → milk ejection (*let-down reflex*).
  4. *Engorgement*—due to venous and lymphatic stasis
     - **a.** Immediately precedes lactation.
     - **b.** Lasts about 24 hr.
     - **c.** Frequent feeding reduces engorgement.

II. Assessment
- **A.** *Colostrum* (yellowish fluid)—continues for first 2–3 days; may have some antibiotic, immunologic, and nutritive value.
- **B.** Milk (bluish-white, thin, consistency)—secreted on about third day.

III. Analysis/nursing diagnosis
- **A.** *Knowledge deficit* related to breastfeeding techniques.
- **B.** *Pain* related to engorgement.
- **C.** *Personal identity disturbance* related to problems in breastfeeding.
- **D.** *Sleep pattern disturbance* related to discomfort and/or infant care needs.

IV. Nursing care plan/implementation
- **A.** Goal: *promote successful breastfeeding*
  1. Encourage first feeding right after giving birth.
  2. Encourage emptying both breasts at each

feeding and before engorgement to stimulate milk production, prevent mastitis.
  3. Encourage rest, relaxation, fluids.
  🍎 4. *Nutritional* counseling (see Chapter 2)
     - **a.** Additional 500 calories/d (per baby; i.e., for twins, mother increases intake by 1000 calories). May be supplied via one extra pint of milk, one extra egg, and one extra serving of meat, citrus fruit, and vegetable.
     - **b.** *Increase* fluid intake to 3000 mL/d.
- **B.** Goal: *prevent or relieve engorgement*
  ☞ 1. Pain: relieved by warm packs, emptying breasts.
  2. Suggest she wear good, supportive bra.
  💊 3. Administer analgesics, as ordered/necessary.
- **C.** Goal: *health teaching*
  ☞ 1. Instruct, demonstrate rooting reflex and putting infant to breast. Infant must grasp nipple and areola over location of milk sinuses.
  ☞ 2. Demonstrate burping techniques, what to do if infant chokes; removing infant from breast.
  ☞ 3. Instruct in *basic nipple care.*
     - ✋ **a.** Use good handwashing.
     - **b.** Nurse on each breast making sure areola is in mouth, alternating position of infant.
     - **c.** Alternate "beginning" breast.
     - **d.** Break suction before removing infant from breast.
     - **e.** Air-dry nipples after each feeding and apply lanolin if abraded. NOTE: Creams, lotions, and ointments block secretion of a natural bacteriostatic oil by Montgomery's glands—and infant may refuse breast until it is washed. Instead, expressed milk may be massaged gently around nipple.
     - **f.** Provide daily hygiene of breasts.
  ☞ 4. Instruct in care of *cracked or fissured nipples*
     - **a.** Encourage and support mothers.
     - **b.** Air-dry nipples after each feeding.
     - **c.** Use nipple shield if nipples extremely sore.
     - **d.** Discontinue nursing for 48 hr; maintain milk supply by expressing milk with pump.
  5. Discuss *avoiding* use of any drugs except under medical supervision—may affect infant or suppress lactation.
  6. Discuss possibility of sexual stimulation during breastfeeding.
     - **a.** Validate normalcy and acceptability.
     - **b.** NOTE: During orgasm, milk may squirt from nipples.
  7. Explain that contraceptive value of nursing is unpredictable; time ovulation is inhibited varies widely.
  ! 8. Explain *contraindications to breastfeeding*
     - **a.** Active tuberculosis.
     - **b.** Severe chronic maternal disease.
     - **c.** Mastitis (temporary interruption may be necessary).
     - **d.** Breast cancer.
     - **e.** Narcotic addiction, therapeutic drug dependence.

    f. Severe cleft lip or palate in newborn (may pump and give in special bottles).

    g. HIV-positive status; AIDS.

    h. Drug abusers (must be drug free 3 mo).

⋈ V. Evaluation/outcome criteria

  A. Woman verbalizes understanding of breastfeeding techniques, nutritional requirements for successful lactation.

  B. Woman successfully demonstrates breastfeeding; infant nurses well.

  C. Woman demonstrates appropriate burping techniques; clears excessive mucus from infant's mouth without incident.

  D. Woman verbalizes understanding of basic breast-care techniques

    1. Self-examination.

    2. Clear water bath.

    3. Drying nipples after bathing, feeding.

    4. Care of cracked or irritated nipples.

Formula Feeding

  A. A successful alternative to breast feeding in certain instances:

    1. Parental choice.

    2. Maternal active infection, e.g., tuberculosis, syphilitic breast lesions, AIDS or HIV positive.

    3. Adoption.

☞ **B.** *Feeding skills*

    1. Baby needs to be wide awake.

    2. During feedings, parent should assume an *en face* position, hold infant closely and securely; parent can talk, sing or just enjoy a time of peaceful relaxation with baby.

    3. Hold bottle like a pencil so that fluid fills the nipple to avoid air bubbles.

    4. A tight bottle cap and small nipple hole makes infant work very hard so that he or she may fall asleep before satiation. The bubbles in the bottle are tiny. *Solution:* loosen the bottle cap and enlarge nipple hole.

    5. If, as the baby sucks, the bubbles in the bottle are large, too much air is entering the baby and stomach cramping and regurgitation may occur. *Solution:* tighten the bottle cap.

    6. *Signs that baby has had enough:* baby falls asleep, turns head aside, ceases to suck; baby voids six or more times per day.

    7. *Test temperature* of formula on feeder's wrist; if comfortably warm, it is correct temperature.

    8. To *test size of nipple hole*, hold bottle of formula upside down. Formula should drip. If hole is too big, formula runs in a stream; if too little, bottle needs to be shaken to get a drop.

    9. To *enlarge* hole in nipple, heat a needle stuck in a cork (used as a handle) and insert hot needle into the nipple. Soften new nipples by boiling for 5 minutes before using.

    10. Most newborns need to be *"burped"* or *"bub-*

bled". Burp before feeding, then after every ounce of formula.

    11. To *feed* baby, place the nipple in the infant's mouth over the tongue to rest against the roof of the mouth; this stimulates the sucking reflex.

    12. Baby's stools are soft but formed, yellow with a characteristic odor; usually stool is passed during feeding or immediately after. Change diaper immediately because stool is irritating to baby's skin.

  C. *Safety tips*

    1. *Never* prop the bottle—nipple may fall against the throat and block the air, or baby could drown in the formula or aspirate any that is regurgitated. If continued in later months, bottle propping has been implicated in causing *nursing bottle caries* or decay of teeth from continuous bathing of teeth with carbohydrate-containing fluid.

    2. *Never* leave baby alone while feeding until he or she is old enough to remove bottle from the mouth.

    3. At end of feeding and burping, place baby in crib on *right side* so air can come up easily.

Critical Path/Case Management

  I. Definition: *Critical path* refers to the exact timing of all key incidents that must occur to achieve the standard outcomes within the DRG-specific length of stay. *"Key incidents"* refers to physical, emotional, and teaching and discharge planning needs.

  A. Developed to implement care needed by patients who have a time limit for hospital stay: 6, 12, to 24 hr for most new mothers.

  B. Examples: nursing responsibilities for a 24-hr stay

    1. *Between 3 and 8 hr after birth*

☞   **a.** Assist with ambulation.

      b. Teach (and observe return demonstration of, prn) self-perineal care, handwashing, assessment and massage of uterine fundus, assessment of lochia character and amount.

☞   **c.** Teach about newborn (and observe return demonstration, prn): holding, techniques for positioning for feeding and burping.

    2. *During second 8-hr period*

      a. *Maternal self-care:* teach (and observe return demonstration, prn) about diet, activity/rest, elimination, sitz bath, medication.

☞   **b.** *Newborn care:* teach (and observe return demonstration, prn) about diaper changes, cord care, circumcision care, feedings and burping.

      c. *Parental concerns:* teach about bonding and attachment, normal newborn characteristics including crying, use of water feedings, pacifiers, and suckling patterns.

☞   **3.** *During third 8-hr period:* teach/review *warning signs* for mother and newborn to report stat; observe *return demonstration* of infant bath, cord care, circumcision care; refer, prn, e.g., lactation consultant; teach *safety*, e.g., baby positioning, car seat, need for baby to be attended to at all times and no propping of baby bottles; discuss *sibling rivalry*. Provide *anticipatory guidance* regarding baby's crying, sneezing, jaundice, etc.

   C. *Implications:* During any one shift, a nurse's assignment may include a newly recovered mother who needs frequent checks, women in different 8-hr periods following giving birth, new admissions, discharges, and the occasional emergency (e.g., hemorrhage, convulsion); in addition, the nurse may be caring for antenatal patients with various medical conditions.

   D. Standard plans of care and check lists to individualize care to meet woman's unique needs
      1. Standard care plan check lists: lochia, fundus, etc.
      2. A check list for each woman to fill out indicating her particular teaching priorities; e.g., woman may prefer to learn about infant illness first, etc. (Woman must be able to read and comprehend; provide lists in woman's language, prn.)

II. *Criteria for early discharge*

Criteria for Early Discharge

Mother
Uncomplicated pregnancy, labor, birth, and postpartum course
No evidence of premature rupture of membranes
Stable blood pressure; temperature < 100.4°F (38°C)
Ability to ambulate
Ability to void without difficulty
Intact perineum without third- or fourth-degree perineal laceration
Hemoglobin > 10 g
No significant vaginal bleeding

Infant
Term infant (38–41 wk) with birth weight of 2500–4500 g°
Normal findings on physical assessment performed by physician°
Normal laboratory data, including negative *Coombs* test result and hematocrit 40–65%°
Stable vital signs°
Temperature stability°
Successful feeding (normal sucking and swallowing)°
Apgar score > 7 at 1 and 5 min
Normal voiding and stooling
PKU and thyroid screening tests completed; repeat of PKU test scheduled for 2 wk°

General
Attendance at classes that include maternal and infant care, with an emphasis on problems of the first week at home°
Presence of a support person in the home to assist with care°
Presence of a strategy for follow-up°

Uncomplicated pregnancy, labor, birth, and postpartum course for mother and baby°
Demonstration of skill by mother in feeding, providing skin and cord care, measuring temperature with a thermometer, assessing infant well-being and signs of illness, and providing emergency care°

PKU-phenylketonuria.
°Recommendations of American Academy of Pediatrics. Criteria for early infant discharge and follow-up evaluation. *Pediatrics* 65:651, 1980.
From IM Bobak, DL Lowdermilk, MD Jensen. *Maternity Nursing* (4th ed). St. Louis: Mosby, 1995. P 507.

III. Maternal warning signs: Mother (family) is given this postpartum discharge list of signs that require reporting stat.

Temperature	More than 100.4°F (38°C) after the first 24 hr
Pulse	Tachycardia, marked bradycardia
Blood pressure	Hypotension or hypertension
Energy level	Lethargy, extreme fatigue
Uterus	Deviated from the midline, boggy, remains above the umbilicus after 24 hr
Lochia	Odor: heavy, foul
Perineum	Pronounced edema, not intact, signs of infection, marked discomfort
Legs	*Homans'* sign positive; painful, reddened area; warmth on posterior aspect of calf
Breasts	Redness, heat, pain, cracked and fissured nipples, inverted nipples, palpable mass
Appetite	Lack of appetite
Elimination	*Urine:* inability to void, urgency, frequency, dysuria; *bowel:* constipation, diarrhea
Rest	Inability to rest or sleep

From IM Bobak, DL Lowdermilk, MD Jensen. *Maternity Nursing* (4th ed). St. Louis: Mosby, 1995.

🏠 Home Care Following Early Discharge

I. *Definition:* service developed in response to consumers' need for continued assistance following early discharge from hospital to meet limits of DRG-specific length of stay
   A. The most critical period for a new mother is the *first 24 hr*, specifically because of her need to be monitored for *postpartum hemorrhage*.
   B. The need for services occurs when the new mother is asked to return home, often to her full responsibilities, following 9 mo of gestation; has experienced hours of physical/emotional stress of labor; has not had adequate sleep/rest while in the hospital; needs to learn about self-care, recover

physically, learn about baby care, and begin attachment/bonding and integrating the new addition with her (their) family structure.

⋈ **II. Assessment,** initial
   A. Review of woman's progress through her critical path and what remains to be done; what are her preferences for teaching?
   B. Components of discharge planning covered before discharge; what remains to be done (or redone)?
III. Services offered
   A. Home visits—planned collaboratively with family.
   B. Telephone follow-up
      1. Assessment.
      2. Health teaching.
      3. Identify complications to facilitate timely interventions, including referrals.
   C. "Warm" line/help line: not a "crisis" hot line; provides consultation for crisis prevention on such issues as postpartum depression, the infant's crying, care of hemorrhoids, breastfeeding or suppression of lactation, etc.
   D. Support groups (e.g., LaLeche League).
IV. Care providers: many home care services are developed and implemented with nurse practitioners who are experts in nursing; telephone follow-up and warm lines/help lines may by staffed by knowledgeable volunteers as well.

Summary

The nurse's knowledge of the postpartum patient's physical, emotional, and social needs lays the foundation for the nursing process with the woman (and family) during this period, the *"fourth trimester"* of the childbearing cycle. The nurse's skill and dedication are put to the test in trying to achieve high standards of care within the time limits of the DRG-specific requirements. To that end, nurses have developed *critical paths, early discharge classes* and discharge plans, *check lists,* and *home care services* (e.g., telephone follow-up, warm lines/ help lines) and support groups. Used individually or in combination, these services are effective in preventing crises and facilitating physiologic and psychological adjustments in the postpartum period.

💡 Study and Memory Aids

Definition

Decidua—from Latin, "cast off" or "shed"

Normal Lochia—Assessment

Rubra	Birth—day 3 or 4
Serosa	Days 3–7
Alba	Weeks 2–6

Goal: Prevent Hemorrhage

Hemorrhage remains the No. 1 cause of maternal mortality.

Psychological/Behavioral Changes: Maternal Role-Taking (Reva Rubin)

Taking-in
↓
Taking-hold
↓
Letting-go

Breastfeeding Foundations

Prolactin → milk production
Oxytocin → milk ejection

Postpartum Home Care Services with Early Discharge

Home visits
Telephone follow-up
Warm line/help line
Support groups

Questions

1. Postbirth, a new mother begins to bleed excessively. The *first* nursing action is to:
   1. Start an IV with Pitocin.
   2. Administer the oxytocic order per os.
   3. Massage the fundus until firm.
   4. Assess for lacerations.
2. A young mother is concerned because someone told her her uterus weighs 2 pounds now, but will get smaller by "involution." She wonders if involution is a form of weight loss that she can use to lose weight in general. The nurse's response is based on knowledge that uterine involution is accomplished by:
   1. Autolysis.
   2. Inversion.
   3. Regeneration of the three layers of the endometrium.
   4. Scarring at the placental site.
3. In assessing involution of the woman's uterus, the nurse determines that it is normal involution when the uterus is:
   1. Firm, 3 cm above the umbilicus.
   2. Firm, below the umbilicus, in the midline.
   3. Slightly boggy, 2 cm above the umbilicus.

4. Slightly boggy, below the umbilicus, in the midline.

4. The nurse applies a covered ice pack to a new mother's episiotomy area several hours after childbirth to reduce discomfort by:
1. Numbing the area to increase comfort.
2. Minimizing the amount of edema.
3. Helping her focus on the cold rather than on the pain.
4. Increasing circulation to the area for more rapid healing.

5. A new mother complains of "afterpains." The nurse's first action is to:
1. Administer ordered analgesics.
2. Advise her to stop breastfeeding until "afterpains" cease.
3. Encourage relaxation and breathing exercises.
4. Assess her for bladder filling.

6. The nurse gathers the following data: A woman gave birth to a daughter instead of a much-desired son. Now, the morning after giving birth, she seems withdrawn, is staying in bed and staring at the wall. Analysis indicates that which action is necessary?
1. No action, since this is a natural "let-down" after giving birth.
2. Referral for psychiatric consult.
3. Reassurance that her baby is beautiful and healthy.
4. Helping the mother to verbalize her disappointment.

7. In the "taking-hold" phase of postpartum recovery, the nurse can expect the new mother to:
1. Express concern about her behavior during labor.
2. State she will assume full care of the baby "tomorrow."
3. Order extra helpings of food at each mealtime.
4. Ask to take care of her baby herself.

8. During a postpartum home visit to a new mother on the day after discharge, the nurse's most therapeutic teaching intervention regarding sexual activity is to explain that:
1. She should use vaseline for lubrication.
2. She may begin sexual intercourse any time after the first week.
3. She should use the female-superior position when resuming sexual intercourse.
4. She can expect to have the same speed and intensity of response to sexual stimulation as she had before pregnancy.

9. The nurse is teaching a lactation class. A woman confides that she is surprised to learn from the nurse that one of the following is *not* related to successful breastfeeding. That one factor is:
1. Maternal nutrition.
2. Rest and relaxation.
3. Breast size.
4. Father's/partner's attitude.

10. A new mother tells the nurse, "I want to breastfeed as long as I can because I don't want to use contraceptives." The nurse's best response would be:
1. "That's right; while breastfeeding, you will not ovulate."
2. "You do not need to worry as long as you do not menstruate."

3. "Wait to resume intercourse until your periods start, then use the symptothermal method of contraception."
4. "It is best to use some type of contraceptive, like foam and condoms."

11. Nursing care for a new mother with engorged breasts who is not breastfeeding includes:
1. Frequent manual expression of milk, ice bags, analgesics.
2. Pumping breasts, restriction of fluids, ice bags.
3. Firm support, ice bags, analgesics.
4. Application of a tight binder, administering drugs to suppress lactation.

12. Which is the appropriate initial nursing action for a woman with an elevated temperature 4 hr after vaginal birth?
1. Push fluids by mouth (PO).
2. Do nothing, since it is a normal finding this soon after giving birth.
3. Check physician's orders for medication for infection.
4. Medicate her for pain, since temperature elevation is one sign of pain.

13. Around the third postpartum day, the nurse would describe normal lochia as:
1. Rubra.
2. Alba.
3. Serosa.
4. Menstra.

14. A woman gave birth 1½ hr ago. She is alert and physically active in bed. She states that she needs to urinate. The nurse's *most therapeutic* response is
1. "I'll walk you to the bathroom and stay with you."
2. "You can get up any time you want to, now."
3. "Make sure you wash your hands before and after, and wipe yourself once with each tissue, from front to back."
4. "Lean forward a little as you void. This will keep the urine off your stitches and be more comfortable."

15. Which laboratory finding would the nurse note as normal for a new mother following birth?
1. A drop in hematocrit.
2. A drop in white blood cell count.
3. Trace to 1+ proteinuria.
4. A decrease in coagulation factors.

16. Which new mother would the nurse expect to be an acceptable candidate for safe early discharge?
1. 17 hr after vaginal birth, third-degree perineal laceration, hemoglobin 12 g.
2. 32 hr after cesarean, voiding and ambulating.
3. 12 hr after vaginal birth, temperature 100°F, scant lochia rubra.
4. 28 hr after vaginal birth, membranes ruptured 30 hr before birth, spinal headache.

17. The trend toward early discharge following birth carries with it the caution that assessment parameters should be within normal limits for the number of postpartum hours. Which nursing assessment finding would require a delay of a planned discharge at 14 hr postpartum?
1. Lochia rubra, moderate.
2. Fundus at umbilicus, firm.

3. Pulse 62.
4. Three voidings in 14 hr, total 490 mL.
18. During the fourth stage of labor, which patient-centered goal is accurately stated and *takes priority?*
    1. Perineal edema is prevented by application of a covered ice pack.
    2. The woman will verbalize increased comfort.
    3. The woman will saturate no more than one peripad per hour.
    4. The woman is encouraged to void.
19. The postpartum nurse plans nursing care based on the knowledge that in the immediate postpartum period, the most serious consequence likely to occur from bladder distention is
    1. A urinary tract infection.
    2. Excessive uterine bleeding.
    3. Afterpains.
    4. Bladder wall atony.
20. Which one of the following conditions would alert the nurse to a possible postbirth hemorrhage?
    1. Precipitate birth.
    2. A full stomach.
    3. Preterm birth.
    4. Pudendal block anesthesia.
21. The nurse is especially alert for postpartum hemorrhage in the woman who:
    1. Had numerous vaginal examinations during labor.
    2. Was recently catheterized for bladder distention.
    3. Gave birth following a 26-hr labor augmented with exogenous oxytocin.
    4. Has diabetes mellitus, well controlled.
22. A woman who gave birth 8 hr ago appears anxious and says she feels "light-headed." A perineal pad has been in place for 15 min and contains clots and a heavy flow of lochia rubra. Which action would the nurse take *first?*
    1. Call the physician.
    2. Assess her vital signs.
    3. Get supplies to start an IV.
    4. Lift both of her legs high.
23. To safely administer ergonovine (Ergotrate) or methylergonovine (Methergine) to a postpartum woman, the nurse should know the woman's:
    1. Blood pressure.
    2. Pulse.
    3. Blood type and Rh.
    4. Method of feeding.
24. During an in-service presentation, nurses are discussing their beliefs about rubella vaccination. The nurse in charge knows that intervention is needed when some of the nurses state that:
    1. Women allergic to duck eggs may develop a hypersensitivity reaction.
    2. Lactating mothers should not receive the live attenuated virus.
    3. A transient arthralgia or rash may develop, but is benign.
    4. Women should practice contraception for 2–3 mo after vaccination.
25. A mother is feeding formula to her newborn. She says that he seems to get full fast and that he has regurgitated some of the formula already. She adds, "Maybe I just don't know how to feed him." As the baby sucks on the nipple, large bubbles are seen in the bottle. The nurse suggests:
    1. "Tighten the bottle cap a little."
    2. "Hold the baby in a more upright position."
    3. "Bubble (burp) him after every half ounce."
    4. "Let me show you how. Then you can try again."
26. A female nurse breastfeeding her 6-wk-old infant has returned to work in the newborn nursery. She notices that her nipples leak milk whenever she hears any newborn cry. A more experienced nurse suggests that the new mother (like all lactating women) needs to wear a breast pad because the let-down reflex in the lactating woman is stimulated by:
    1. Oxytocin.
    2. Estradiol.
    3. Pregnanediol.
    4. Luteinizing hormone (LH).
27. Which statement by a breastfeeding mother shows correct understanding of the nurse's initial instructions?
    1. "I'll call softly to him to get him to turn toward the breast."
    2. "A 15-min application of ice, followed by the electric pump and nursing, repeated until my breasts soften, will help my engorgement."
    3. "Tapping the baby on the cheek will make him let go of the nipple."
    4. "He will need to be fed less often than a formula-fed baby."

Answers/Rationale

1. **(3)** The nurse should massage the fundus until firm and expel any clots. If bladder is filling, ask her to void. Then reassess for continued uterine tone. If bleeding is excessive or uterine tone cannot be maintained, *then* an IV with the ordered amount of Pitocin (usually 40 μ in 1000 mL Ringer's solution) is started **(1)**; this may need to be done by another nurse while the first nurse continues to compress the relaxed uterus. Option **2** is incorrect: Any oral preparation requires time to contract the uterus, and is given *only* if uterine tone is not maintained by other means. Assessment for internal vaginal/perineal lacerations **(4)** may be warranted if continued bleeding is noted *after* the fundus is firmed with gentle massage. **IMP, 6, HPM**

2. **(1)** Involution is accomplished by autolysis of some tissue, contraction of stretched muscle fibers, and

---

Key to Codes

Nursing process: AS, assessment; **AN**, analysis; **PL**, planning; **IMP**, implementation; **EV**, evaluation. (See Appendix I for explanation of nursing process steps.)

Category of human function: 1, protective; **2**, sensory-perceptual; **3**, comfort, rest, activity, and mobility; **4**, nutrition; **5**, growth and development; **6**, fluid-gas transport; **7**, psychosocial-cultural; **8**, elimination. (See Appendix K for explanation.)

Client need: SECE, safe, effective care environment; **PhI**, physiologic integrity; **PsI**, psychosocial integrity; **HPM**, health promotion/maintenance. (See Appendix L for explanation.)

sloughing of the decidua. Inversion (**2**) is the turning inside-out of the uterus. Only the upper two-thirds of the endometrium are regenerated, *not* the bottom layer (**3**). *No* scarring of the placental site (**4**) takes place because regeneration occurs upward from the bottom third of the endometrium. **IMP, 5, HPM**

3. (**2**) Firm, below the umbilicus, in the midline describes the uterus in normal involution. In option **1**, the fundus is *high*, possibly indicating a filling bladder, which could soon cause the uterus to relax and hemorrhage to occur. A boggy fundus (**3** and **4**) indicates uterine *atony*, the No. 1 cause of postpartum hemorrhage. **EV, 5, HPM**

4. (**1**) Numbing the area will increase comfort *several hours* after birth. After the first 2 hr, ice packs have *little* effect on edema formation (**2**). Distraction (**3**) does *not* decrease discomfort. Ice packs *decrease* circulation to the area, rather than increasing it (**4**). **PL, 1, SECE**

5. (**4**) A filling bladder presses up on the lower uterine segment, causing the uterus to relax; the uterus tries to maintain tone by contracting. Analgesics (**1**) are appropriate only after other comfort measures fail. Mild analgesics given 40 min before the mother breastfeeds, and reassurance that this discomfort is transitory (about 2 days), usually is sufficient for most women. Cessation of breastfeeding (**2**) is *not* warranted. Encouraging relaxation and breathing exercises (**3**) is appropriate only *after* ensuring an empty bladder. **IMP, 1, HPM**

6. (**4**) The nurse should help the mother to verbalize her disappointment. The new mother must accept the reality of the child who was born and let go of the fantasy (or dream) child that she held during the pregnancy. Sometimes, the woman is disappointed and must resolve this response before she can bond with the newborn. This woman's response is *not* suggestive of the natural "letdown" after giving birth or of "baby blues" (**1**). A psychiatric referral (**2**) is *not* necessary at *this* time. The response in option **3** does *not* address the new mother's *feelings* at this time; it may be viewed as a "put-down" by the new mother. **PL, 7, PsI**

7. (**4**) Asking to take care of her baby herself indicates that she has moved out of the "taking-in" phase and into the "taking-hold" phase (per Reva Rubin). The behaviors in options **1**, **2**, and **3** are all expected of a new mother in the *"taking-in"* phase. NOTE: Progression through these phases is not seen today primarily because many women are discharged within hours (6–24) after giving birth. **EV, 7, PsI**

8. (**3**) The female-superior position is more comfortable for the woman since she can control the depth and angle of penile penetration.

Option **1** is incorrect because petroleum jelly (vaseline) may clog pores or damage condoms or diaphragms. In the postpartum period hormone-poor vaginal mucosa does not provide good lubrication, so dyspareunia is common; the woman should use contraceptive cream (which provides both contraception and lubrication) or a water-soluble product (such as K-Y Jelly). Option **2** is incorrect because most couples are ready to resume sexual intercourse after healing occurs and when lochia stops, usually by about 3 wk postpar-

tum. Option **4** is incorrect because the woman's physiologic response is *slower* and less intense during the early postpartum period. **IMP, 3, HPM**

9. (**3**) Breast size is not related to successful lactation. Breast size is genetically determined and is related to amount of fat in the breast. The factors in options **1**, **2**, and **4** all *are* directly related to the new mother's success with lactation. **AN, 4, HPM**

10. (**4**) Breastfeeding is unreliable as a contraceptive method. Foam can be recommended, since the postpartum hormone-poor mucosa does not provide good lubrication and dyspareunia is common; foam with nonoxynol-9 has an antimicrobial action as well as contraceptive value. Condoms decrease the likelihood of transmission of sexually transmitted disease as well as provide contraception.

Option **1** is incorrect because some women who breastfeed *have* been known to ovulate as early as the 39th day after giving birth. Option **2** is incorrect because women ovulate before menstruation, and therefore conception *may* occur even before the first menstruation. Option **3** is incorrect because people are usually ready to resume intercourse *sooner* than the time menstruation resumes. Also, although the sympto-thermal method does provide one method to determine when ovulation resumes, it has a higher failure rate than use of spermicide and condoms. **IMP, 5, HPM**

11. (**3**) Firm support, ice bags, and analgesics may be all that are required for comfort during the transient period (24–36 hr) of engorgement. Emptying the breasts (**1** and **2**) is the stimulus that is needed for the *continued production* of milk. A tight binder (**4**) is uncomfortable, and there are no universally accepted antilactogenic drugs (Parlodel was taken off the market early in 1995). **IMP, 3, HPM**

12. (**2**) An elevated temperature is secondary to the work and dehydrating effects of labor and birth. It would only be cause for concern in the presence of *other* signs of infection. She should take only sips of water to meet thirst; if she takes gulps or takes large amounts of water rapidly (**1**), she will vomit! Elevated temperature, by itself, does not indicate the need for medication (**3** and **4**). **IMP, 5, HPM**

13. (**3**) Lochia serosa is usually seen by the third postpartum day. The amount of blood decreases, and the placental site exudes serous material and lymph. Lochia rubra (**1**) is red and made up of blood, endometrial decidua, and fetal lanugo, vernix, and sometimes meconium and small shreds of placental tissue and membranes; it is usually seen for the *first 2* days. Lochia alba (**2**) usually appears about the *third week*. As endometrial epithelialization progresses, the amount of lochia decreases markedly and takes on a seromucinous consistency and a gray-white color. Cessation of lochial flow occurs at about 6 wk. There is *no such word* as menstra (**4**). **AS, 5, HPM**

14. (**1**) The nurse should accompany the new mother, due to the dangers of hypotension and fainting caused by splanchnic engorgement (excessive filling or pooling of blood within the visceral vasculature that occurs fol-

lowing the removal of pressure from the abdomen, and happens after the birth of a baby).

Option **2** is incorrect: This suggests that she get up on her own; instead, the nurse should *accompany* the woman for her first ambulation to decrease the possibility of her fainting and falling. Option **3** is incorrect: Although this hygiene measure is correct to prevent infection, it is more important to maintain patient safety during her first ambulation. Option **4** is incorrect: This action would indeed be advisable for increasing comfort during voiding if stitches are painful, but it is more important to protect her from falling during her first ambulation. **IMP, 1, HPM**

15. **(3)**   Proteinuria, trace to 1+, is a common finding for 1–2 days after a woman gives birth, as a result of the catalytic processes of involution (autolysis, or self-digestion, and breakdown of excess protein in the uterine muscle cells). Hematocrit may *rise* for a short time in normal postpartum cases, rather than drop **(1)**, because there is a greater loss in plasma volume than in blood cells during the first 72 hr. An *increase* in white blood cells (leukocytosis of pregnancy), averaging about 12,000/μL (20,000–25,000), is normal during pregnancy, rather than a decrease **(2)**. An extensive *activation* of blood-clotting factors occurs after childbirth, rather than a decrease **(4)**. **As, 8, HPM**

16. **(3)**   This mother meets the criteria for early discharge at 12 hr after vaginal birth: Slight temperature elevation (100°F, 37.8°C) is expected as a normal consequence of labor (an elevation of 100.4°F; 38°C or less is acceptable); lochia is within normal range. The woman should have an intact perineum, *without* third- or fourth-degree perineal laceration **(1)**, to qualify for early discharge. A cesarean birth **(2)** constitutes a *"complicated birth"*; the usual postoperative stay is 2–3 days. Another *deterrent* to early discharge is premature rupture of membranes **(4)**. **AN, 1, SECE**

17. **(4)**   490 mL total output is *insufficient*. The new mother should be experiencing diuresis at this time, voiding about 3000 mL/24 hr on the first postpartum day, as her water metabolism reverts to the nonpregnant state. The findings in options **1, 2,** and **3** all *are* within normal limits at this time. **EV, 8, HPM**

18. **(3)**   The woman who saturates one or more peripads in 1 hr is in danger; postpartum hemorrhage is commonly defined as 500 mL/first 24 hr. Uterine atony is the most common cause of hemorrhage during the fourth stage; hemorrhage remains one of the most life-threatening complications worldwide for new mothers. While the goals in options **1, 2,** and **4** are desirable, they do not *directly* relate to a threat to life and well-being, such as hemorrhage, and do not take priority.

Note: An accurately stated goal contains three elements: who, what, within what time limits. *Who* = the woman; *what* = will saturate no more than one peripad; *what time period* = 1 hr. **PL, 6, HPM**

19. **(2)**   A full bladder presses on the lower uterine segment and raises the uterus in the abdomen; therefore, the living ligature of the uterine fundus cannot contract and excessive uterine bleeding can occur. A distended bladder alone does *not* cause urinary tract infection **(1)**

immediately; uterine atony is the *immediate* consequence. Afterpains **(3)** are caused by uterine contractions (which *prevent* excessive uterine bleeding). Repeated and prolonged bladder distention does cause bladder wall atony **(4)**; however, the *immediate* danger is that even with the first distention, *uterine atony* can occur. **PL, 6, PhI**

20. **(1)**   Precipitate birth causes the uterus to become very tired, so that it does not contract well, resulting in increased risk of hemorrhage. Precipitate birth is birth following very rapid labor. The labor—from the beginning of cervical dilatation and effacement to full dilatation and birth—is 3 hr in length or less. (Rapid labor/birth can also result in lacerations of the cervix, lower uterine segment, vagina, and perineum.)

A full stomach **(2)** does *not* cause postbirth hemorrhage. Preterm birth **(3)** is *not* a cause of postbirth hemorrhage. Pudendal block anesthesia **(4)** does *not* affect uterine muscle tone; the living ligature is not affected by this anesthesia. **AN, 6, PhI**

21. **(3)**   Constant, prolonged stimulation of any muscle leads to fatigue in that muscle; uterine atony and hemorrhage can result from a 26-hr, augmented labor. Numerous vaginal examinations during labor **(1)** can predispose the woman to postpartum ("childbed") fever, but are *not* considered a precipitating factor in postpartum hemorrhage. Catheterization to keep the bladder empty **(2)** is a preventive measure *against* postpartum uterine atony and hemorrhage. A woman with well-controlled diabetes **(4)** usually has a baby whose weight is average for gestational age (AGA) and does *not* experience hydramnios (that is, her uterus has not been overdistended; her muscle tone, and therefore her risk of hemorrhage, should be *similar to that of other* postpartum women). **AN, 6, HPM**

22. **(4)**   Blood flow to the head and heart can be improved by lifting her legs. Then the nurse massages the fundus while calling for help verbally or by pressing the emergency button. Calling the physician first **(1)** would *delay* therapeutic intervention. Assessing her vital signs first **(2)** would *delay* therapeutic intervention; the nurse already knows that the woman's blood pressure has fallen since she complained of light-headedness and is anxious. Getting supplies first **(3)** to start an IV would *delay* therapeutic intervention; a second nurse would start the IV, etc. **IMP, 6, PhI**

23. **(1)**   Ergot products, used to contract the uterus, cause vasoconstriction and can raise blood pressure. Therefore, they are not given to women who have high blood pressure from any cause. Pulse **(2)**, blood type and Rh, **(3)** and method of feeding **(4)** are *not relevant* when safely administering an ergot product to increase uterine tone. **AS, 6, PhI**

24. **(2)**   Lactating mothers *can* receive the live attenuated virus. The statements in options **1, 3,** and **4** are all true regarding rubella vaccination during the early postpartum period and therefore intervention is *not* needed.

NOTE: If the woman receiving rubella vaccination is also Rh negative and is a candidate for RhoGAM, she should be tested within 3 mo to determine if the vaccination "took." The RhoGAM may prevent the vaccination from "taking" and she will not be immune to rubella. Rubella vaccination would then need to be repeated. **EV, 1, SECE**

25. **(1)** A loose cap allows too much air into the bottle. The air bubbles result in a feeling of fullness and discomfort; regurgitation is common. The large bubbles are responsible in this situation, *not* positioning **(2).** Although frequent burping **(3)** is appropriate, it does *not* resolve the problem of air bubbles. The comment in option **4** is a *put-down* for the mother, implying that the nurse "knows better." **IMP, 4, HPM**

26. **(1)** Oxytocin, produced by the posterior pituitary, stimulates the let-down reflex. Stimuli (infant's sucking, mother's emotions) stimulate the hypothalamus, which then stimulates the pituitary gland. Estradiol **(2),** produced by the ovary, is the most potent naturally occurring human female hormone; estrogen *prepares* the breasts for lactation. Pregnanediol **(3)** is a biologically *inactive* compound found in the urine of women during pregnancy or the secretory phase of the menstrual cycle; it is produced by the reduction of progesterone.

LH **(4),** produced by the anterior pituitary, stimulates secretion of sex hormones by the ovary; it is involved in the *maturation of ova.* **IMP, 5, HPM**

27. **(2)** Covered ice packs for no more than 15 min, followed by the electric pump and nursing (repeat as necessary) until the breasts are softened, is one treatment for engorgement in breastfeeding mothers. Application of warm, moist heat may help lessen the engorgement; however, most mothers' breasts are so swollen that heat only brings more blood to an already congested area.

Newborn infants do *not* respond to voice **(1);** the mother needs to bring the baby to the breast with a nipple touching the cheek or lips to elicit the rooting reflex. To break the suction **(3),** the mother needs to gently insert her finger into the corner of the baby's mouth between the gums; pulling the baby away without breaking suction can be painful and lead to sore nipples. Breastfed babies often feed *more* frequently than formula-fed babies, *not* less frequently **(4).** **EV, 4, HPM**

Complications During the Postpartal Period

Chapter Outline

KEY POINTS

- Postpartum hemorrhage is the most common and most serious type of excessive maternal blood loss; *causes:* uterine atony; lacerations of the birth canal; subinvolution of placental site, retained placental tissue, or infection.
- Clotting disorders—hypofibrinogenemia and disseminated intravascular coagulation (DIC)—are associated with a number of pregnancy-related conditions.
- Postpartum infection is a significant cause of maternal morbidity; its origin may be a continuation from the antepartum period or a result of intrapartal events.
- Sequelae of childbirth trauma include alterations in pelvic support, uterine displacement, and genital fistulas.

Key Words

Disseminated intravascular coagulation (DIC)
Hypofibrinogenemia
Postpartum hemorrhage
  Uterine atony
  Lacerations
  Subinvolution
Postpartum infection
  "Childbed fever"
  Endometritis
  Pelvic cellulitis or parametritis
  Perineal infection
  Mastitis
  Thrombophlebitis
Postpartum psychosis
Sheehan's syndrome

General overview: Postpartum complications arise from many sources. Some problems that the new mother may experience in the postpartum period result from high-risk medical conditions that predate the pregnancy, e.g., heart disease, diabetes mellitus, and infections. Others have antecedents during pregnancy, e.g., preeclampsia/eclampsia and HELLP syndrome. Intrapartum events can give rise to postpartum infections, e.g., placenta previa, saddle block (spinal) anesthesia, or a long, difficult labor with many vaginal examinations. These conditions have been covered in previous chapters.

I. Disorders affecting fluid-gas transport

A. Postpartum hemorrhage

1. *Definition*—loss of 500 mL of blood or more during first 24 hr postpartum in *vaginal* birth; 1000 mL in *cesarean* birth.

2. **Pathophysiology**—excessive loss of blood secondary to trauma, decreased uterine contractility; results in hypovolemia.

3. **Etiology** (in order of frequency):
   a. Uterine atony
      (1) Uterine overdistention (multiple pregnancy, hydramnios, fetal macrosomia).
      (2) Multiparity.
      (3) Prolonged or precipitous labor.
      (4) Anesthesia—deep inhalation or regional (particularly saddle block).
      (5) Myomata (fibroids).
      (6) Oxytocin induction of labor.
      (7) Overmassage of uterus in postpartum.
      (8) Distended bladder.
   b. Lacerations—cervical, vagina, perineal.
   c. Retained placental fragments—usually delayed postpartum hemorrhage.
   d. Hematoma—deep pelvic, vaginal, or episiotomy site.

4. **Assessment** (review *warning signs*, Chapter 6, p. 145)
   a. Uterus—boggy, flaccid; excessive vaginal bleeding (dark; seepage, large clots)—due to uterine atony, retained placental fragments.
   b. Signs of shock—air hunger; anxiety/apprehension, tachycardia, tachypnea, hypotension.
   c. Blood values (admission and postpartal) Hgb, Hct, clotting time.
   d. Estimated blood loss: during labor/birth; in early postpartum.
   e. Pain: vulvar, vaginal, perineal.
   f. Perineum: distended—due to edema; discoloration—due to hematoma.
   g. Vaginal hematoma: "feeling of fullness"; assessed when woman is *side lying* with knees drawn up, bearing down; a dark purple-blue mass seen at the vaginal introitus is characteristic. Woman may also complain of rectal pressure.
   h. Lacerations—bright-red vaginal bleeding with firm fundus.

5. **Analysis/nursing diagnosis**
   a. *Fluid volume deficit* related to excessive blood loss secondary to uterine atony, retained placental fragments.
   b. *Anxiety/fear* related to unexpected complication.
   c. *Altered tissue perfusion* related to decreased oxygenation secondary to blood loss.
   d. *Activity intolerance* related to fatigue.

6. **Nursing care plan/implementation**
   a. *Medical management*
      (1) Intravenous oxytocin infusion; intravenous or oral ergot preparations (*ergonovine* [*Ergotrate Maleate*], *methylergonovine* [*Methergine*]); *carboprost* (*Prostin/M15*), an *oxytocic; prostaglandin*. (See *Pharmacology Box* 6.1).
      (2) Order blood work: clotting time, platelet count, fibrinogen level, hemoglobin, hematocrit, CBC.
      (3) Type and cross-match for blood replacement.
      (4) Surgical:
         (a) Repair of lacerations.
         (b) Evacuation, ligation of hematoma.
         (c) Curettage—retained placental fragments.
   b. *Nursing management*
      (1) Goal: *minimize blood loss*
         (a) Notify physician promptly of abnormal assessment findings.
         (b) Order laboratory work stat, as directed—to determine blood loss and etiology.
         (c) Fundal massage.
         (d) Administer medications to stimulate uterine tone.
      (2) Goal: *stabilize status*
         (a) Establish IV line—to enable administration of medications and rapid absorption/action. Administer whole blood (with larger catheter).
         (b) Administer medications, as ordered —to control bleeding, combat shock.
         (c) Prepare for surgery, as ordered.
      (3) Goal: *prevent infection*. Strict aseptic technique; use universal precautions.
      (4) Goal: *continual monitoring*. Vital signs, bleeding (do pad count or weigh pads), fundal status.
      (5) Goal: *prevent sequelae* (Sheehan's syndrome).
      (6) Goal: *health teaching*—after episode: reinforce appropriate perineal care and handwashing techniques.

7. **Evaluation/outcome criteria**
   The woman's:
   a. Vital signs are stable.
   b. Bleeding has diminished or is absent.
   c. Assessment findings are within normal limits.

B. Subinvolution—delayed return of uterus to normal size, shape, position.

1. **Pathophysiology**—inability of inflamed uterus (endometritis) to contract effectively → incomplete uterine involution; failure of contractions to effect closure of vessels in site of placental attachment → bleeding.

2. Etiology

a. Premature or prolonged rupture of membranes (PROM) with secondary amnionitis, endometritis.

b. Retained placental fragments.

c. Oxytocin stimulation or augmentation of labor of overdistended uterine muscle may interfere with involution.

3. Assessment

a. Uterus: large, flabby; lack of uterine tone; failure to progressively shrink.

b. Discharge: persistent lochia; painless fresh bleeding, hemorrhagic episodes.

4. Analysis/nursing diagnosis

a. *Pain* related to tender, inflamed uterus secondary to endometritis.

b. *Anxiety/fear* related to change in physical status.

c. *Knowledge deficit* related to diagnosis, treatment, prognosis.

d. *High risk for injury* related to infection.

e. *Fluid volume deficit* related to excessive bleeding.

5. Nursing care plan/implementation

a. *Medical management*

(1) Have woman void or catheterize; massage uterus gently.

(2) Surgical (curettage)—to remove placental fragments.

(3) Antibiotic therapy—to treat intrauterine infection.

(4) Oxytocics—to stimulate/enhance uterine contractions.

b. *Nursing management*

(1) Goal: *health teaching*

(a) Explain condition and treatment.

(b) Describe, demonstrate perineal care, pad change, handwashing.

(2) Goal: *emotional support.* encourage verbalization of anxiety regarding recovery, separation from newborn.

(3) Goal: *promote healing*

(a) Encourage rest, compliance with medical/nursing regimen.

(b) Administer oxytocics, antibiotics, as ordered.

6. Evaluation/outcome criteria:

The woman

a. Verbalizes understanding of condition and treatment.

b. Complies with medical/nursing regimen.

c. Demonstrates normal involutional progress.

d. Has assessment findings (vital signs, fundal height and consistency, lochial discharge) that are within normal limits.

e. Expresses satisfaction with care.

C. Hypofibrinogenemia

1. **Pathophysiology**—decreased clotting factors, fibrinogen; may be accompanied by disseminated intravascular coagulation (DIC).

2. Etiology

a. Missed abortion (retained dead fetus syndrome).

b. Fetal death, delayed emptying of uterine contents.

c. Abruptio placentae; Couvelaire uterus.

d. Amniotic fluid (pulmonary) embolism.

e. Hypertension.

3. Assessment

a. Observe for bleeding from injection sites, epistaxis, purpura.

b. See *DIC assessment* (following, p. 156).

c. Maternal vital signs, color.

d. I&O.

e. Medical evaluation—procedures

(1) Thrombin clot test—important: size and persistence of clot.

(2) Prothrombin time (PT)—prolonged.

(3) Bleeding time—prolonged.

(4) Platelet count—decreased.

(5) Activated partial thromboplastin time—prolonged.

(6) Fibrinogen (factor I concentration)—decreased.

(7) Fibrin degradation products—present.

4. Analysis/nursing diagnosis

a. *Fluid volume deficit* related to uncontrolled bleeding secondary to coagulopathy.

b. *Anxiety/fear* related to unexpected critical emergency.

c. *Altered tissue perfusion* related to decreased oxygenation secondary to blood loss.

5. Nursing care plan/implementation

a. *Medical management*

(1) Replace platelets.

(2) Replace blood loss.

(3) IV heparin—to inhibit conversion of fibrinogen to fibrin.

b. *Nursing management*

(1) Goal: *continuous monitoring*

(a) Vital signs.

(b) I&O hourly.

(c) Skin: color, emergence of petechiae.

(d) Note, measure (as possible), record and report blood loss.

(2) Goal: *control blood loss*

(a) Establish IV line, administer fluids or blood products as ordered.

(b) *Position:* side-lying—to maintain blood supply to vital organs.

(3) Goal: *emotional support*

(a) Encourage verbalization of anxiety, fear, concerns.

(b) Explain all procedures.

(c) Remain with woman continuously.

(d) Keep woman and family informed.

6. Evaluation/outcome criteria

The woman's

a. Bleeding is controlled.

b. Laboratory studies are returning to normal values.

c. Status is stable.

D. Disseminated intravascular coagulation (DIC): diffuse or widespread coagulation initially within arterioles and capillaries leading to hemorrhage.

    1. Pathophysiology: activation of coagulation system from tissue injury → fibrin microthrombin form in brain, kidneys, lungs → microinfarcts, tissue necrosis → red blood cells, *platelets*, prothrombin, other clotting factors trapped, destroyed in process → excessive clotting → release of fibrin split products → inhibition of platelet clotting → bleeding.

    2. Risk factors

      a. Obstetric complications (see Hypofibrinogenemia etiology, p. 155).

      b. Neoplastic disease.

      c. Low perfusion states, e.g., severe preeclampsia.

    3. Assessment—*objective data:*

      a. Skin, mucous membranes: petechiae, ecchymosis.

      b. Extremities (fingers, toes): cyanosis.

      c. Bleeding: venipuncture sites, wound, oral, rectal, vaginal.

      d. Urine output: oliguria → anuria.

      e. Level of consciousness: convulsions, coma.

      f. Laboratory data: *prolonged*—PT (>15 sec); *decreased*—platelets, fibrinogen level.

    4. Analysis/nursing diagnosis

      a. *Altered tissue perfusion* related to peripheral microthrombi.

      b. *High risk for injury* (death) related to bleeding.

      c. *High risk for impaired skin integrity* related to ischemia.

      d. *Altered urinary elimination* related to renal tubular necrosis.

    5. Nursing care plan/implementation: goal: *prevent and detect further bleeding*

      a. Carry out nursing measures designed to alleviate underlying problem (e.g., shock, birth of fetus).

      b. Medications: heparin SO₄ IV, 1000 U/hr, if ordered, to reverse abnormal clotting (controversial).

      c. IVs: blood to lessen shock; platelets, cryoprecipitate, fresh plasma to restore clotting factors, fibrinogen.

      d. Observe: vital signs, central venous pressure (CVP; normal 5–15 mm Hg), pulmonary artery pressure (PAP) (normal 20–30 systolic and 8–12 diastolic), and intake and output for signs of shock or fluid overload from frequent infusions; specimens for occult blood (urine, stool).

      e. Precautions: *avoid* IM injections if possible; apply pressure 5 min to venipuncture sites; *no* rectal temperatures.

    6. Evaluation/outcome criteria

      a. Clotting mechanism restored (increased platelets, normal PT).

      b. Renal function restored (urine output >30 mL/hr).

      c. Circulation to fingers, toes; no cyanosis.

      d. No irreversible damage from renal, cerebral, cardiac, or adrenal hemorrhage.

II. Disorders affecting protective functions: postpartal infection (Table 7.1).

  A. General aspects

    1. *Definition*—reproductive system infection occurring during the postpartal period.

    2. Pathophysiology—bacterial invasion of birth canal; most common: localized infection of the lining of the uterus (*endometritis*).

    3. Etiology

      a. Anaerobic nonhemolytic streptococci.

      b. *Escherichia coli.*

      c. *Chlamydia trachomatis* (bacteroides).

      d. Staphylococci.

    4. Predisposing conditions

      a. Anemia.

      b. Premature or prolonged rupture of membranes (PROM).

      c. Prolonged labor.

      d. Repeated vaginal examinations during labor.

      e. Intrauterine manipulation—e.g., manual extraction of placenta.

      f. Retained placental fragments.

      g. Postpartum hemorrhage.

    5. Assessment

      a. Fever 38°C (100.4°F) or more on two or more occasions after first 24 hr postpartum. Warning: puerperal infection.

      b. Other signs of infection: pain, malaise, dysuria, subinvolution, foul odor to lochia.

    6. Analysis/nursing diagnosis

      a. *Fluid volume deficit* related to excessive blood loss, anemia.

      b. *Knowledge deficit* related to danger signs of postpartum period.

      c. *High risk for injury* related to infection.

    7. Nursing care plan/implementation: prevention

      a. Goal: *prevent anemia*

        (1) Minimize blood loss—accurate postpartal assessment and management of bleeding.

        (2) *Diet:* high protein, high vitamin.

        (3) Vitamins, iron—suggest continuing prenatal pattern until postpartum check-up.

      b. Goal: *prevent entrance/transport of microorganisms*

        (1) Strict aseptic technique during labor, birth and postpartum (universal precautions).

        (2) Minimize vaginal examinations during labor.

TABLE 7.1 POSTPARTUM INFECTIONS

Condition/Etiology	✉ Assessment: Signs/Symptoms	✉ Nursing Interventions

Postpartum infection
 	
Traumatic labor and birth and postpartum hemorrhage make woman more vulnerable to infection by such bacteria as nonhemolytic streptococci, *Escherichia coli,* and *Staphylococcus* species
	1. Dependent on location and severity of infection
	2. Usually include fever, pain, swelling, and tenderness
	3. Temperature ≥ 100.4°F (38°C) *after first 24 hr postbirth on 2 or more occasions* indicates puerperal infection ("childbed fever")
		1. *Monitor:*
		   Signs and symptoms
		   Drainage, e.g., uterine
		2. Obtain culture and sensitivity
		3. Administer antimicrobial agents and analgesic agents
		4. Assure comfort; encourage rest
		5. Use *universal* precautions
		6. *Force fluids* and provide *high-calorie diet*
		7. Keep family informed of mother's and newborn's progress
		8. Promote maternal-infant contact as soon as possible
		9. Plan and implement discharge and follow-up care

Endometritis Microorganisms invade placental site, and may spread to entire endometrium	1. Fever 2. Chills 3. Anorexia 4. Malaise 5. Boggy uterus 6. Foul-smelling lochia 7. Uterine cramps	1. Administer *antimicrobial* agents and *analgesic* agents 2. Encourage *Fowler's position* to promote drainage 3. Force fluids 4. Use universal precautions
Pelvic cellulitis or parametritis Microorganisms spread via lymphatics and invade tissues surrounding uterus	1. Fever 2. Chills 3. Lower abdominal pain 4. Tenderness	1. Administer *antimicrobial* agents and *analgesic* agents 2. Encourage bedrest 3. *Force fluids*
Perineal infection Trauma to perineum makes woman more vulnerable to infection	1. Localized pain 2. Fever 3. Swelling 4. Redness 5. seropurulent drainage	1. Administer *antimicrobial* agents and *analgesic* agents 2. Provide sitz baths or other heat/cold applications 3. Use *universal* precautions

(continued)

☞ **(3)** Perineal care.

c. Goal: *health teaching*

✋ **(1)** Handwashing—before and after each pad change, after voiding and/or defecating.

☞ **(2)** Perineal care—wipe from front to back; use clear, warm water or mild antiseptic solution as a cascade; do *not* separate labia.

☞ **(3)** Maintain sterility of pads; apply from front to back.

(4) *Avoid* use of tampons until normal menstrual cycle resumes.

✉ **8. Evaluation/outcome criteria**

TABLE 7.1   POSTPARTUM INFECTIONS (*Continued*)

Condition/Etiology	◄ Assessment: Signs/Symptoms	◄ Nursing Interventions
Mastitis		
Lesions or fissures on nipples allow entry of microorganisms (e.g., *Staphylococcus aureus*) from nose/mouth of infant or mother's unwashed hands (breast milk is a good medium for growth of organism)	1. Marked engorgement 2. Pain 3. Chills 4. Fever 5. Tachycardia If untreated, single or multiple breast abscesses may form	1. Order culture and sensitivity studies of mother's milk 2. Administer *antimicrobial* agents and *analgesic* agents 3. Apply heat or cold therapy 4. Assist with incising and draining abscesses 5. Use *universal* precautions and perform meticulous handwashing
Thrombophlebitis		

Infected pelvic or femoral thrombi
Increased tendency to clot formation during pregnancy
Trauma to tissues
Hemorrhage decreases new mother's resistance to infection
	1. Pain
	2. Chills and fever
	Femoral: stiffness of affected area or part and *positive Homan's sign*
	
	Pelvic: severe chills and wide fluctuations in temperature
		Femoral
		  1. Rest and *elevate* leg
		  2. Administer *antimicrobial* agents, *analgesic* agents, and *anticoagulants*
		Pelvic
		  1. Encourage bedrest
		  2. *Force fluids*
		  3. Administer *antimicrobial* agents and *anticoagulants*

a. The woman's assessment findings are within normal limits
  (1) Vital signs.
  (2) Rate of involution (fundal height, consistency).
  (3) Lochia: character, amount, odor.
  b. The woman avoids infection.
B. **Endometritis**—infection of lining of uterus
  1. **Pathophysiology**—see *General aspects*, II.A (p. 156).
  2. **Etiology**—most common: invasion by normal body flora (e.g., anaerobic streptococci).
  3. **Characteristics:**
    a. *Mild*, localized—asymptomatic, or low-grade fever.
    b. *Severe*—may lead to ascending infection, parametritis, pelvic abscess, pelvic thrombophlebitis.
    c. If remains localized, self-limiting; usually resolves within 10 days.
  ◄ 4. **Assessment**
    a. *Signs of infection:* fever, chills, malaise, anorexia, headache, backache.
    b. *Uterus:* large, boggy, extremely tender
      (1) Subinvolution.
      (2) Lochia: dark brown; foul odor.
  ◄ 5. **Analysis/nursing diagnosis**
    a. *Anxiety/fear* related to effects on self and newborn.

b. *Self-esteem disturbance and altered role performance* related to inability to meet own expectations regarding parenting, secondary to unexpected hospitalization.
  c. *Pain* related to inflammation/infection.
  d. *Ineffective individual coping* related to physical discomfort and psychological stress associated with self-concept disturbance; worry, guilt, concern regarding newborn at home.
  e. *Altered family processes*—interruption of adjustment to altered life pattern related to postpartal infection/hospitalization.
◄ 6. **Nursing care plan/implementation**
  a. Goal: *prevent cross-contamination.* Contact-item isolation; use universal precautions.
  b. Goal: *facilitate drainage. Position:* semi-Fowler's.
  c. Goal: *nutrition/hydration*
    (1) *Diet:* high calorie, high protein, high vitamin.
    (2) Push *fluids* to 4000 mL/d (oral and/or IV, as ordered).
    (3) I&O.
  d. Goal: *increase uterine tone/facilitate involution.* Administer medications, as ordered (e.g., oxytocics, antibiotics).

e. Goal: *minimize energy expenditure, as possible*
  (1) Bedrest.
  (2) Maximize rest, comfort.
f. Goal: *emotional support*
  (1) Encourage verbalization of anxiety, concerns.
  (2) Keep informed of progress.
7. Evaluation/outcome criteria: The woman responds to medical/nursing regimen
  a. Vital signs stable, within normal limits.
  b. All assessment findings within normal limits.
  c. Unable to recover organism from discharge.

C. Urinary tract infections (UTIs)
  1. Pathophysiology—normal physiologic changes associated with pregnancy (e.g., ureteral dilatation) and the postpartal period (e.g., diuresis, increased bladder capacity with diminished sensitivity of stretch receptors) → increased susceptibility to bacterial invasion and growth → ascending infections (cystitis, pyelonephritis).
  2. Etiology: usually bacterial.
  3. Predisposing factors:
    a. Birth trauma to bladder, urethra, or meatus.
    b. Bladder hypotonia with retention (due to intrapartal anesthesia or trauma).
    c. Repeated or prolonged catheterization, or poor technique.
  4. Assessment
    a. Maternal vital signs (fever, tachycardia).
    b. Dysuria, frequency (flank pain—with pyelonephritis).
    c. Feeling of "not emptying" bladder.
    d. Cloudy urine; frank pus.
  5. Analysis/nursing diagnosis
    a. *Altered urinary elimination* related to diuresis, dysuria, inflammation/infection.
    b. *Pain* related to dysuria secondary to cystitis.
    c. *Knowledge deficit* related to self-care (perineal care).
  6. Nursing care plan/implementation
    a. Goal: *minimize perineal edema*
      (1) Perineal ice pack in fourth stage—to limit swelling secondary to trauma, facilitate voiding.
      (2) Perineal ice pack after first 2 hr—to provide comfort.
    b. Goal: *prevent overdistention of bladder*
      (1) Monitor level of fundus, lochia, bladder distention. (NOTE: Distended bladder displaces uterus, limits its ability to contract → boggy fundus, increased vaginal bleeding.)
      (2) Encourage *fluids* and voiding; I&O.
      (3) Aseptic technique for catheterization.
      (4) Slow emptying of bladder on catheterization—to maintain tone.

c. Goal: *identification of causative organism*—to facilitate appropriate medication (antibiotics). Obtain clean-catch (or catheterized) specimen for culture and sensitivity.
d. Goal: *health teaching.* See previous discussion re fluids, general hygiene, diet, and medications.
7. Evaluation/outcome criteria
The woman responds to medical/nursing regimen:
  a. Voiding: quantity sufficient (although small, frequent output may mean overflow with retention).
  b. Urine character: clear, amber, or straw-colored.
  c. Vital signs: within normal limits.
  d. No complaints of frequency, urgency, burning on urination, flank pain.

D. Mastitis—inflammation of breast tissue
  1. Pathophysiology—local inflammatory response to bacterial invasion; suppuration may occur; organism can be recovered from breast milk.
  2. Etiology—most common: *Staphylococcus aureus;* source—most common: infant's nose, throat.
  3. Assessment
    a. Signs of infection (may occur several weeks postpartum).
      (1) Fever.
      (2) Chills.
      (3) Tachycardia.
      (4) Malaise.
      (5) Abdominal pain.
    b. Breast
      (1) Reddened area(s).
      (2) Localized/generalized swelling.
      (3) Heat, tenderness, palpable mass.
  4. Analysis/nursing diagnosis
    a. *Impaired skin integrity* related to nipple fissures, cracks.
    b. *Pain* related to tender, inflamed tissue secondary to infection.
    c. *Disturbance in body image, self-esteem* related to association of breastfeeding with female identity and role.
    d. *Anxiety/fear* related to sexuality; impact on breastfeeding, if any.
  5. Nursing care plan/implementation
    a. Goal: *prevent infection.* Health teaching in early postpartum
      (1) Handwashing.
      (2) Breast care—wash with warm water only (*no soap*)—to prevent removing protective body oils.
      (3) Let breast milk dry on nipples to prevent drying of tissue.
      (4) Clean bra (with no plastic pads or liners) to support breasts, reduce friction, minimize exposure to microorganisms.
      (5) Good breastfeeding techniques (see p. 143).

(6) Alternate position of infant for nursing to change pressure areas.

b. Goal: *comfort measures*

(1) Encourage bra or binder—to support breasts, reduce pain from motion.

☞ (2) Local heat or ice packs as ordered—to reduce engorgement, pain.

● (3) Administer analgesics, as necessary.

c. Goal: *emotional support*

(1) Encourage verbalization of feelings, concerns.

(2) If breastfeeding discontinued, reassure woman that she will be able to resume breastfeeding.

d. Goal: *promote healing*

☞ (1) Maintain lactation (if desired) by manual expression or breast pump, every 4 hr.

● (2) Administer antibiotics as ordered.

⋈ **6. Evaluation/outcome criteria**

The woman:

a. Promptly responds to medical/nursing regimen

(1) Symptoms subside.

(2) Assessment findings within normal limits.

b. Successfully returns to breastfeeding.

E. Thrombophlebitis

1. Pathophysiology—inflammation of a vein secondary to lodging of a clot.

2. Etiology

a. Extension of endometritis with involvement of pelvic and femoral veins.

b. Clot formation in pelvic veins following cesarean birth.

c. Clot formation in femoral (or other) veins secondary to poor circulation, compression, and venous stasis.

⋈ **3. Assessment**

a. Pelvic—pain: abdominal or pelvic tenderness.

b. Calf—pain: positive *Homans'* sign (pain elicited by flexion of foot with knee extended).

c. Femoral

(1) Pain.

(2) Malaise, fever, chills.

(3) Swelling—"milk leg."

⋈ **4. Analysis/nursing diagnosis**

a. *Pain* in affected region related to local inflammatory response.

b. *Anxiety/fear* related to outcome.

c. *Ineffective individual coping* related to unexpected postpartum complications, hospitalization, separation from newborn.

d. *Impaired physical mobility* related to imposed bedrest to prevent the formation and dislodging of a clot (embolus).

⋈ **5. Nursing care plan/implementation**

a. Goal: *prevent clot formation*

(1) Encourage early ambulation.

(2) *Position: avoid* prolonged compression of popliteal space, use of knee gatch.

☞ (3) Apply TED hose, as ordered, preoperatively and/or postoperatively for cesarean birth.

b. Goal: *reduce threat of emboli*

(1) *Bedrest,* with cradle to support bedding.

(2) Discourage massaging "leg cramps."

● c. Goal: *prevent further clot formation.* Administer anticoagulants, as ordered.

d. Goal: *prevent infection*

☞● (1) Administer antibiotics, as ordered.

(2) Push *fluids.*

☞ e. Goal: *facilitate clot resolution.* Heat therapy, as ordered.

⋈ **6. Evaluation/outcome criteria**

The woman responds to medical/nursing regimen:

a. Symptoms subside; all assessment findings within normal limits.

b. No evidence of further clot formation.

III. Disorders affecting psychosocial-cultural functions: postpartum psychosis

A. General aspects

1. Can occur in both new parents.

2. Usually occurs within 2 wk of birth.

3. Increased incidence among single parents.

4. Most common symptomatology: affective disorders.

5. Psychiatric intervention required in small percentage of cases; if underlying cause unresolved, increased risk in subsequent pregnancies.

B. Etiology—theory: birth of child may emphasize:

1. Unresolved role conflicts.

2. Unachieved normal development tasks.

⋈ **C. Assessment**

1. Onset of postpartum psychosis is abrupt and occurs within days of childbirth.

2. A major depressive condition is one that continues for more than 2 wk.

3. A major depressive condition is one that includes at least four of the following:

a. Change in appetite—anorexia.

b. Change in sleep.

c. Psychomotor agitation.

d. Loss of interest in usual activities.

e. Decrease in sexual drive.

f. Increased fatigue.

4. Additional findings may include withdrawal, paranoia, mood swings; depression may alternate with manic behavior.

5. Differentiated from *"baby blues" (postpartum blues)* because the "blues," usually transient and affecting 75–80% of women giving birth, often elicits crying spells and is characterized by feelings of loneliness or rejection, anxiety, confusion, restlessness, exhaustion, forgetfulness, and inability to sleep.

D. Analysis/nursing diagnosis
1. *High risk for injury,* to self or child (abuse/neglect) related to postpartum psychosis.
2. *Ineffective individual coping* related to perceived inability to meet role expectations ("mother") and ambivalence related to dependence/independence.
3. *Self-esteem disturbance and altered role performance* related to "femaleness" and reaction to responsibility for care of newborn.
4. *High risk for violence,* self-directed or directed at newborn related to anger or depression.
5. *Ineffective family coping* related to lack of support system in early postpartum.
6. *Altered family processes* related to psychological stress, interruption of bonding.
7. *Altered parenting* related to hormonal changes and stress.

E. Nursing care plan/implementation
1. Goal: *emotional support*
   a. Encourage verbalization of feelings, fears, anxiety, concerns.
   b. Support positive self-image, feelings of adequacy, self-worth.
      (1) Reinforce appropriate comments and behaviors.
      (2) Encourage active participation in self-care, comment on accomplishments.
      (3) Reduce threat to self-image, fear of failure. Maintain support, gradually increase tasks.
2. Goal: *safeguard status of mother/newborn*
   a. Unobtrusive, protective environment.
   b. Stay with woman when she is with infant.
3. Goal: *nutrition/hydration*
   a. Encourage selection of favorite foods—to aid security in decision making; counteract anorexia, refusal to eat by tempting appetite.
   b. Push *fluids* (juices, soft drinks, milkshakes)—to maintain hydration.
4. Goal: *minimize stress, facilitate effective coping.* Administer therapeutic medications, as ordered
   a. Schizophrenia—*phenothiazines.*
   b. Depression—*mood elevators.*
   c. Manic behaviors—*sedatives, tranquilizers.*

F. Evaluation/outcome criteria
The woman responds to medical/nursing regimen:
1. Increases interaction with infant.
2. Expresses interest in learning how to care for infant.
3. Evidences no agitation, depression.
4. Actively participates in caring for self and infant.
5. Demonstrates increasing comfort in mothering role.
6. Demonstrates positive family interactions.

IV. Sequelae to trauma sustained during childbirth
A. A delayed, but direct, result of childbearing is the weakening and lengthening (overstretching of the supporting tissues of the perineum) of fascial supports of the pelvic organs, termed **pelvic relaxation.** Symptoms most often appear during the perimenopausal period. Symptoms are related to the structure involved: urethra, bladder, uterus, vagina, cul-de-sac, or rectum. *Common symptoms:* pulling, dragging sensations, pressure, protrusions, fatigue, and low backache, and sometimes, urinary stress incontinence.
B. **Rectocele:** herniation or protrusion of the rectum into the posterior vaginal wall. *Complaints:* disturbance in bowel functioning, sensation of "bearing-down." Usually repaired surgically.
C. **Cystocele:** bladder hernia into the vagina is a sequel to injury to the vesicovaginal fascia. Often complicated by recurrent cystitis and ascending UTI. Often occurs along with rectocele. Complete emptying is difficult.
D. **Urinary stress incontinence:** secondary to injury to bladder neck structures—angle between the urethra and the base of the bladder is lost or increased, if the supporting pubococcygeus muscle is injured. Mild stress incontinence may be relieved by strengthening the pubococcygeus muscle with *Kegel's* exercises.
E. **Uterine displacement:** uterine prolapse—falling, sinking, or sliding of the uterus from its normal position.
F. **Pelvic fistula problems:** urethrovaginal, perineovaginal, vesicovaginal, rectovaginal, vesicocervical. Nursing care requires great sensitivity because the woman's reactions are often intense. The nurse suggests tactfully the hygienic practice of *douching and irrigating external perineal* structures with a deodorizing solution such as 1 tsp chlorine household bleach to 1 qt water. Before leaving the house, the woman can give herself *high enemas,* which provide temporary relief from oozing of fecal material in the preoperative period. Genitals should be thoroughly washed with unscented, uncolored, mild soap and warm water to avoid adding chemical irritation and/or allergy to her symptoms.

Summary

Nursing care of the new mother challenges the nurse with a variety of medical-surgical, psychiatric, and pediatric conditions. Disorders discussed in this chapter relate to *postpartum hemorrhage, infections, mental illness,* and *sequelae to trauma* sustained during childbirth. In addition, the nurse must confront the *sequelae* of conditions that arose during the *antepartum* (Chapter 3) and *intrapartum* periods (Chapter 5).

Study and Memory Aids

Causes of Postpartum Hemorrhage

Uterine atony
Lacerations
Retained placental fragments
Hematoma

Nursing Management of Postpartum Hemorrhage: Alert

Ergot products and carboprost: monitor BP.

Hypofibrinogenemia Assessment

Check for predisposing conditions for DIC.

UTI—Prevent Bladder Overdistention

A full bladder → uterine atony → hemorrhage.

Prevention of Infections

HANDWASHING—for nurse *and* mother—cannot be overemphasized!

Prevention of Mild Stress Incontinence

Remember Kegel's exercises!

Questions

1. The nurse notes that a pregnant woman's rubella titer is 1 : 6. This means that she:
   1. Has had rubella at some time in her life.
   2. Has just been exposed to rubella.
   3. Should receive rubella vaccination after giving birth.
   4. Must wait until she weans the baby before receiving vaccination for rubella.
2. After a woman has given birth, the nurse gives her Rh_o (D) immune globulin before discharge, if needed, to prevent her from:
   1. Isoimmunization.
   2. Autoimmunization.
   3. Developing AB antibodies.
   4. Becoming Coombs negative.

3. Before administering Rh_oGAM (Rh_o [D] immune globulin) to a new mother, the nurse explains that it is a drug that:
   1. Removes Rh + antibodies from maternal blood.
   2. Destroys fetal Rh_o erythrocytes in maternal blood.
   3. Deactivates maternal Rh + antibodies in fetal blood.
   4. Destroys fetal Rh + erythrocytes in maternal blood.
4. A new mother, who is drug dependent, requests information about breastfeeding. The nurse's response is based on knowledge that breastfeeding:
   1. Should be encouraged, to increase bonding.
   2. Is encouraged, to wean the baby from the substance.
   3. May need to be discouraged.
   4. May be safe, because most substances do not pass into breast milk.
5. A worried lactating mother tells the nurse that she has been exposed to "some PCB" (polychlorinated biphenyl). Her breast milk is tested and found to have a trace of PCB. The nurse advises her to:
   1. Discontinue breastfeeding immediately.
   2. Avoid crash diets that mobilize her fat stores.
   3. Drink up to 2 liters of water every day to facilitate its elimination.
   4. Feel free to do whatever she wishes regarding breastfeeding, fluid intake, and diet.
6. At 8 hr postpartum, a new mother has an oral temperature of 100°F. The nurse's evaluation of her status is:
   1. Anemia.
   2. Breast engorgement.
   3. Dehydration.
   4. Infection.
7. After a long and difficult labor, a woman had a spontaneous vaginal birth, assisted with low forceps. Since she is at risk for postpartum infection, the nurse should watch for which sign?
   1. Laboratory value: increased RBC sedimentation rate.
   2. Decreased pulse rate.
   3. Decreased lochia flow.
   4. Temperature: 38°C (100.4°F) 30 hr postpartum.
8. The postpartum recovery room nurse recognizes that a new mother is particularly vulnerable to postpartum hemorrhage if she:
   1. Is an older primipara.
   2. Experienced hydramnios during pregnancy and labor.
   3. Experienced a third stage that lasted 30 min.
   4. Gained excessive weight during pregnancy.
9. Before developing a plan of care for a woman who has just given birth, the nurse reviews her pregnancy and intrapartal record to identify possible risk factors. The nursing plan of care is based on knowledge that the most common cause of postpartum hemorrhage is:
   1. Lacerations of the birth canal.
   2. Subinvolution of the placental site.
   3. Retained placental fragments.
   4. Uterine atony.
10. All of the following are appropriate nursing interventions for uterine atony. The initial intervention should be:
    1. Expulsion of clots.

2. Gentle massage until the fundus is firm.
3. Administration of an oxytocic medication.
4. Ambulation to empty the urinary bladder.

11. A nursing plan of care includes therapeutic interventions for common conditions expected when a woman has just given birth. After evaluating results of unsuccessful nonpharmacologic measures to restore uterine tone, the nurse can expect to prepare and administer:
    1. Parlodel (bromocriptine).
    2. Methergine (methylergonovine maleate).
    3. Vitamin K (AquaMEPHYTON).
    4. Rh$_o$GAM (Rh$_o$[Du] immune globulin).

12. During a woman's first hour postbirth, the nurse notices a continuous trickle of bright-red vaginal bleeding; the fundus remains firm. Based on analysis of these data, the nurse:
    1. Does nothing; this is normal.
    2. Prepares the woman for exploration of her vaginal vault for possible lacerations.
    3. Administers an oxytocic medication to stimulate the living ligature in the lower uterine segment.
    4. Examines the woman for possible vaginal hematoma.

13. The nurse would *not* administer Rh$_o$(D) immune globulin to a new mother if:
    1. The mother is Rh$_o$(D) negative.
    2. The infant is Rh$_o$(D) positive.
    3. Coombs test on the cord blood is negative.
    4. Coombs test on the mother's blood is positive.

14. A pregnant woman has just arrived at the emergency room after suffering a spontaneous miscarriage at home. Which of the following assessment data alerts the nurse that this woman may be a candidate for receiving Rh$_o$(Du) immune globulin?
    1. Woman is Rh negative; pregnancy of 11 wk gestation.
    2. Woman's religion forbids the use of blood products.
    3. Woman is Rh negative and states that the father is also Rh negative.
    4. Woman's Coombs test is positive.

15. The nurse would help expel intrauterine blood and clots from a postpartum woman by using:
    1. Gentle pressure on a firm fundus, supporting the base of the uterus just above the symphysis.
    2. Vigorous massage of the boggy uterus, supporting the base of the uterus just above the symphysis.
    3. Firm pressure downward on the uterine fundus, in the direction of the vagina.
    4. Gentle pressure on the boggy fundus in the direction of the vagina.

16. A new mother was discharged 24 h after giving birth. Eight hours later, she calls the maternity unit concerned about a "flabby womb" (uterus) that doesn't contract well and episodes of painless bleeding." The nurse's response is based on knowledge that the mother:
    1. Is describing *uterine atony*, which is managed with keeping the bladder empty, gentle massage, and expulsion of clots.
    2. Is describing *subinvolution*, which is managed with curettage, antibiotics, and oxytocin.
    3. Is describing *hypofibrinogenemia*, which is managed with IV infusion of heparin, platelets, and blood.

4. Is describing *normal involution*, which is managed with rest and reassurance.

Answers/Rationale

1. **(3)** Rubella immunity is present if the titer is 1 : 8 or higher; because her titer is 1 : 6, this woman should receive rubella vaccination after giving birth. A titer of 1 : 6 indicates a *lack* of immunity, *not exposure* to rubella or a *history* of the disease (**1** and **2**). Breastfeeding (**4**) *can* continue after vaccination. NOTE: Before vaccination, the woman may be asked to sign an informed consent and verbalize that she understands that she must refrain from conceiving before 3 mo after vaccination, since rubella is teratogenic. Immune response may be inhibited if the woman has also received Rh$_o$GAM; her rubella titer must be rechecked at 3 mo to confirm that she has indeed developed antibodies against rubella, and she may need to be revaccinated. **EV, 1, HPM**

2. **(1)** Isoimmunization refers to the development of sensitivity in the human to antigens commonly found in other humans. Autoimmunization (**2**) refers to the development of antibodies against constituents of one's own tissues (e.g., a man may develop antibodies against his own sperm). AB antibodies (**3**) refer to blood type, not to the Rh factor. The immune globulin is given to prevent her from becoming Coombs *positive* (**4**), that is, to keep her from developing Rh antibodies. **PL, 1, SECE**

3. **(4)** Rh$_o$GAM destroys fetal Rh + erythrocytes in maternal blood. Once the woman is sensitized to the Rh factor, *nothing* will remove the antibodies (**1**); she will continue to be Coombs positive. It destroys fetal Rh +, *not* Rh$_o$ RBCs (**2**). *Nothing* deactivates maternal antibodies to the Rh factor (**3**); antibodies in fetal blood can *only* be removed with an exchange blood transfusion. **IMP, 6, HPM**

4. **(3)** Drugs used in substance abuse are not pure. The drugs are often mixed with a variety of other substances. The single or mixed combination of drugs is likely to pass into breast milk. Methods other than breastfeeding are to be used to encourage bonding (**1**). Babies are *not* weaned from the substance (**2**) by taking breastfeedings from their drug-dependent mothers. Most substances *do* pass into breast milk (**4**). **IMP, 4, HPM**

Key to Codes

Nursing process: AS, assessment; **AN,** analysis; **PL,** planning; **IMP,** implementation; **EV,** evaluation. (See Appendix I for explanation of nursing process steps.)

Category of human function: 1, protective; **2,** sensory-perceptual; **3,** comfort, rest, activity, and mobility; **4,** nutrition; **5,** growth and development; **6,** fluid-gas transport; **7,** psychosocial-cultural; **8,** elimination. (See Appendix K for explanation.)

Client need: SECE, safe, effective care environment; **PhI,** physiological integrity; **PsI,** psychosocial integrity; **HPM,** health promotion/maintenance. (See Appendix L for explanation.)

5. **(2)** Crash diets mobilize fats (where PCB is stored). If the level in milk is *high*, then breastfeeding should be discontinued, but discontinuation is unnecessary at trace levels **(1)**. Increased fluid intake **(3)** does *not* facilitate elimination of PCB. There *is* a recommended restriction **(4)**: She should *avoid* crash diets. **IMP, 4, SECE**

6. **(3)** The body attempts to rid itself of excess fluids, and fluids may be restricted during labor and birth; due to these dehydrating effects, the woman may develop a slight temperature elevation after giving birth. Anemia **(1)** and breast engorgement **(2)** (which would not occur until the *3rd* day) would *not* cause a rise in temperature. It is *too early* for a postpartum infection **(4)** to cause a rise in temperature. **AN, 6, HPM**

7. **(4)** A temperature of 38°C within the first 10 postpartum days, *excluding the first 24 hr,* is an indication of postpartum infection, and should be investigated. An increased sedimentation rate **(1)** is seen in *normal* pregnancy/postpartum period (a *decreased* rate is a sign of infection in the nonpregnant woman). The pulse **(2)** becomes *rapid*, weak, and easily compressible with infection. Lochia flow **(3)** *increases.* **EV, 1, SECE**

8. **(2)** Hydramnios (polyhydramnios) refers to amniotic fluid in excess of 1.5 liters; this excess fluid stretches the uterine muscle, decreasing its ability to retain its tone after birth. *None* of the histories in options **1, 3,** and **4** reflects a probable cause of postpartum hemorrhage. **AN, 6, HPM**

9. **(4)** The *most* common cause of postpartum hemorrhage is uterine atony. Lacerations **(1)** constitute the *second* most common cause of postpartum hemorrhage, and retained placental fragments **(3)** are the *third* most common cause. Subinvolution of the placental site **(2)** is an *infrequent* cause of postpartum hemorrhage; it is characterized by persistent lochia and episodes of brisk, painless bleeding. **PL, 6, HPM**

10. **(2)** Gentle massage will stimulate the living ligature to contract. Expulsion of clots **(1)** is only attempted *after* the fundus is firm; the lower part of the uterus is supported (with the nurse's other hand), to prevent turning the uterus inside out. Ambulation **(4)** to empty the bladder is the *third* step, after massage and expulsion of clots. An oxytocic **(3)** is given *only* when all other measures fail. **IMP, 6, PhI**

11. **(2)** Methergine (Ergotrate, ergonovine maleate) has an oxytocic effect. Parlodel (bromocriptine) **(1)** is an *antilactogenic* formerly used by some women who did not choose to breastfeed (it was taken *off the market* in 1995). Vitamin K **(3)** is given to *prevent hemolytic* disease in the newborn during the first 8 days of life (after that, the newborn's gut has sufficient bacteria to produce his or her own vitamin K). Rh$_o$GAM **(4)** is an immune globulin given to *Rh-negative mothers* who give birth to Rh-positive infants, and who are *Coombs negative,* to prevent Rh immunization. **IMP, 6, PhI**

12. **(2)** This type of bleeding suggests vaginal lacerations. Option **1** is incorrect because this type of bleeding *requires* further investigation. Option **3** is incorrect because, if the fundus is already firm, she does *not* need an oxytocic medication. Option **4** is incorrect because hematomas result from bleeding into an enclosed space; *no external* bleeding would be evident. **IMP, 1, SECE**

13. **(4)** A positive Coombs test means that the mother has been sensitized to the Rh factor; that is, she has already developed antibodies. An Rh-negative mother **(1)** may be a candidate for receiving Rh$_o$ (D) immune globulin. The Rh-negative mother who gives birth to an Rh-positive baby **(2)** *may* be a candidate to receive Rh$_o$ (D) immune globulin. An Rh-negative mother *may* be a candidate for receiving Rh$_o$ (D) immune globulin if a Coombs test on her Rh-positive baby is negative **(3)**. **AN, 1, SECE**

14. **(1)** If the pregnancy is at 8 wk or more, the Rh-negative woman is a candidate for Rh$_o$ (Du) immune globulin if she is Coombs negative (no titer of antibodies), even if this was her first pregnancy. Rh$_o$ (Du) immune globulin *is* a blood product **(2)**; the woman must be informed of this fact so that she can decide for herself. (NOTE: The process of preparing the immune globulin destroys any infectious microorganism the donor may have.) If both parents are Rh negative **(3)** and she has never had a blood transfusion, she will probably *not* need the medication. If her Coombs test is positive **(4)**, she has already been sensitized to the Rh factor; since the medication *cannot* reverse the sensitization, no medication is given. **AN, 6, PhI**

15. **(1)** Using gentle pressure on a firm fundus while supporting the uterus prevents the uterus from being turned inside out. *Vigorous* massage of the uterus **(2)** tires the muscle and results in relaxation of the living ligature and hemorrhage. Firm pressure downward on the uterine fundus **(3)** without supporting the base of the uterus can turn the uterus inside out, even if the fundus is firm. Pressure on a boggy fundus **(4)** can result in turning the uterus inside out. **IMP, 6, PhI**

16. **(2)** Subinvolution is the delayed return of the uterus to normal tone, size, shape, and position. The uterus is large and flabby, and lacks good tone; there is painless fresh bleeding with hemorrhagic episodes. Management consists of curettage, antibiotics, and oxytocin. The symptoms as given do *not* describe uterine atony **(1)**, which would include intermittent uterine relaxation with some "after pains"; uterine tone is achieved with gentle massage. The symptoms also do *not* describe hypofibrinogenemia **(3)**, which does not affect uterine tone. Symptoms of hypofibrinogenemia would be emergence of petechiae and bleeding gums; management would include IV infusion of heparin, platelets, and blood. With normal involution **(4)**, the uterus *does* contract with gentle massage; lochia gradually changes to serosa and amount decreases. **EV, 6, PhI**

The Newborn Infant

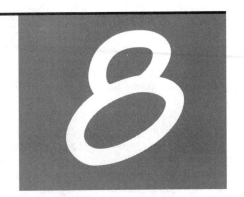

Chapter Outline

⚷ KEY POINTS

- At term gestation, the newborn's *anatomic* and *physiologic* systems have reached a level of development and functioning that supports a physical existence apart from the mother, and *sensory* capabilities that indicate a state of readiness for social interactions.
- Newborns require a *protective* environment, e.g., correct identification procedures, *safe restraining* techniques (including car seats), measures to *prevent infection*, and *support of physiologic functions*.
- Parents need to learn techniques to *safeguard* their newborns: CPR, maintaining a *patent airway*, knowledge of their *developmental/behavioral* characteristics, hygiene, *nutrition, cord* and *circumcision* care, and *prevention of infection* (including emphasis on *immunizations* and keeping scheduled medical appointments).
- Parents are entitled to know about newborn *nutrition and feeding:* the benefits of both breastfeeding and formula feeding; the powerful effect the partner's attitude toward breastfeeding has on achieving successful lactation; the need to avoid use of honey in home-prepared formulas (can be fatal if newborn is infected with botulism).

Key Words
(With definitions to facilitate reading of Table 8-1)

Acrocyanosis peripheral cyanosis; blue color of hands and feet in most infants at birth that may persist for *7–10* days.

Agenesis *A:* a prefix meaning un-, -less, lack, not; *-genesis:* a combining form denoting origination, development, evolution.

Caput succedaneum swelling of the tissue over the presenting part of the fetal head caused by pressure during labor; fluid is serum; swelling *crosses* suture lines.

Cephalohematoma extravasation of blood from ruptured vessels between a skull bone and its external covering, the periosteum; fluid is blood; swelling limited by the margins of the cranial bone affected; does *not* cross suture lines.

Ductus arteriosus in fetal circulation, an anatomic shunt between the pulmonary artery and arch of the aorta.

Erythema toxicum innocuous, pink, papular neonatal rash of unknown cause, appearing within *24–48* hr after birth and resolving spontaneously within a few days.

Foramen ovale septal opening between the atria of the fetal heart.

Imperforate without the normal opening.

Lanugo downy, fine hair characteristic of the fetus between *20 wk* gestation and birth that is most noticeable over the shoulder, forehead, and cheeks but is found on nearly all parts of the body (except the palms of the hands, soles of the feet, and the scalp).

Milia unopened sebaceous glands appearing as tiny, white, pinpoint papules on forehead, nose, cheeks, and chin of a neonate that disappear spontaneously in a *few days* or *weeks.*

Mongolian spot bluish-gray or dark, nonelevated pigmented area usually found over the lower back and buttocks, present at birth in some infants, primarily nonwhite.

Mottling variability of coloration (with distinct pattern) of newborn skin, secondary to an immature vascular system; a normal variation.

Periods of reactivity *first period* (within *30 min* after birth): brief cyanosis, flushing with crying; crackles, nasal flaring, grunting, retractions; heart sounds loud, forceful, irregular; alert; mucus; no bowel sounds; followed by period of sleep. *Second period* (*4–8 h* after birth): swift color changes; irregular respiratory and heart rates; mucus with gagging; meconium passage; and stabilizing temperature (Figure 8.1).

Phenylketonuria (PKU) recessive hereditary disease that results in a defect in the metabolism of the amino acid phenylalanine, caused by the lack of an enzyme, *phenylalanine hydroxylase*, that is necessary for the conversion of the amino acid phenylalanine into *tyrosine*. If untreated, brain damage may occur, causing severe mental retardation.

Physiologic jaundice hemolysis of excessive fetal RBCs in the early neonatal period; jaundice not apparent during first 24 h; nontoxic.

Pseudomenstruation bloody discharge from the newborn girl's vagina in response to maternal hormones during intrauterine life.

Pulmonary surfactant a phosphoprotein necessary for normal respiratory function that prevents alveolar collapse (*atelectasis*). (see also *lecithin* and *L/S ratio*).

Vernix caseosa protective gray-white fatty substance of cheesy consistency covering the fetal skin.

Vitamin K a necessary component for blood clotting; produced in the GI tract after the introduction of bacteria, starting at about *8 days* after birth.

Wharton's jelly white, gelatinous material surrounding the umbilical vessels within the cord.

Witch's milk secretion of a whitish fluid for about a *week* after birth from enlarged mammary tissue in the neonate, presumably resulting from maternal hormonal influences.

Wry neck (torticollis) congenital or acquired stiff neck caused by shortening or spasmodic contraction of the neck (sternocleidomastoid) muscles that draws the head to one side with the chin pointing in the other direction.

General overview: Effective nursing care of the newborn infant is based on: (1) knowledge of the conditions present during fetal life; (2) requirements for independent extrauterine life; and (3) alterations needed for successful transition (Figure 8.1). *The first 24 hr are the most hazardous.*

I. Biologic foundations of neonatal adaptation—*general aspects*
  A. Fetal anatomy and physiology
    1. *Fetal circulation*—four intrauterine structures, which differ from extrauterine structures (Figure 8.2)
      a. *Umbilical vein*—carries oxygen and nutrient-enriched blood from placenta to ductus venosus and liver. (*Ductus venosus*

—connects to inferior vena cava; allows most blood to bypass liver.)
      b. *Foramen ovale*—allows fetal blood to bypass fetal lungs by shunting it from right atrium into left atrium.
      c. *Ductus arteriosus*—allows fetal blood to bypass fetal lungs by shunting it from pulmonary artery into aorta.
      d. *Umbilical arteries* (two)—allow return of deoxygenated blood to the placenta.
    2. *Umbilical cord*—extends from fetus to center of placenta; usually 50 cm (18–22 in.) long and 1–2 cm (½–1 in.) in diameter. Contains:
      a. *Wharton's jelly*—protects umbilical vessels from pressure, cord "kinking," and interference with fetal-placental circulation.
      b. Umbilical vein—carries oxygen and nutrients from placenta to fetus.
      c. Two umbilical arteries—carry deoxygenated blood and fetal wastes from fetus to placenta. NOTE: Absence of one artery indicates need to rule out intraabdominal anomalies.
    3. *Characteristics of fetal blood*
      a. Fetal hemoglobin (Hb_f)
        (1) Higher oxygen-carrying capacity than adult hemoglobin.
        (2) Releases oxygen easily to fetal tissues.
        (3) Ensures high fetal oxygenation.
        (4) *Normal range at term: 12–22 g/dL; average: 15–20 g/dL.*
      b. Total blood volume at term: 85 mL/kg body weight; Hct: 38–62%, average 53%; RBC 3–7 million, average 4.9 million/unit.
  B. Extrauterine adaptation: tasks
    1. Establish and maintain ventilation, successful gas transfer—requires patent airway and adequate **pulmonary surfactant.**
    2. Modify circulatory patterns—requires closure of fetal structures.
    3. Absorb and utilize fluids and nutrients.
    4. Excrete body wastes.
    5. Establish and maintain thermal stability.
  C. Nursing care plan
    1. Facilitate successful transition to independent life.
    2. Protect infant from physiologic stress and environmental hazards.
    3. Encourage development of a strong family unit.

II. Normal newborn experience
  A. Assessment of normal, term neonate
    1. Review antepartum, intrapartum, and recovery period events.
    2. Color and reactivity.
    3. General appearance, symmetry.
    4. Length and weight.
    5. Head and chest circumference.
    6. Vital signs
      a. Axillary temperature.

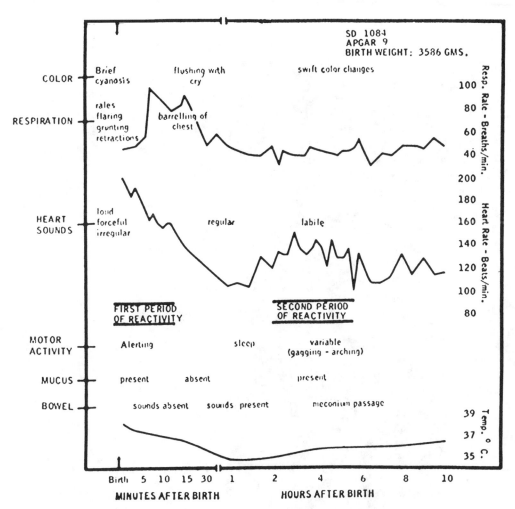

SD 1084
APGAR 9
BIRTH WEIGHT: 3586 GMS.

FIGURE 8.1 **NORMAL TRANSITION PERIOD.** (From M Desmond, A Rudolph, P Phitakspharaiwan. *Pediatr Clin North Am* 13:651, 1996.)

   b. Respirations (check rate, character, rhythm).

   Respiratory warning signs
   (1) Abnormal rate
      Bradypnea: respirations $\leq$ 25/min.
      Tachypnea: respirations $\geq$ 60/min.
   (2) Abnormal breath sounds: crackles (rales), wheezes (rhonchi), expiratory grunt.
   (3) Respiratory distress: nasal flaring, retractions, chin tug, costal breathing, cyanosis.

   c. Apical pulse.
7. General physical assessment (Table 8.1; see *Glossary* at front of chapter for selected terms and their definitions) and *reflexes* (Table 8.2).
8. Estimate of gestational age (Table 8.3).
B. Analysis/nursing diagnosis
   1. *Altered health maintenance* related to separation from maternal support system.
   2. *Impaired skin integrity* related to umbilical stump; incontinence of urine and meconium

stool; skin penetration by scalp electrode, injections, heel stick, scalpel during cesarean birth; abrasion from obstetric forceps.
3. *Ineffective airway clearance* related to excessive mucus.
4. *Pain* related to environmental stimuli.
5. *Ineffective thermoregulation* related to immature temperature regulation mechanism.
C. Nursing care plan/implementation
   1. Goal: *promote effective gas transport*
      a. Maintain patent airway—to promote effective gas exchange and respiratory function.
      b. *Position:* right side lying, head dependent (gravity drainage of fluid, mucus).
      c. Suction for mucus, prn, with bulb syringe or DeLee suction (Figure 8.3), which meets protocol for universal precautions.
   2. Goal: *establish/maintain thermal stability*
      a. *Avoid* chilling—to prevent metabolic acidosis.
      b. Dry, wrap, and apply hat.
      c. Place in heated crib.

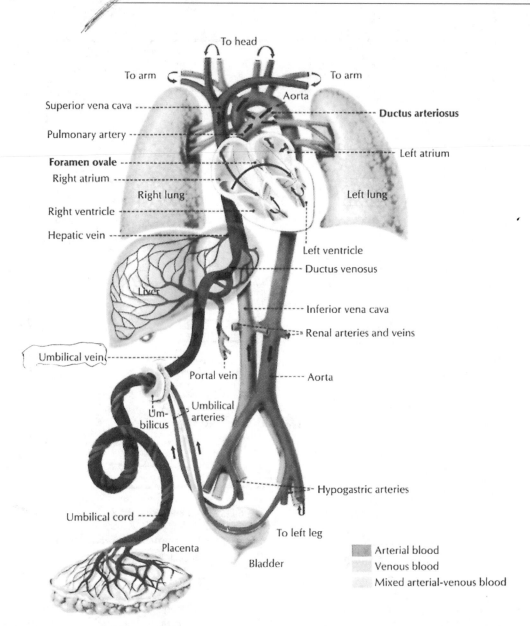

FIGURE 8.2 **FETAL CIRCULATION:** The *foramen ovale and the ductus arteriosus act as bypass channels,* allowing a large part of the combined cardiac output to perfuse body tissues without flowing through the lungs. (Courtesy Ross Laboratories, Columbus, OH.)

  d. Monitor vital signs hourly until stable.
3. Goal: *reduce possibility of blood loss*
  a. Check cord clamp for security.
  b. Administer vitamin K injection, as ordered, in anterior or lateral thigh muscle—to stimulate blood coagulability (Figure 8.4).
4. Goal: *prevent infection*
  a. Administer antibiotic treatment to eyes (if not performed in birth room)—to prevent ophthalmia neonatorum.
  b. Treat cord stump (alcohol, Triple Dye antibiotic ointment), as ordered.
  c. Use universal precautions.

5. Goal: *promote comfort and cleanliness.* Admission bath when temperature stable.
6. Goal: *promote nutrition, hydration, elimination.*
  a. Encourage breastfeeding immediately after birth.
  b. Check blood sugar (Dextrostix or Chem-strip) at 30 min, 1, 2, and 4 hr for infants at risk for hypoglycemia (e.g., small for gestational age [SGA], large for gestational age [LGA]). See Figure 8.5 for acceptable puncture sites for heel stick.
  c. First feeding at 1–4 hr of age with *sterile*

TABLE 8.1 ⋈ Physical Assessment of the Term Neonate[a]

Criterion	Average Values and Normal Variations	Deviations from Normal
Vital signs		
Heart rate	120–140/min, irregular, especially when crying, and functional murmur	Faint sound—pneumomediastinum; and heart rate <100 or >180/min
Respiratory rate	30–60/min with short periods of apnea, irregular; cry—vigorous and loud	Distress—flaring of nares, retractions, tachypnea, grunting, excessive mucus, <30 or >60/min; cyanosis
Temperature	Stabilizes about 8–10 hr after birth; 36.5–37°C (97.7–98.6°F) axillary	Unreliable indicator of infection
Blood pressure	80/46; varies with change in activity level	Hypotension: with RDS Hypertension: coarctation of aorta
Measurements		
Weight	3400 g (7½ lb)	Birth weight <2500 g: preterm or SGA infant; >4000 g: LGA infant, evaluate mother for gestational diabetes
Length	50 cm (20 in.)	
Chest circumference	2 cm (¾ in.) less than head circumference	If relationship varies, check for reason
Head circumference	33–35 cm (13–14 in.)	Check for microcephalus and macrocephalus
General assessment		
Muscle tone	Good tone and generalized flexion; full range of motion; spontaneous movement	Flaccid, and persistent tremor or twitching; movement limited; asymmetric
Skin color	Mottling, *acrocyanosis*, and physiologic jaundice; petechia (over presenting part), milia, mongolian spotting, lanugo, and vernix caseosa; erythema toxicum ("newborn rash")	Pallor, cyanosis, or jaundice within 24 hr of birth Pethechiae or ecchymoses elsewhere; all rashes, except erythema toxicum; pigmented nevi; hemangioma; and yellow vernix
Head	Molding of fontanels and suture spaces; comprises ¼ of body length	*Cephalohematoma, caput succedaneum,* sunken or bulging fontanels, closed sutures; excessively wide sutures
Hair	Silky, single strands; lies flat; grows toward face and neck	Fine, wooly; unusual swirls, patterns, hair line; coarse
Eyes	Edematous eyelids, conjunctival hemorrhage; grayish-blue to grayish-brown in color; *blink reflex;* usually no tears; uncoordinated movements may focus for a few seconds; good placement on face; cornea is bright and shiny; pupillary reflex equal and reactive to light; eyebrows distinct	Epicanthal folds (in non-Asians); discharges; agenesis; opaque lenses; lesions; strabismus; *"doll's eyes"* beyond 10 days; absence of reflexes Gonorrhea: *Ophthalmia neonatorum* appears about 3–4 d after birth *Chlamydia trachomatis:* Conjunctivitis (congestion and edema) with minimal drainage develops 5 d–2 wk after birth
Nose	Appears to have no bridge; should have no discharge; preferential nose breathers; sneezes to clear nose	Discharge and choanal atresia; malformed; flaring of nares beyond first few moments of life
Mouth	*Epstein's pearls* on gum ridges; tongue does not protrude and moves freely, symmetrically; uvula in midline; reflexes present: sucking, rooting, gag, extrusion	*Cleft lip or palate;* teeth; cyanosis, circumoral pallor; asymmetric lip movement; excessive saliva; *thrush;* incomplete or absent reflexes
Ears	Well formed, firm; notch of ear should be on straight line with outer canthus	Low placement, clefts; tags; malformed; lack of cartilage
Face	Symmetric movements and contours	Facial palsy (7th cranial nerve); looks "funny"

(continued)

TABLE 8.1   PHYSICAL ASSESSMENT OF THE TERM NEONATE[a] (Continued)

Criterion	Average Values and Normal Variations	Deviations from Normal
Neck	Short, freely movable; some head control	Wry neck, webbed neck; restricted movement; masses; distended veins; absence of head control
Chest	Enlarged breasts, "witch's milk"; barrel-shaped; both sides move synchronously; nipples symmetrical	Flattened, funnel-chested, asynchronous movement; lack of breast tissue; fracture of clavicle(s); supernumerary or widely spaced nipples; bowel sounds
Abdomen	Dome-shaped, abdominal respirations; soft; may have small umbilical hernia; umbilical cord well formed, containing 3 vessels; dry around base; bowel sounds within 2 hr of birth; voiding; passage of meconium	Scaphoid-shaped, omphalocele, diastasis recti, and distention; umbilical cord containing 2 vessels; redness or drainage around base of cord
Genitalia		
Female	Large labia; may have pseudomenstruation, smegma; vaginal orifice open; increased pigmentation; ecchymosis and edema following breech birth; pink-stained urine (uric acid crystals)	Agenesis and imperforate hymen; ambiguous labia widely separated, fecal discharge per vagina; epispadias or hypospadias
Male	Pendulous scrotum covered with rugae, and testes usually descended; voids with adequate stream; increased pigmentation; edema and ecchymosis following breech birth	Phimosis, epispadias, or hypospadias; ambiguous; scrotum smooth and testes undescended
Hydrocele: collection of fluid in the sac surrounding the testes
Extremeties	Synchronized movements, freely movable through full range of motion; legs appear bowed, and feet appear flat; attitude of general flexion; arms longer than legs; grasp reflex; palmar and sole creases; normal contour	Fractures, Erb-Duchenne paralysis (Flaccid arm with elbow extended), brachial nerve palsy, clubbed foot, phocomelia or amelia, unusual number or webbing of digits, and abnormal palmar creases; poor muscle tone; asymmetry; hypertonicity; unusual hip contour and click sign (hip dysplasia); hypermobility of joints
Back	Spine straight, easily movable, and flexible; may have small pilonidal dimple at base of spine; may raise head when prone	Fusion of vertebrae; pilonidal dimple with tuft of hair; spina bifida, agenesis of part of vertebral bodies; limitation of movement; weak or absent reflexes
Anus	Patent, well placed; "wink" reflex	Imperforate, and absence of "wink" (absence of sphincter muscle); fistula
Stools	Meconium within 24 hr; transitional—days 2–5; breastfed: loose, golden yellow; bottlefed: formed, light yellow	Light-colored meconium (dry, hard), or absent with distended abdomen (cystic fibrosis or Hirschsprung's disease); diarrhetic
〰 Laboratory values		
Hemoglobin (cord)	13.6–19.6 g/dL	Evaluate for anemia and persistent polycythemia
Serum bilirubin	2–6 mg/dL	Hyperbilirubinemia (term: 12 mg or more; preterm: 15 mg or more)
Blood glucose	>30–40 mg/dL for term; >20 mg/dL for preterm	Identify hypoglycemia before overt or asymptomatic hypoglycemia—do blood glucose on all suspects (large- or small-for-gestational-age neonates, or neonates of diabetic mothers)

(continued)

TABLE 8.1   PHYSICAL ASSESSMENT OF THE TERM NEONATE[a] (*Continued*)

Criterion	Average Values and Normal Variations	Deviations from Normal
Neurologic examination[b]	Specific to gestational age and state of wakefulness	
1. Behavioral patterns		
a. Feeding	Variations in interest, hunger; usually feeds well within 48 hr	Lethargic; poor suck, poor coordination with swallow, choking, cyanosis
b. Social	Crying is lusty, strong, and soon indicative of hunger, pain, attention-seeking; responds to cuddling, voice by quietness and increased alertness	Absent; no focusing on person holding him/her; unconsolable
c. Sleep-wakefulness	Two periods of reactivity: at birth, and 6–8 h later; stabilization, with wakeful periods about every 3–4 hr	Lethargy, drowsiness Disorganized pattern

d. Elimination	Stooling: see *Stools*
	Urination:
	  first few days: 3–4 qd
	  end of first week: 5–6 qd
	  later: 6–10 qd, with adequate hydration
		See *Stools*
		Diminished number: dehydration

2. Reflex response	Bilateral, symmetric response (see Table 8.2)	Absent, hyperactive, incomplete, asynchronous
3. Sensory capabilities		
a. Vision	Limited accomodation, with clearest vision within 7–8 in; focuses and follows by 15 min of age; prefers patterns to plain	Absence of these responses may be due to absence of or diminished acuity or to sensory deprivation
b. Hearing	By 2 min of age, can move in direction of sound: responds to high pitch by "freezing," followed by agitation; to low pitch (crooning) by relaxing	Absence of response: deafness
c. Touch	Soothed by massaging, warmth, weightlessness (as in water bath)	Unable to be comforted: possible drug dependence Cocaine-addicted newborns avoid eye contact
d. Smell	By 5th day, can distinguish between mother's breasts and those of another woman	
e. Taste	Can distinguish between sweet and sour	
f. Motor	Coordinates body movement to parent's voice and body movement	Absence

RDS = respiratory distress syndromes; SGA = small for gestational age; LGA = large for gestational age.

[a]**See Glossary at front of chapter for definitions of selected terms used in this table.**

[b]Based on Brazelton's method.

---

water if permissible, and if not breast-feeding.

  d. Note voiding and/or meconium stool; report failure to void or defecate within 24 hr.

 🍎 **e.** Teach parents newborn's *nutrient* and *fluid* needs

    (1) Calories—115 kcal/kg/d.*

    (2) Protein—3.5 g/kg/d (1 g protein = 1 oz milk).

    (3) Fluids—3.5 oz (105 mL)*/kg/24 hr.

    (4) Vitamin D—400 IU/d for bottle-fed babies after week 2.

    (5) Fluoride—0.25 mg/d regardless of content in local water supply.

7. Goal: *promote bonding*

  a. Encourage parent-infant interaction (holding, touching, eye contact, talking to infant).

  b. Encourage breastfeeding within 1 h of birth, if applicable.

  c. Encourage parent participation in infant care—to develop confidence and competence in caring for newborn

*1 oz = 30 mL; 2.2 pounds = 1 kg.

TABLE 8.2   ☛ ASSESSMENT: NORMAL NEWBORN REFLEXES*

Reflex	Description	Implications of Deviations from Normal Pattern
Moro (startle)	Symmetric *abduction* and *extension* of arms with fingers extended in response to sudden movement or loud noise	Asymmetric reflex may indicate brachial (*Erb's*) palsy or fractured clavicle
Tonic neck (fencing)	When head turned to one side, arm and leg on *that* side *extend,* and *opposite* arm and leg *flex*	Asymmetry may indicate cerebral lesion, if persistent
Rooting and sucking	With stimulus to cheek, turns *toward* stimulus, opens mouth, sucks	Absence of response may indicate prematurity, neurologic problem, or depressed infant (or not hungry)
Palmar grasp	If palm stimulated, fingers *curl;* holds adult finger briefly	Asymmetry may indicate neurologic involvement
Plantar grasp	Pressure on sole will elicit *curling* of toes	Absence/asymmetry associated with defects of lower spinal column
Stepping/dancing	If held in upright position with feet in contact with hard surface, alternately raises feet	Asymmetry may indicate neurologic problem
Babinski	Stroking the sole in an upward fashion elicits *hyperextension* of toes	Same as for plantar grasp
Crawling	When placed in prone position, attempts to crawl	Absence may indicate prematurity or depressed infant

*NOTE: Reflexes are good indicators of the neurologic system in well infants but not in sick neonates. Infants with infections may not show normal reflexes yet have an intact neurologic system.

☛ (1) Assist with initial efforts at feeding.
☛ (2) Discuss and demonstrate positioning and burping techniques.
☛ (3) Demonstrate/assist with basic care procedures, as necessary
    (a) Bath.
    (b) Cord care.
    (c) Diapering.
    (d) Aid parents in distinguishing normal versus abnormal newborn characteristics.

8. Goal: *health teaching*—to provide anticipatory guidance for discharge
  a. Facilitate sibling bonding.
  b. Describe/discuss normal newborn behavior
    (1) *Sleeping*—almost continual (wakes only to feed) or 12–16 h/d.
    (2) *Feeding*—from every 2–3 h to longer intervals; establish own pattern; breast-fed babies feed more often.
    (3) *Weight loss*—5–10% in first few days; regained in 7–14 days.
    (4) *Stools*—see Table 8.4.
    (5) *Physiologic jaundice*—occurs 24–72 h postbirth
      (a) Nonpathologic.
      (b) Need for hydration.
  c. Demonstrate **cord care**—drops off in 7–10 d.
    (1) Keep clean and dry.

    (2) Alcohol to stump.
    (3) Human immunodeficiency virus (HIV) precautions.
  d. Demonstrate **circumcision care**
    (1) Keep clean and dry; heals rapidly.
    (2) Watch for bleeding.
    (3) Petroleum jelly, gauze, prn, if ordered.
    (4) Do *not* remove yellowish exudate.
  e. Identify need for biochemical tests for inborn errors of metabolism—see Figure 8.5, *Heel stick.* (These tests are mandatory in most states; if parents prefer these tests not be done, they need to sign an informed consent.)
    (1) Phenylketonuria (PKU), after ingestion of milk.
    (2) Galactosemia.
    (3) Thyroxine (T_4) for hypothyroidism.
  f. Describe suggested sensory *stimulation* modalities (mobiles, color, music).
  g. Discuss *safety* precautions
    (1) Infant seat for travel and home safety.
    (2) Maintaining contact/control over infant to prevent falls, drowning in bath.
    (3) Instruct parents in infant CPR (Figure 8.6, p. 177)
☛   • Place mouth over mouth and nose of newborn; repeat word *ho* as you gently puff volume of air from your cheeks into infant; *do not force air.*

TABLE 8.3   ESTIMATION OF GESTATIONAL AGE—COMMON CLINICAL PARAMETERS

Characteristic	*Preterm*	*Term*
Head	Oval—narrow biparietal; large in proportion to body; face looks like "old man"; soft, flat, shapeless	Square-shaped biparietal prominences; ¼ body length
Ears: form, cartilage	Soft, flat, shapeless	Pinna firm; erect from head
Hair: texture, distribution	Fine, fuzzy, or wooly; clumped; appears at 20 wk	Silky; single strands apparent
Sole creases	Starting at ball of foot, ⅓ covered with creases by 36 wk; ⅔ by 38 wk	Entire sole heavily creased
Breast nodules	0 mm at 36 wk; 4 mm at 37 wk	10 mm or more
Nipples	No areolae	Formed; raised above skin level
Genitalia		
Female	Clitoris large, labia gaping	Labia larger, meet in midline
Male	Small scrotum, rugae on inferior surface only, and testes undescended	Scrotum pendulous, covered with rugae; testes usually descended
Skin: texture, opacity	Visible abdominal veins; thin, shiny	Few indistinct larger veins; thick, dry, cracked, peeling
Vernix	Covers body by 31–33 wk	Small amount or absent at term; postterm: dry, wrinkled
Lanugo	Apparent at 20 wk; by 33–36 wk, covers shoulders	Minimal or no lanugo
Muscle tone	Hypotonia; extension of arms and legs	Hypertonia; well flexed
Posture	Froglike	Attitude of general flexion
Head lag	Head lags; arms have little or no flexion	Head follows trunk; strong arm flexion
Scarf sign	Elbow can extend to opposite axilla	Elbow to midline only; infant resists
Square window	90 degrees	0 degrees
Ankle dorsiflexion	90 degrees	0 degrees
Popliteal angle	180 degrees	<90 degrees
Heel-to-ear maneuver	Touches ear easily	90 degrees
Ventral suspension	Hypotonia; "rag-doll"	Good caudal and cephalic tone
Reflexes		
Moro	Apparent at 28 wk; good, but no adduction	Complete reflex with adduction; disappears 4 mo postterm
Grasp	Fair at 28 wk; arm is involved at 32 wk	Strong enough to sustain weight for a few seconds when pulled up; hand, arm, shoulder involved
Cry	24 wk: weak; 28 wk: high-pitched; 32 wk: good	Lusty; can persist for some time
Length	Under 47 cm (18½ in.), usually	50 cm (20 in.)
Weight	Under 2500 g (5 lb 5 oz)	3400 g (7½ lb)

- *Compressions:* using two or three fingers, compress sternum to depth of ½–¾ in.; repeat at a rate of at least 100 times/min; five compressions in 3 sec or less, pausing at end of each compression to allow chest to fall by passive recoil; one breath. Reassess after every 20 cycles of 5:1.
- *Discontinue:* when infant's spontaneous heart rate reaches or exceeds 80 beats/min.

 (4) Instruct parents in relieving airway obstruction for infants of 1 yr of age or younger (Figure 8.7, p. 178) *NO HEIMLICH MANEUVER. USE NO BLIND FINGER SWEEPS.* Initiate back blows and chest thrusts.

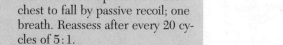

- *Back blows:* deliver up to five back blows forcefully between infant's shoulder blades with heel of free hand. Turn infant over (while supporting neck and head) and provide up to five quick, downward chest thrusts to same location as chest compressions.

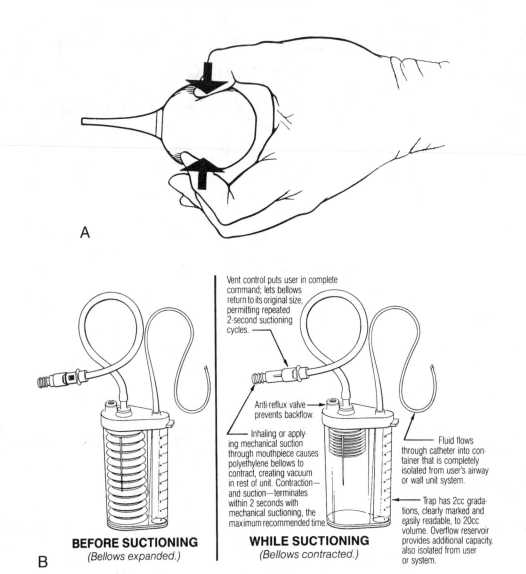

FIGURE 8.3   **Suction devices.** (A) Bulb syringe. Compress bulb before inserting. (From NL Caroline. *Emergency Care in the Streets* (5th ed). Boston: Little, Brown, 1995. P 865.) (B) (Isolated) DeLee suction method with catheter and mucus trap. (Courtesy Busse Hospital Disposables, PO Box 011067, Hauppauge, NY 11788-0920.)

- *Open airway:* head-tilt/chin lift, and ventilate.
- *Discontinue:* signs of recovery— palpable peripheral pulses, return of pupils to normal size and responsiveness, and disappearance of mottling and cyanosis.

    h. Describe signs of *common health problems,* to be reported promptly:
      (1) Diarrhea, constipation.
      (2) Colic, vomiting.
      (3) Fever.
      (4) Signs of inflammation and/or infection at cord stump.

      (5) Bleeding at circumcision site.
      (6) Rash, jaundice.
      (7) Deviation from normal patterns.
    D. Evaluation/outcome criteria
     1. *Infant* demonstrates successful transition to independent life:
      a. Nurses well.
      b. Normal feeding, sleeping, elimination patterns.
      c. No evidence of infection or abnormality.
     2. *Mother/family* evidence bonding
      a. Eye contact.
      b. Stroking, cuddling.
      c. Crooning, calling baby by name, talking to infant.

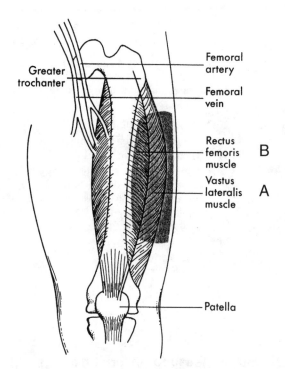

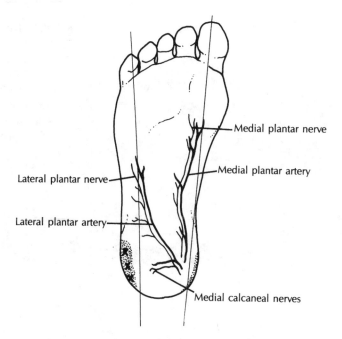

FIGURE 8.4 **ACCEPTABLE INTRAMUSCULAR INJECTION SITE:** Lateral aspect of muscle mass in middle third of distance between greater trochanter and patella. (A) Preferred injection site in vastus lateralis muscle. (B) Alternate injection site in rectus femoris muscle. (From IM Bobak, MD Jensen. *Maternity and Gynecologic Care: The Nurse and the Family* (5th ed). St. Louis: Mosby, 1993. P 599.)

FIGURE 8.5 **PUNCTURE SITES** (*x*) on infant's foot for heel stick samples of capillary blood. The newborn's foot is wrapped for warmth to increase blood flow to extremity before heel stick. (From IM Bobak, DL Lowdermilk, MD Jensen. *Maternity Nursing* (4th ed). St. Louis: Mosby, 1995, P 390.)

3. *Mother* demonstrates comfort and skill in basic newborn care.
4. *Mother* verbalizes understanding of subjects discussed:
   a. Safety precautions.
   b. Health maintenance actions.
   c. Signs of normal infant behavior and health.
5. Evaluate: *Criteria for early discharge* (see also *Criteria for early discharge, mother,* in Chapter 6, p. 145).

Criteria for Early Discharge

Infant

Term infant (38–41 wk) with birth weight of 2500–4500 g°

Normal findings on physical assessment performed by physician°

Normal laboratory data, including negative *Coombs* test result and hematocrit 40–65%°

Stable vital signs°

Temperature stability°
Successful feeding (normal sucking and swallowing)°
Apgar score >7 at 1 and 5 min
Normal voiding and stooling
PKU and *thyroid* screening tests completed; repeat of PKU test scheduled for 2 wk°

General

Attendance at classes that include maternal and infant care, with an emphasis on problems of the first week at home°

Presence of a support person in the home to assist with care°

Presence of a strategy for follow-up°

Uncomplicated pregnancy, labor, birth, and postpartum course for mother and baby°

Demonstration of skill by mother in feeding, providing skin and cord care, measuring temperature with a thermometer, assessing infant well-being and signs of illness, and providing emergency care°

°Recommendations of American Academy of Pediatrics: Criteria for early infant discharge and follow-up evaluation. *Pediatrics* 65:651, 1980.
From IM Bobak, DL Lowdermilk, MD Jensen. *Maternity Nursing* (4th ed). St. Louis: Mosby, 1995. P 507.

TABLE 8.4   INFANT STOOL CHARACTERISTICS

Age	Bottle-fed	Breastfed	Implications of Abnormal Patterns
1 day	Meconium	Meconium	Absence may indicate obstruction, atresia
2–5 days (transitional)	Greenish-yellow; loose	Greenish-yellow; loose, frequent	NOTE: At any time: *Diarrhea*—greenish, mucus or blood-tinged, or forceful expulsion, may indicate infection *Constipation*—dry, hard stools or infrequent or absent stools may indicate obstruction
>5 days	Yellow to brown; firm; 2–4/d; foul odor	Bright golden yellow, loose; 6–10/d	

Summary

It is of utmost importance that the nursery nurse be highly skilled in assessment of the neonate—the life and the quality of life of this child can be affected for years to come by the timely identification and treatment of deviations from the norm. The biologic foundations of *neonatal adaptation, fetal anatomy and physiology, extrauterine adaptations,* and nursing goals are presented in this chapter. The nursing process as implemented with the newborn includes guidelines for nurses' hands-on care and teaching the parents about the new member of the family. Teaching topics include *CPR* and relieving *airway obstruction* in the infant of 1 yr of age or less. *Criteria for early discharge* are listed.

Study and Memory Aids

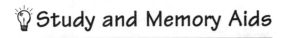

Newborn Nutrient Needs—Recommended Energy Intake

Newborns, 0–6 mo 115 kcal/kg
Infants, 6–12 mo 105 kcal/kg

Newborn—Fluid Maintenance Requirements

Age	Qty/Feeding	Feedings/24 h
Birth–3 wk	2–3 oz (60–90 mL)	6–10
3 wk–2 mo	5 oz (150 mL)	5–8
2–3 mo	5–7 oz (150–210 mL)	5–6

Newborn—Tests for Inborn Errors of Metabolism

PKU
Galactosemia
Hypothyroidism

Questions

1. During a prenatal class for adolescents, the discussion turns to concerns about how the unborn baby breathes "under water." The nurse's reassurance is based on knowledge that during fetal circulation, two fetal structures allow fetal blood to bypass fetal lungs; these are the:
   1. Umbilical vein and ductus venosus.
   2. Foramen ovale and ductus arteriosus.
   3. Umbilical artery and atrial septal shunt.
   4. Ductus venosus and ductus arteriosus.
2. Risk management, a standard for nursing care, requires the nurse to evaluate all assessment findings. The nurse must know that within 3 min of birth, the normal newborn's heart rate may range from:
   1. 100–130.
   2. 110–180.
   3. 120–160.
   4. 130–170.
3. The nurse assesses the Apgar score of a newborn at 1 and 5 min of age based on the following findings: heart rate—118; muscle tone—maintains attitude of general flexion; respirations—lusty cry; reflex response—active at +2; color—pink with some acrocyanosis. What score should the nurse enter on the newborn's records?

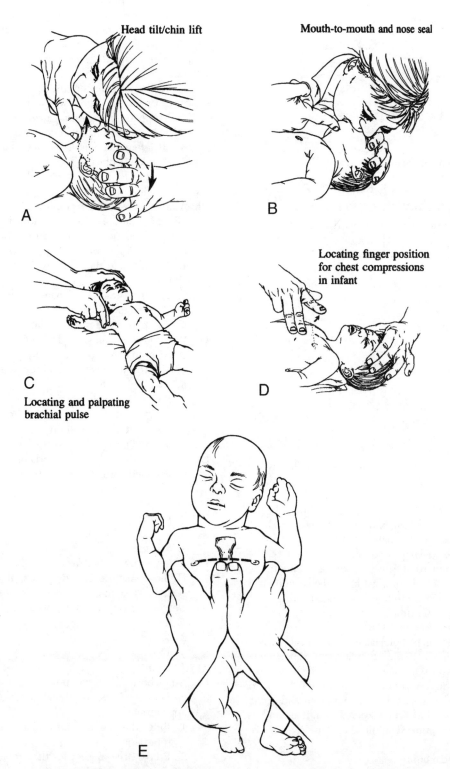

FIGURE 8.6 **(A–D) PROCEDURES FOR CARDIOPULMONARY RESUSCITATION.** (From Guidelines for cardiopulmonary resuscitation [CPR] and emergency cardiac care [ECC]. *JAMA* 286:2171, 1992. (E) When two rescuers are present, use your thumbs side by side, placed just below an imaginary line drawn between the two nipples. (From N Caroline. *Emergency Care in the Streets* (5th ed). Boston: Little, Brown, 1995. P 885.)

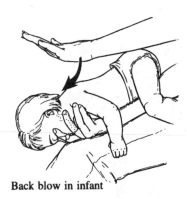

Back blow in infant

FIGURE 8.7 **BACK BLOW IN INFANT FOR CLEARING AIRWAY OBSTRUCTION.** (From Guidelines for cardiopulmonary resuscitation [CPR] and emergency cardiac care [ECC]. *JAMA* 286:2171, 1992.)

    1. 7.
    2. 8.
    3. 9.
    4. 10.

4. The nurse tests the newborn's Babinski reflex by:
    1. Touching the corner of the newborn's mouth or cheek.
    2. Changing the newborn's equilibrium.
    3. Placing a finger in the palm of the newborn's hand.
    4. Stroking the lateral aspect of the sole from the heel upward and across the ball of the foot.

5. The nurse tests a newborn for the rooting reflex by:
    1. Touching the corner of the newborn's mouth or cheek.
    2. Placing a finger in the palm of the newborn's hand.
    3. Stroking the lateral aspect of the sole from the heel upward and across the ball of the foot.
    4. Changing the newborn's equilibrium.

6. To meet the standard of care for risk management, the nurse assessing a newborn must know that asymmetric Moro reflex responses are often associated with:
    1. Injury to the cerebrum or cerebellum.
    2. Injury to cranial nerve VII.
    3. Injury to the brachial plexus, clavicle, or humerus.
    4. Poor muscle tone secondary to a genetic aberration such as Down's syndrome.

7. A new mother questions the nurse about the "lump" on her baby's head. She says that the physician told her it was "a collection of blood between a skull bone and its covering" (periosteum). The nurse explains that this is called:
    1. Caput succedaneum.
    2. Molding.
    3. Cephalohematoma.
    4. Subdural hematoma.

8. The home health nurse notices that a newborn has developed purulent conjunctivitis on the sixth day. At this time, the nurse:
    1. Calls the physician for an order to test the infant for allergy.

    2. Assesses the infant for signs of pneumonia.
    3. Demonstrates for the mother how to bathe the infant's eyes with tepid boric acid solution.
    4. Asks the mother if an older sibling has a cold.

9. The nurse must intervene when, after checking the parent's understanding regarding circumcision, the parent states:
    1. "Yellowish crusting (exudate) is normal within 24 hr of the circumcision, so I won't worry if I see any."
    2. "Applying petrolatum gauze wrap will keep the healing wound from sticking to the diaper."
    3. "Brief application of a wrapped ice pack is recommended if bleeding is seen."
    4. "Using cloth diapers will help me see if there is any bleeding."

10. A neonate weighed 7 pounds, 15 oz (3600 g) at birth; at discharge on the second day after birth, the neonate weighs 7 pounds, 8 oz (3402 g). What would be a valid interpretation of the neonate's current condition?
    1. The neonate should show weight gain instead of loss.
    2. The new mother is having trouble breastfeeding.
    3. The weight loss is within normal limits.
    4. The neonate is retaining fluid.

11. When parents question the need for a newborn to receive an injection of vitamin K soon after birth, the nurse's response is based on the knowledge that vitamin K_1 is given to:
    1. Promote hematopoiesis.
    2. Promote synthesis of clotting factors.
    3. Stimulate the formation of platelets.
    4. Stimulate the release of stored iron.

12. Which of the following criteria of gestational age must be assessed within 2 hr of birth for the results to be valid?
    1. Breast tissue.
    2. Posture.
    3. Sole of feet creases.
    4. Scarf sign.

13. A newborn weighed 7 pounds, 8 oz at birth 3 days ago. He now weighs 6 pounds, 12 oz; his mother is concerned. The nurse can assure his mother that her son's weight loss is still within normal limits if he loses up to:
    1. 9 oz.
    2. 12 oz.
    3. 15 oz.
    4. 18 oz.

14. A newborn's head circumference is 34 cm; chest circumference is 32 cm. Which nursing action would be appropriate?
    1. Refer the newborn for evaluation for psychomotor retardation.
    2. Prepare the mother for the probability that the physician will want to transilluminate the cranial vault.
    3. Measure the occipitofrontal circumference daily.
    4. Record the findings and take no further action.

15. A newborn is admitted to the nursery 15 min after birth. He is moderately cyanotic, has a mottled trunk and active movements of the extremities, and is wrapped in a cotton blanket. The *primary* assessment by the nurse would be to check:

1. The umbilical stump for bleeding.
2. The baby's temperature.
3. For visible abnormalities.
4. For a patent airway.

16. Suctioning the newborn should follow which procedure?
    1. Suction mouth first, then nose.
    2. Suction nose first, then mouth.
    3. Milk the trachea first, then proceed with suctioning.
    4. Smartly slap the infant's back, then proceed with a bulb syringe or catheter.

17. If bleeding is noted from a newly circumcised penis, the nurse's initial response should be to:
    1. Apply a diaper tightly over the penis to maintain a steady pressure.
    2. Notify the physician immediately.
    3. Apply gentle pressure to the bleeding site with a folded gauze pad.
    4. Wrap the glans penis in a fresh sterile petrolatum gauze and observe for 2 hr.

18. A 5-hr-old newborn boy wakes up in his mother's room, spits up some mucus and has a gagging episode. The nurse's *first* action is to:
    1. Sit him upright and pat his back.
    2. Immediately take him to the nursery for suctioning.
    3. Help his mother hold him face down with his head lower than his buttocks.
    4. Reassure his mother that this is normal at this age, and the baby needs no assistance.

Answers/Rationale

1. **(2)** The foramen ovale and ductus arteriosus are the two fetal structures that allow fetal blood to bypass the fetal lungs; oxygen is obtained from maternal circulation to placenta to umbilical vein. Because only these structures allow fetal blood to bypass fetal lungs, options **1, 3,** and **4** each contain at least one incorrect structure. **IMP, 5, HPM**

2. **(3)** The normal range is 120–160. The rate varies with activity, increasing to 160 while crying and decreasing to 120 when in deep sleep. Bradycardia, rates below 120 (**1** and **2**), and tachycardia, rates above 160 (**2** and **4**), are *not normal* and require further evaluation and intervention. **EV, 5, HPM**

3. **(3)** 9 is recorded because the heart rate (>100), muscle tone, respirations, and reflex response each receive a score of 2, and color pink with acrocyanosis (bluish

---

Key to Codes

Nursing process: AS, assessment; **AN,** analysis; **PL,** planning; **IMP,** implementation; **EV,** evaluation. (See Appendix I for explanation of nursing process steps.)

Category of human function: 1, protective; **2,** sensory-perceptual; **3,** comfort, rest, activity, and mobility; **4,** nutrition; **5,** growth and development; **6,** fluid-gas transport; **7,** psychosocial-cultural; **8,** elimination. (See Appendix K for explanation.)

Client need: SECE, safe, effective care environment; **PhI,** physiologic integrity; **PsI,** psychosocial integrity; **HPM,** health promotion/maintenance. (See Appendix L for explanation.)

hands and feet) is scored as 1. Options **1, 2,** and **4** represent *inaccurate* scores. **IMP, 6, HPM**

4. **(4)** The Babinski reflex is elicited by stroking the lateral aspect of the sole from the heel upward and across the ball of the foot. A positive test (in neonates) of fanning the toes and dorsiflexing the big toe is an indication of fetal well-being. Touching the corner of the newborn's mouth or cheek (**1**) elicits the *rooting reflex*. Changing the newborn's equilibrium (**2**) elicits the *Moro reflex*. Placing a finger in the palm of the newborn's hand (**3**) elicits the *palmar grasp reflex.* **IMP, 5, HPM**

5. **(1)** The rooting reflex is elicited by touching the corner of the newborn's mouth or cheek. Placing a finger in the palm of the newborn's hand (**2**) elicits the *palmar grasp* reflex. Stroking the lateral aspect of the sole from the heel upward and across the ball of the foot (**3**) elicits the *Babinski* reflex. Changing the newborn's equilibrium (**4**) elicits the *Moro* reflex. **IMP, 5, HPM**

6. **(3)** An asymmetric Moro reflex response is often associated with injury to the brachial plexus, clavicle, or humerus, preventing abductive and adductive movements of the upper extremities. Injuries to the cerebrum or cerebellum (**1**) could result in *symmetric* loss of the reflex. Cranial VII nerve (**2**) is the facial nerve; even if it is paralyzed, there is *no* effect on the Moro response. Down's syndrome (**4**) is *not* responsible for an asymmetric Moro response. **AN, 3, HPM**

7. **(3)** Cephalohematoma is a collection of blood between a skull bone and its covering (periosteum). Caput succedaneum (**1**) is a swelling of the tissue over the presenting part of the fetal head caused by pressure during labor. Molding (**2**) refers to the overlapping of cranial bones or shaping of the fetal head to accommodate and conform to the bony and soft parts of the mother's birth canal during labor. Subdural hematoma (**4**) refers to bleeding between the dural and arachnoid membranes of the brain. **IMP, 5, HPM**

8. **(2)** Purulent conjunctivitis that first appears 5 days–2 wk after birth is symptomatic of *Chlamydia trachomatis* infection; this organism causes pneumonia in the untreated child. If untreated, chronic follicular conjunctivitis, with conjunctival scarring and corneal neovascularization, may result. Purulent conjunctivitis is neither a sign of allergy (**1**), nor related to an older child's cold (**4**). To bathe the eyes with anything (**3**), a physician's order is required. (See treatment note, below.)

    NOTE: Signs of pneumonia include prolonged staccato cough, tachypnea, mild hypoxemia, and eosinophilia. Prevention of conjunctivitis: ophthalmic ointment of erythromycin or tetracycline. Treatment of pneumonia: oral erythromycin for 2–3 wk, and irrigation of the eye with saline or buffered ophthalmic solution daily. **IMP, 1, SECE**

9. **(3)** The nurse *must* intervene if the parent thinks that a wrapped ice pack is to be applied to the healing site if bleeding occurs, because the ice pack can injure the glans penis. Parents should use a sterile Teflon gauze (to avoid sticking) to apply gentle intermittent pressure to stem the bleeding. If bleeding continues, the pedia-

trician should be notified stat. In options **1, 2,** and **(4)** is *correct* regarding circumcision and its care, so *no intervention* is needed. **EV, 1, SECE**

10. **(3)**   The weight loss is within normal limits. The normal neonate may lose up to 10% of the birth weight (in this case, 12.7 oz or 360 g). This loss is usually the extra fluid the neonate has at birth until the mother's milk comes in on day 3. Option **1** is the *opposite* of the correct interpretation. Option **2** is incorrect because the mother's milk is not yet in; nature has helped compensate for this by the extra fluid most neonates have at birth. Option **4** is incorrect because the neonate is *losing* fluid, at a rate within normal limits. **EV, 5, HPM**

11. **(2)**   Vitamin K's function is to promote synthesis of clotting factors. It is produced in the GI tract by microorganisms, but the newborn's GI tract is sterile; vitamin K is not produced by the newborn until about the eighth day of life. It is given by IM injection, into the vastus lateralis muscle preferably; an alternate injection site is the rectus femoris muscle. Options **1, 3,** and **4** are all unrelated to vitamin K_1, since its only purpose is to promote synthesis of clotting factors. **IMP, 1, HPM**

12. **(3)**   After 2 hr, the edema of tissues present in most newborns begins to resolve and creases appear; these creases do not have the same predictive value as those assessed before resolution of newborn edema. All of the criteria in options **1, 2,** and **4** remain predictive *beyond* the first 2 hr after birth. **AS, 5, HPM**

13. **(2)**   Normal term newborns whose weight averages from 2500–4000 g (5 lb 8 oz–8 lb 13 oz) can lose about 10% of their birth weight in the first few days of life. This baby can lose 12 oz (7 lb 8 oz = 120 oz × 0.10 = 12 oz) and be within normal limits. This is due to the excretion of fluids through the lungs, urinary bladder, and bowels, and to the small amount of intake during this time. Newborns begin to regain their birth weight by 10–14 days of age. The amounts in options **1, 3,** and **4** are due either to *inaccurate* calculations or to use of the *wrong* formula. **EV, 5, HPM**

14. **(4)**   Record the findings and take no further action; this finding is normal. The actions in options **1, 2,** and **3** are *unnecessary* since the finding is within normal limits. **IMP, 5, HPM**

15. **(2)**   These symptoms reflect a cold body temperature. These symptoms are *not* associated with bleeding from the umbilical stump **(1)**, congenital abnormalities **(3)**, or respiratory distress **(4)**; rather, they *are* the usual symptoms of cold stress **(2)**. **AS, 3, HPM**

16. **(1)**   The newborn will commence breathing when the nose is stimulated; clearing the mouth first clears oral mucus that might otherwise be aspirated when breathing starts. Stimulating breathing before the mouth is clear **(2)** can lead to aspiration of oral mucus. The trachea should *never* be milked **(3)**; this action is ineffective and wastes valuable time. Slapping the infant **(4)** would cause the baby to gasp and aspirate oral and nasopharyngeal contents (and the nurse should *never* hit an infant!). **IMP, 1, SECE**

17. **(3)**   Gentle pressure to the bleeding site will usually stop the bleeding. Only enough pressure should be exerted to stop the flow of blood; excessive pressure can compromise needed blood flow to the structure. Option **1** is incorrect since bleeding can continue unseen, and too tight a diaper can *obstruct* flow of blood to the diaper area. Option **2** is incorrect because it is *unnecessary at this time,* although it may be necessary if the gentle pressure for a short time does not suffice. Option **4** is incorrect because it does *not* assist with stopping the hemorrhage. **IMP, 1, HPM**

18. **(3)**   The mother needs to learn what to do when an infant is gagging. The parent(s) should learn how to use a bulb syringe as well. Option **1** is incorrect since this would tend to cause the infant to gasp and *aspirate* mucus. Option **2** is incorrect since this would tell the mother that she is incapable of handling the situation. Option **4** is incorrect since, although this is normal for the second period of reactivity, she needs to know that she can handle the situation herself. **IMP, 1, HPM**

Complications During the Neonatal Period: The High-Risk Newborn

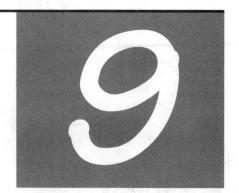

Chapter Outline

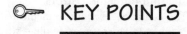 KEY POINTS

- To maintain high standards of care, the nurse must identify risk situations caused by **immaturity, alter**ations in functioning of systems, metabolic imbalances, **developmental** problems (*congenital* anomalies), and **acquired problems,** such as *birth injuries, infections,* and *drug dependence.*
- The alert nurse often is the pivotal link between functional and dysfunctional survival for the infant at risk.
- The earliest clinical *signs of neonatal illness* are char-

acterized by a lack of specificity: lethargy, poor feeding, poor weight gain, or irritability.
- The curative and rehabilitative problems of children with some disorders are often complex, requiring a multidisciplinary approach to the care of such a child and his/her parents.

Key Words

Bronchopulmonary dysplasia (BPD)
Direct Coombs test
Erythroblastosis fetalis
Exchange blood transfusion
Fetal alcohol syndrome (FAS)
Hip dysplasia
Hyperbilirubinemia
Iatrogenic (nosocomial)
Kernicterus
Meconium aspiration syndrome
Necrotizing enterocolitis (NEC)
Pilonidal dimple
Retinopathy of prematurity (ROP)
Scaphoid abdomen

All Infants

I. **General overview**—successful newborn adaptation to the demands of independent extrauterine life may be complicated by environmental insults during the *prenatal* period (see *Chapter 3*) and/or those arising in the period immediately surrounding birth (see *Chapter 5*). The nursing role focuses on minimizing the effect of present and emerging health problems and on facilitating and supporting a successful transition to extrauterine life. Review Table 8.1 for deviations from the norm.
  A. **General aspects**—common neonatal risk factors
    1. Gestational age profile (see Tables 8.1 and 8.3)
      a. Prematurity.
      b. Dysmaturity.
      c. Postmaturity.
    2. Congenital disorders.
    3. Birth trauma.
    4. Infections.
II. **Disorders affecting protective function: neonatal infections**
  A. **Oral thrush** (*mycotic stomatitis*)
    1. **Pathophysiology**—local inflammation of oral mucosa due to fungal infection.
    2. **Etiology**
      a. Organism—*Candida albicans.*
      b. More common in vulnerable newborn, i.e., sick, debilitated; those receiving antibiotic therapy.
    3. Mode of transmission—direct contact with
      a. Maternal birth canal, hands, and linens.
      b. Contaminated feeding equipment, staff's hands.

⋈ 4. **Assessment**
  a. White patches on oral mucosa, gums, and tongue that bleed when touched.
  b. Occasional difficulty in swallowing.
⋈ 5. **Analysis/nursing diagnosis**
  a. *Pain* related to irritation of oral mucous membrane secondary to oral moniliasis.
  b. *Altered nutrition, less than body requirements* related to irritability and poor feeding.
⋈ 6. **Nursing care plan/implementation:** goal: *prevent cross-contamination*
  a. Aseptic technique; good handwashing; use universal precautions.
  b. Chemotherapy, as ordered
    (1) *Aqueous gentian violet,* 1–2%: apply to infected area with swab.
    (2) *Nystatin (Mycostatin)*—instill into mouth with medicine dropper, or apply to lesions with swab, *after* feedings. NOTE: before medicating, feed sterile water to rinse out milk.
⋈ 7. **Evaluation/outcome criteria**
  a. The newborn's oral mucosa is intact, lesions are healed, with no evidence of infection.
  b. The newborn feeds well; maintains weight or regains weight lost, if any.
B. **Neonatal sepsis**
  1. **Pathophysiology**—generalized infection; may overwhelm infant's immature immune system.
  2. **Etiology**
    a. Prolonged rupture of membranes.
    b. Long, difficult labor.
    c. Resuscitation procedures.
    d. Maternal infection (i.e., beta-hemolytic streptococcus vaginosis).
    e. Aspiration—amniotic fluid, formula, mucus.
    f. **Iatrogenic (nosocomial)**—caused by infected health personnel or equipment.
⋈ 3. **Assessment**
  a. Respirations—irregular, periods of apnea.
  b. Irritability or lethargy.
⋈ 4. **Analysis/nursing diagnosis**
  a. *Fatigue* related to increased oxygen needs.
  b. *High risk for infection* related to septic condition.
⋈ 5. **Nursing care plan/implementation**
  a. Order cultures (spinal, urine, blood).
  b. Check vitals.
  c. Monitor respirators.
⋈ 6. **Evaluation/outcome criteria**
  a. The newborn responds to medical/nursing regimen (all assessment findings within normal limits).
  b. Parent(s) verbalize understanding of diagnosis, treatment; demonstrate appropriate techniques in participating in care (as possible).

c. Parent(s) demonstrate effective coping with situation; express satisfaction with care.

C. Hepatitis B and herpes simplex type II viral infections

1. Hepatitis B virus (HBV) infection
    a. Mode of transmission—from the mother to the newborn in about 90% of cases.
    b. HBV is associated with about a 32% increase in preterm birth.
    c. *Medical management—infants* who require hepatitis B immune globulin (HBIG) should receive 0.5 mL intramuscularly, as soon as possible after birth.
       (1) The *protocol* for injections of the vaccine is
           Dose 1: within the first 12 h of birth.
           Dose 2: at 1 mo.
           Dose 3: at 6 mo.

2. **Herpes virus** infection
    a. Precautions—while a mother is awaiting the results of cultures for diagnosis of *Herpes virus* infection; both *gown and gloves* should be worn by persons in contact with the infant.
    b. Medical management
       (1) *Vidarabine ophthalmic ointment* is administered for 5 days for prevention of keratoconjunctivitis.
       (2) As long as no suspicious lesions are found on the mother's breasts, breast-feeding is allowed.
       (3) The infant should be seen by the pediatrician *every week* for the *first month* after birth.

III. Disorders affecting nutrition: infant of the diabetic mother (IDM)

A. **Pathophysiology**—hyperplasia of pancreatic beta cells → increased insulin production → excessive deposition of glycogen in muscles, subcutaneous fat, and tissue growth. Results in fetal:
   1. *Macrosomia*—large for gestational age (LGA).
   2. *Enlarged internal organs*—common
       a. Cardiomegaly.
       b. Hepatomegaly.
       c. Splenomegaly.
   3. Neonatal—inadequate carbohydrate reserve to meet energy needs.
   4. Associated with *increased incidence of*
       a. *Congenital anomalies* (5 times average incidence)—includes cardiac, pelvic, and spinal anomalies.
       b. *Preterm birth.* Respiratory distress syndrome (RDS). Increased insulin needs prenatally lead to decreased surfactant production.
       c. *Maternal dystocia*—due to cephalopelvic disproportion (CPD).
       d. *Neonatal metabolic problems*
           (1) Hypoglycemia.
           (2) Hypocalcemic tetany.

(3) Metabolic acidosis.
(4) Hyperbilirubinemia.

B. **Etiology**—high circulating maternal glucose levels during fetal growth and development; loss of maternal glucose supply following birth; decreased hepatic gluconeogenesis.

C. **Assessment**
   1. Characteristics of IDM: see III.A. *Pathophysiology.*
   2. Hypoglycemia—apply Dextrostix or Chemstrip to heel stick at
       a. 30 min.
       b. 1, 2, 4, 6, 9, 12, and 24 hr of age.
       c. Hypoglycemia laboratory values for *term* infant: under 30–40 mg/dL.
       d. Hypoglycemia laboratory values for *preterm* infant: under 20 mg/dL.
       e. Behavioral signs—tremors, twitching, hypotonia, seizures.
   3. Gestational age, since macrosomia may mask prematurity.
   4. *Hypocalcemia*—usually within first 24 hr
       a. Irritability.
       b. Coarse tremors, twitching, convulsions.
   5. *Birth injuries*
       a. Fractures: clavicle, humerus, skull.
       b. Brachial palsy, Erb-Duchenne paralysis
       c. Intracranial hemorrhage/signs of *increased intracranial pressure* (ICCP).
           (1) Widening of fontanels and sutures.
           (2) Bulging fontanels at rest.
           (3) High-pitched, whiny cry.
       d. Cephalohematoma.
   6. *Respiratory distress in the newborn*
       a. Nasal flaring.
       b. Sternal retraction.
       c. Costal breathing.
       d. Cyanosis.
       e. Expiratory grunt.
   7. *Jaundice.*

D. **Analysis/nursing diagnosis**
   1. *High risk for injury* related to CPD, dystocia.
   2. *Altered cardiopulmonary tissue perfusion* related to placental insufficiency, RDS.
   3. *Impaired gas exchange* related to RDS.
   4. *Altered nutrition, less than body requirements,* related to hypoglycemia, hypocalcemia.
   5. *Risk for altered endocrine/metabolic processes* related to hyperbilirubinemia and kernicterus.

E. **Nursing care plan/implementation**
   1. Hypoglycemia—administer oral or intravenous *glucose,* as ordered (may cause rebound effect).
   2. Premature/immature—institute premature care, prn.
   3. Hypocalcemia—administer oral or intravenous calcium gluconate, as ordered.
   4. Inform pediatrician immediately of signs of:
       a. Jaundice.
       b. Hyperirritability.
       c. Birth injury.

       d. Increased intracranial pressure/hemorrhage.

✖ **F. Evaluation/outcome criteria**

   The newborn:

    1. Makes successful transition to extrauterine life.

    2. Responds to medical/nursing regimen. Experiences minimal or no metabolic disturbances (e.g., hypoglycemia, hypocalcemia, hyperbilirubinemia).

    3. Exhibits normal respiratory function and gas exchange.

IV. Hypoglycemia in the newborn

   A. Pathophysiology—low serum-glucose level → altered cellular metabolism → cerebral irritability, cardiopulmonary problems.

   B. Etiology

    1. Loss of maternal glucose supply.

    2. Normal physiologic activities of respiration, thermoregulation, and muscular activity exceed carbohydrate reserve.

    3. Decreased hepatic ability to convert amino acids into glucose.

    4. More common in

      a. Infants of diabetic mothers (**IDM**).

      b. Preterm, postterm infants.

      c. Small for gestational age (**SGA**).

      d. Smaller twin.

      e. Infant of preeclamptic mother.

      f. Birth asphyxia.

✖ **C. Assessment**

    1. Jitteriness, tremors, convulsions; lethargy and hypotonia.

    2. Sweating; unstable temperature.

    3. Tachypnea; apneic episodes; cyanosis.

    4. High-pitched, shrill cry.

    5. Difficulty in feeding.

✖ **D. Analysis/nursing diagnosis**

    1. *Altered tissue perfusion (fetal)* related to placental insufficiency associated with maternal diabetes, preeclampsia, renal and/or cardiac disorders; erythroblastosis.

    2. *Risk for altered endocrine/metabolic processes* related to high incidence of morbidity associated with birth asphyxia.

    3. *Impaired gas exchange* related to coexisting RDS.

    4. *Altered nutrition, less than body requirements,* related to hypoglycemia.

    5. *High risk for injury* related to coexisting infection, metabolic acidosis.

✖ **E. Nursing care plan/implementation:** see III. *Infant of the diabetic mother.*

✖ **F. Evaluation/outcome criteria:** see III. *Infant of the diabetic mother.*

V. Disorders affecting psychosocial-cultural function: drug-dependent (heroin) neonate

   A. General aspects

    1. Maternal drug addiction has been associated with

      a. Prenatal malnutrition and vitamin deficiencies.

      b. Increased risk of antepartal infections.

      c. Higher incidence of antepartal and intrapartal complications.

    2. Infant at risk for

      a. Intrauterine growth retardation (**IUGR**).

      b. Prematurity.

      c. Congenital anomalies.

      d. Fetal distress.

      e. Perinatal death.

      f. Child abuse.

   B. Pathophysiology—withdrawal of accustomed drug levels → physiologic deprivation response.

   C. Etiology—repeated intrauterine absorption of heroin/cocaine/methadone from maternal bloodstream → fetal drug dependency.

✖ **D. Assessment**—degree of newborn drug dependence (withdrawal) depends on type and duration of addiction, and maternal drug levels at birth.

    1. Irritability, hyperactivity, hypertonicity, exaggerated reflexes, tremors, high-pitched cry, difficult to comfort

      a. *"Step" reflex* (dancing)—infant places both feet on surface; assumes rigid stance—does not "step" or dance.

      b. *"Head-righting" reflex*—holds head rigid; fails to demonstrate head lag.

    2. Nasal stuffiness and sneezing; respiratory distress, tachypnea, cyanosis and/or apnea.

    3. Exaggerated acrocyanosis and/or mottling in the warm infant.

    4. Sweating.

    5. Hunger—sucks on fists; feeding problems—regurgitation, vomiting, poor feeding, diarrhea and increased mucus production.

    6. Convulsions with abnormal eye-rolling and chewing motions.

    7. Developmental lags/mental retardation.

✖ **E. Analysis/nursing diagnosis**

    1. *Risk for injury* related to convulsions secondary to physiologic response to withdrawal, CNS hyperirritability.

    2. *Impaired gas exchange* related to respiratory distress secondary to inhibition of reflex clearing of fluid by the lungs.

    3. *Altered nutrition, less than body requirements,* related to feeding problems secondary to respiratory distress and GI hypermotility.

    4. *High risk for impaired skin integrity* related to scratching secondary to withdrawal symptoms.

✖ **F. Nursing care plan/implementation**

    1. Goal: *prevent/minimize respiratory distress*

      a. *Position:* side lying, head dependent—to facilitate mucus drainage.

   ☞ **b.** Suction, prn, with bulb syringe for excess mucus—to maintain patent airway.

      c. Monitor respirations and apical pulse.

    2. Goal: *minimize possibility of convulsions*

      a. Decrease environmental stimuli—quiet, touch only when necessary, offer pacifier.

b. Keep warm, swaddle for comfort.

3. Goal: *maintain nutrition/hydration*
   a. Food/fluids—oral or IV, as ordered.
   b. I&O.
   c. Daily weight.

☞ **4.** Goal: *assist in diagnosis of drug and drug level.* Collect all urine during first 24 hr for toxicologic studies.

5. Goal: *maintain/promote skin integrity*
   a. Mitts over hands—to minimize scratching.
   b. Keep clean and dry.
   💊 **c.** Medicated ointment/powder, as ordered, every 2–4 hr, to excoriated areas.
   d. Expose excoriated areas to air.

💊 **6.** Goal: *minimize withdrawal symptoms.* Administer medications, as ordered.
   a. *Paregoric elixir*—to wean from drug.
   b. *Phenobarbital*—to reduce CNS hyperirritability, hyperbilirubinemia.
   c. *Chlorpromazine (Thorazine), diazepam (Valium)*—to tranquilize, reduce hyperirritability. NOTE: Valium is **contraindicated** for jaundiced neonate because it predisposes to hyperbilirubinemia.
   d. *Methadone.*

7. Goal: *emotional support to mother.*
   a. Encourage verbalization of feelings of guilt, anxiety, fear, concerns.
   b. Refer to social service.

🔀 **G. Evaluation/outcome criteria**
   The newborn:
   1. Responds to medical/nursing regimen
      a. Maintains adequate respirations.
      b. Feeds well, gains weight.
      c. No evidence of CNS hyperirritability, convulsions; demonstrates normal newborn reflexes.
   2. Evidences bonding with parent(s). Responsive to mother's voice.

VI. Disorders affecting psychosocial-cultural function: *fetal alcohol syndrome (FAS). General aspects:*
   A. Maternal alcohol abuse has been associated with:
      1. Malnutrition, vitamin deficiencies.
      2. Bone marrow suppression.
      3. Liver disease.
      4. Child abuse.
   ⚡ **B.** Infant at risk for:
      1. Congenital anomalies.
      2. Mental deficiency.
      3. IUGR, (intrauterine growth retardation).
   C. Pathophysiology—permanent damage to developing embryonic/fetal structures; cardiovascular anomalies (*ventricular septal defects*).
   D. Etiology—*high* circulating alcohol levels are lethal to the embryo; *lower* levels cause permanent cell damage.
   🔀 **E. Assessment**
      1. Characteristic *craniofacial abnormalities:*
         a. Short, palpebral fissure.
         b. Epicanthal folds.
         c. Maxillary hypoplasia.

d. Micrognathia (abnormal smallness of mandible or chin).
   e. Long, thin upper lip.
2. Short stature.
3. Irritable, hyperactive, poor feeding.
4. High-pitched cry, difficult to comfort.

🔀 **F. Nursing care plan/implementation**
   1. Goal: *reduce irritability*
      a. Reduce environmental stimuli.
      b. Wrap, cuddle.
   💊 **c.** Administer sedatives, as ordered.
   2. Goal: *maintain nutrition/hydration.*
   3. Goal: *emotional support to mother.*

🔀 **G. Evaluation/outcome criteria:** see *Drug-dependent (heroin) neonate,* p. 182
   1. No respiratory distress.
   2. Infant feeding properly.
   3. Maternal bonding apparent.
   4. Social service—home involvement.

VII. Classification of infants by weight and gestational age
   A. Terminology
      1. *Preterm, or premature*—37 wk gestation or less [usually 2500 g (5 lb) or less].
      2. *Term*—38–42 wk gestation.
      3. *Postterm*—over 42 wk.
      4. *Postmature*—gestation greater than 42 wk.
      5. *Appropriate for gestational age (AGA)*—for each week of gestation, there is a normal range of expected weight
         a. Term infants weighing 2500 g or more are usually mature in physiologic functions.
         b. If respiratory distress occurs, it is usually related to *meconium aspiration syndrome.*
      6. *Small for gestational age (SGA), or dysmature* —weight falls below normal range for age. *Etiology:*
         a. Preeclampsia.
         b. Malnutrition.
         c. Smoking.
         d. Placental insufficiency.
         e. Alcohol syndrome.
         f. Rubella.
         g. Syphilis.
         h. Multifetal gestation (twins, etc.).
         i. Genetic.
         j. Cocaine abuse.
      7. *Large for gestational age (LGA)*—above expected weight for age. NOTE: If **preterm,** at risk for **respiratory distress syndrome.** If **postterm,** at risk for **meconium aspiration** and **sudden intrauterine death.**
         a. *Etiology*
            (1) Maternal diabetes or prediabetes.
            (2) Maternal weight gain over 35 pounds.
            (3) Maternal obesity.
            (4) Genetic.
         b. *Associated problems:*
            (1) Hypoglycemia.
            (2) Hypocalcemia.
            (3) Hyperbilirubinemia.

(4) Birth injury, e.g., fractures; conditions secondary to type of birth (scalpel wounds during cesarean; Erb-Duchenne paralysis due to shoulder dystocia during vaginal birth)

B. *Estimation of gestational age*—planning appropriate care for the newborn requires accurate assessment to differentiate between premature and term infants.

Preterm/Premature Infant

Definition: born at 37 wk gestation or less.

I. General aspects
A. Pathophysiology—anatomic and physiologic immaturity of body systems compromises ability to adapt to extrauterine environment and independent life
  1. *Interference with* **protective** *functions*
    a. Temperature *regulation*—unstable, due to:
      (1) Lack of subcutaneous fat.
      (2) Large body surface area in proportion to body weight.
      (3) Small muscle mass.
      (4) Absent sweat or shiver responses.
      (5) Poor capillary response to changes in environmental temperature.
    b. *Resistance to infection*—low, due to:
      (1) Lack of immune bodies from mother (these cross placenta *late* in pregnancy).
      (2) Inability to produce own immune bodies (immature liver).
      (3) Poor white blood cell response to infection.
    c. *Immature liver*
      (1) Inability to conjugate bilirubin liberated by normal breakdown of red blood cells → increased susceptibility to hyperbilirubinemia and kernicterus.
      (2) Immature production of clotting factors and immune globulins.
      (3) Inadequate glucose stores → increased susceptibility to hypoglycemia.
  2. *Interference with* **elimination:** immature *renal* function—unable to concentrate urine → precarious fluid/electrolyte balance.
  3. *Interference with* **sensory-perceptual functions:** central nervous system—immature → weak or absent reflexes and fluctuating primitive control of vital functions.
B. Etiology: (often unknown); preterm labor
  1. *Iatrogenic*—estimated date of birth (EDB) miscalculated for repeat cesarean birth.
  2. *Placental factors*
    a. Placenta previa.
    b. Abruptio placentae.
    c. Placental insufficiency.
  3. *Uterine factors*
    a. Incompetent cervix.

b. Overdistention (multifetal gestation, hydramnios).
c. Anomalies (e.g., myomas).
  4. *Fetal factors*
    a. Malformations.
    b. Infections (e.g., rubella, toxoplasmosis, human immunodeficiency virus [HIV]-positive status, AIDS, cytomegalic inclusion disease).
    c. Multifetal gestations (e.g., twins, triplets).
  5. *Maternal factors*
    a. Severe physical or emotional trauma.
    b. Coexisting disorders (e.g., preeclampsia, hypertension, heart disease, diabetes, malnutrition).
    c. Infections (e.g., strepococcus, syphilis, pyelonephritis, pneumonia, influenza, leukemia).
  6. *Miscellaneous factors*
    a. Close frequency of pregnancies.
    b. Advanced parental age.
    c. Heavy smoking.
    d. High-altitude environment.
    e. Cocaine use.
  7. *Factors influencing* survival
    a. Gestational age.
    b. Lung maturity.
    c. Anomalies.
    d. Size.
  8. *Causes of mortality* (in order of frequency):
    a. Abnormal pulmonary ventilation.
    b. Infection
      (1) Pneumonia.
      (2) Septicemia.
      (3) Diarrhea.
      (4) Meningitis.
    c. Intracranial hemorrhage.
    d. Congenital defects.

II. Disorders affecting fluid-gas transport: respiratory distress syndrome (RDS)
A. Pathophysiology—insufficient pulmonary surfactant (lecithin) and insufficient number/maturity of alveoli predispose to atelectasis; alveolar ducts and terminal bronchi become lined with fibrous, glossy membrane.
B. Etiology
  1. Primarily associated with prematurity.
  2. Other *predisposing* factors:
    a. *Fetal hypoxia*—due to decreased placental perfusion secondary to maternal bleeding (e.g., abruptio) or hypotension.
    b. *Birth asphyxia.*
    c. *Postnatal hypothermia, metabolic acidosis, or hypotension.*
C. Factors *protecting* neonate from RDS
  1. Chronic fetal stress—due to maternal hypertension, preeclampsia, or heroin addiction.
  2. Premature rupture of membranes (PROM).
  3. Maternal steroid ingestion (i.e., *betamethasone*).
  4. Low-grade chorioamnionitis.

D. Assessment

1. Usually appears during first or second day after birth.
2. Signs of *respiratory distress:*
   a. Nasal flaring.
   b. Sternal retractions.
   c. Tachypnea (60/min or more).
   d. Cyanosis.
   e. Expiratory grunt.
   f. Increasing number and length of apneic episodes.
   g. Increasing exhaustion.
3. *Respiratory acidosis*—due to hypercapnia and rising carbon dioxide level.
4. *Metabolic acidosis*—due to increased lactic acid levels and falling pH.

E. Analysis/nursing diagnosis

1. *Impaired gas exchange* related to lack of pulmonary surfactant secondary to preterm birth, intrapartal stress and hypoxia, infection, postnatal hypothermia, metabolic acidosis, or hypotension.
2. *Altered nutrition, less than body requirements,* related to poor feeding secondary to respiratory distress.

F. Nursing care plan/implementation

1. Goal: *reduce metabolic acidosis, increase oxygenation, support respiratory efforts*
   a. Ensure warmth (*isolette at 97.6 °F*).
   b. Warmed, humidified oxygen at lowest concentration required to relieve cyanosis, through hood, nasal prongs, or endotracheal tube.
   c. *Monitor continuous positive airway pressure (CPAP)*—oxygen-air mixture administered under pressure during inhalation *and* exhalation to maintain alveolar patency.
   d. *Position:* side lying or supine with neck slightly extended ("sniffing" position); arms at sides.
   e. Suction, prn, with bulb syringe—for excessive mucus.
2. Goal: *modify care for infant with endotracheal tube*
   a. Disconnect tubing at adapter.
   b. Inject 0.5 mL sterile normal saline.
   c. Insert sterile suction tube, start suction, rotate tube, withdraw.
   d. Suction up to 5 sec.
   e. Ventilate with bag and mask during procedure.
   f. Reconnect tubing securely to adapter.
   g. Auscultate for breath sounds and pulse.
3. Goal: *maintain nutrition/hydration*
   a. Administer: fluids, electrolytes, calories, vitamins, minerals PO or IV, as ordered.
   b. I&O.
4. Goal: *prevent secondary infections*
   a. Strict aseptic technique.
   b. Handwashing.

5. Goal: *emotional support of infant*
   a. Gentle touching.
   b. Soft voices.
   c. Eye contact.
   d. Rocking.
6. Goal: *emotional support of parents*
   a. Keep informed of status and progress.
   b. Encourage contact with infant—to promote bonding, understanding of treatment.
7. Goal: *minimize possibility of iatrogenic disorders associated with oxygen therapy* (see below, *Iatrogenic [oxygen toxicity] disorders:* retinopathy of prematurity).

G. Evaluation/outcome criteria

1. The infant's respiratory distress is treated successfully; infant breathes without assistance.
2. The infant completes successful transition to extrauterine life.

III. Iatrogenic (oxygen toxicity) disorders: *retinopathy of prematurity* (ROP)

   A. Pathophysiology—intraretinal hemorrhage → fibrosis → retinal detachment → loss of vision.
   B. Etiology—prolonged exposure to high concentrations of oxygen.
   C. Assessment—only perceptible retinal change is vasoconstriction.

   NOTE: arterial blood (PaO$_2$) gas readings less than 50 or more than 70 mm Hg.

   D. Nursing care plan/implementation: goal: *prevent disorder.* Maintain PaO$_2$ of 50–70 mm Hg.
   E. Evaluation/outcome criteria
   1. The infant demonstrates successful recovery from respiratory distress.
   2. No evidence of disorder.

IV. Iatrogenic (oxygen toxicity) disorders: *bronchopulmonary dysplasia (BPD)*

   A. Pathophysiology—damage to alveolar cells results in focal emphysema.
   B. Etiology—positive pressure ventilation (CPAP) and positive end-expiratory pressure (PEEP) and prolonged administration of high concentrations of oxygen.
   C. Assessment—monitor for signs of:
   1. Tachypnea.
   2. Increased respiratory effort.
   3. Respiratory distress.
   D. Nursing care plan/implementation: goal: *prevent disorder*
   1. Use of positive pressure devices (CPAP, PEEP)
   2. Maintain oxygen concentration *below* 70%.
   3. Supportive care.
   4. Wean off ventilator, as possible.
   E. Evaluation/outcome criteria
   The infant demonstrates:
   1. Successful recovery from respiratory distress.
   2. No evidence of disorder.

V. Intraventricular hemorrhage

   A. Pathophysiology—rupture of thin, fragile capillary walls within ventricles of the brain (more common in preterm).

B. Etiology
1. Hypoxia.
2. Respiratory distress.
3. Birth trauma.
4. Birth asphyxia.
5. Hypercapnia.

C. Assessment
1. Hypotonia.
2. Lethargy.
3. Hypothermia.
4. Bradycardia.
5. Bulging fontanels.
6. Respiratory distress or apnea.
7. Seizures.
8. Cry: high-pitched whining.

D. Nursing care plan/implementation: goal: *supportive care*—to promote healing
1. Monitor vital signs.
2. Maintain thermal stability.
3. Assure adequate oxygenation (may be placed on CPAP).

E. Evaluation/outcome criteria
The infant demonstrates:
1. Condition stable, all assessment findings within normal limits.
2. No evidence of residual damage.

VI. Disorders affecting nutrition
A. **Pathophysiology**—underdeveloped feeding abilities, small stomach capacity, immature enzyme system, fat intolerance.
B. **Etiology**—immature body systems associated with preterm birth.
C. Assessment
1. Weak suck, swallow, gag reflexes—tendency to aspiration.
2. Signs of malabsorption and fat intolerance (abdominal distention, diarrhea, weight loss, or failure to gain weight).
3. Signs of vitamin E deficiency (edema, anemia).
D. Analysis/nursing diagnosis
1. *Altered nutrition, less than body requirements,* related to poor feeding reflexes, reduced stomach capacity, inability to absorb needed nutrients.
2. *Impaired gas exchange* related to aspiration.
E. Nursing care plan/implementation: goal: *maintain/increase nutrition*
1. Frequent, small feedings—to *avoid* exceeding stomach capacity, facilitate digestion.
2. Frequent "burping" during feeding—to *avoid* regurgitation/aspiration.
3. Supplement vitamin E (alpha-tocopherol) intake, as ordered, in formula-fed infants (NOTE: intake adequate in breastfed babies.)
   a. *Vitamin E* actions:
      (1) Antioxidant.
      (2) Maintains structure and function of smooth, skeletal, and cardiac muscle.
      (3) Maintains structure and function of

vascular tissue, liver, and red blood cell integrity.
      (4) Coenzyme in tissue respiration.
      (5) Treatment for malnutrition with macrocytic anemia.
4. Encourage parent/family participation.
F. Evaluation/outcome criteria
The infant:
1. Feeds well without regurgitation/aspiration.
2. Maintains/gains weight.
3. Shows no evidence of malabsorption, vitamin deficiency.

VII. Disorders affecting nutrition/elimination: *necrotizing enterocolitis (NEC)*
A. **Pathophysiology**—intestinal thrombosis, infarction, autodigestion of mucosal lining, and necrotic lesions; incidence increased in preterm.
B. **Etiology**—intestinal ischemia, due to blood shunt to brain and heart in response to:
1. Fetal distress.
2. Fetal/neonatal asphyxia.
3. Neonatal shock.
4. After birth, may result from:
   a. Low cardiac output.
   b. Infusion of hyperosmolar solutions.
5. Complicated by action of enteric bacteria on damaged intestine.
C. Assessment—early identification is **vital**
1. Abdominal distention and/or erythema.
2. Poor feeding, vomiting.
3. Blood in stool.
4. Systemic signs associated with sepsis that may need temporary colostomy or iliostomy:
   a. Lethargy or irritability.
   b. Hypothermia.
   c. Labored respirations or apnea.
   d. Cardiovascular collapse.
5. *Medical* diagnosis:
   a. Increased gastric residual.
   b. X-ray shows ileus, air in bowel wall.
D. Analysis/nursing diagnosis
1. *Altered nutrition, less than body requirements,* related to inability to tolerate oral feedings and gastrointestinal dysfunction secondary to ischemia, thrombosis, and/or necrosis.
2. *Constipation* related to paralytic ileus with stasis; diarrhea related to water loss.
3. *High risk for injury* related to infection, thrombosis, metabolic alterations (acidosis, osmotic diuresis, dehydration, hyperglycemia) due to parenteral nutrition.
4. *Altered parenting* related to physiologic compromise and prolonged hospitalization.
5. *Impaired skin integrity* when colostomy is necessary.
E. Nursing care plan/implementation
1. Goal: *supportive care*
   a. Rest GI tract: *no oral intake*—to achieve gastric decompression.
   b. IV fluids, as ordered—to maintain hydration.

2. Goal: *prevent infection.* Administer antibiotics, as ordered.
3. Goal: *prevent trauma to skin surrounding stoma.*

F. Evaluation/outcome criteria
1. The infant:
   a. Tolerates oral feedings.
   b. Demonstrates weight gain.
   c. Demonstrates normal stool pattern.
2. Parents are accepting and knowledgeable about care of infant.

Postterm/Postmature Infant

Definition: over 42 wk gestation.

I. General aspects—labor may be hazardous for mother and fetus because:
   A. Large size of infant contributes to maternal dystocia; diagnosis by ultrasound, X-ray.
   B. Placental insufficiency → fetal hypoxia; diagnosis by:
      1. Contraction stress test.
      2. Nonstress test.
   C. Meconium passage (common physiologic response) increases chance of meconium aspiration.

II. Assessment
   A. If postmature skin: dry, wrinkled—due to metabolism of fat and glycogen reserves to meet in utero energy needs.
   B. Long limbs, fingernails, and toenails—due to continued growth in utero.
   C. Lanugo and vernix—absent.
   D. Expression: wide-eyed, alert—probably due to chronic hypoxia (oxygen hunger).
   E. Placenta—signs of aging.

III. Analysis/nursing diagnosis: *high risk for injury* related to high incidence of morbidity and mortality due to dystocia and/or hypoxia.

IV. Nursing care plan/implementation
   A. During labor
      1. Goal: *emotional support of mother*—may require cesarean birth due to CPD or fetal distress.
      2. Goal: *continuous electronic monitoring of fetal heart rate (FHR).* Report *late* or *variable* decelerations immediately (indicate fetal distress).
   B. After birth
      1. Goal: *if born vaginally, prompt identification of birth injuries, respiratory distress.* Continual observation.
      2. Goal: *early identification/treatment of emerging signs of complications*
         a. *Hypoglycemia*—Dextrostix readings and behavior.
         b. Administer oral or intravenous glucose, as ordered.

V. Evaluation/outcome criterion: successful transition to extrauterine life (all assessment findings within normal limits).

Infant with Congenital Disorders

I. *General overview:* Genetic abnormalities and environmental insults often lead to congenital disorders of the newborn. Successful transition to independent extrauterine life may pose a major challenge to infants compromised by anatomic and/or physiologic disorders. Knowledge regarding the implications of the neonate's structural and/or metabolic problems enables the nurse to identify early signs of health problems and to plan, provide, and evaluate appropriate outcome-directed care to safeguard the status of the infant with a congenital disorder.

II. Disorders affecting fluid-gas transport: *congenital heart disease*
   A. Pathophysiology—altered hemodynamics, due to persistent fetal circulation or structural abnormalities
      1. *Acyanotic defects*—no mixing of blood in the systemic circulation
         a. Patent ductus arteriosus.
         b. Atrial septal defect.
         c. Ventricular septal defect.
         d. Coarctation of the aorta.
      2. *Cyanotic defects*—unoxygenated blood enters systemic circulation
         a. Tetralogy of Fallot.
         b. Transposition of the great vessels.
   B. Etiology—unknown. Associated with maternal:
      1. Prenatal viral disease (e.g., rubella, Coxsackie).
      2. Malnutrition; alcoholism.
      3. Diabetes, poorly controlled.
      4. Ingestion of lithium salts.
   C. Assessment
      1. **Patent ductus arteriosus (PDA)**
         a. Characteristic machine murmur, mid to upper left sternal border (cardiomegaly); persists throughout systole and most of diastole; associated with a "thrill."
         b. Widened pulse pressure.
         c. Bounding pulse, tachycardia, "gallop" rhythm.
      2. **Atrial septal defect (ASD)**
         a. Characteristic crescendo/decrescendo systolic ejection murmur.
         b. Fixed S_2 splitting.
         c. Dyspnea, fatigue on normal activity.
         d. Medical diagnosis—cardiac catheterization, X-ray.
      3. **Ventricular septal defect (VSD)**
         a. Loud, harsh, pansystolic murmur; heard best at left lower sternal border; radiates throughout precordium. (NOTE: may be

absent—due to high pulmonary vascular resistance → equalization of interventricular pressure.)

     b. Medical diagnosis—cardiac catheterization, ECG, chest X-ray.

  4. Coarctation of the aorta
     a. Absent femoral pulse.
     b. Late systolic murmur.
     c. Decreased blood pressure in *lower* extremities.
     d. Medical diagnosis: X-ray.

  5. Tetralogy of Fallot ("blue" baby)
     a. Acute hypoxic/cyanotic episodes.
     b. Limp, sleepy, exhausted; hypotonic extended position—postepisode.
     c. Medical diagnosis—cardiac catheterization.

  6. Transposition of the great vessels
     a. Cyanotic after crying or feeding.
     b. Progressive tachypnea—attempt to compensate for decreased PaO_2, metabolic acidosis.
     c. Heart sounds vary, consistent with defect.
     d. Signs of heart failure.
     e. *Medical* diagnosis—cardiac catheterization, X-ray, ECG.

D. Analysis/nursing diagnosis
  1. *Fluid volume excess* related to persistent fetal circulation, structural abnormalities.
  2. *Impaired gas exchange* related to abnormal circulation, secondary to above pathology.
  3. *Altered nutrition, less than body requirements,* related to exhaustion, dyspnea.

E. Nursing care plan/implementation
  1. Goal: *minimize cardiac workload*
     a. Minimize crying—snuggle; pacifier—to meet psychological needs.
  2. Goal: *maintain thermal stability*—to reduce body need for oxygen. Keep clean and dry.
  3. Goal: *prevent infection.*
     a. Strict aseptic technique; universal precautions.
     b. Handwashing.
  4. Goal: *parental emotional support*
     a. Encourage verbalization of anxiety, fears, concerns.
     b. Keep informed of status.
  5. Goal: *health teaching*—explain, discuss
     a. Diagnostic procedures.
     b. Treatment procedures.
     c. Basic care modalities.
  6. Goal: *promote bonding.* encourage to participate in infant care, as possible.
  7. *Medical/surgical* management: surgical intervention/repair of congenital cardiac abnormality.

F. Evaluation/outcome criteria
  1. The infant experiences no respiratory embarrassment in immediate postnatal period.
  2. The infant completes transfer to high-risk center without incident, if applicable.
  3. Surgical intervention successful, where applicable.

III. Disorders affecting fluid-gas transport: *hemolytic disease of the newborn*

  A. Rh incompatibility
    1. Pathophysiology and **Etiology**—see *Rh isoimmunization,* chapter 3, p. 53.
    2. Assessment
       a. *Prenatal*—maternal Rh titers, amniocentesis.
       b. *Intrapartal*—amniotic fluid color
         (1) Straw colored: *mild* disease.
         (2) Golden: *severe* fetal disease.
       c. Direct Coombs test on cord blood; positive test demonstrates Rh antibodies in fetal blood.

         The newborn's RBCs are "washed" and mixed with Coombs serum. The test result is positive (i.e., maternal antibodies are present) if the infant's blood agglutinates. If the titer is 1 : 64, an exchange transfusion is indicated.

    3. Nursing care plan/implementation—exchange transfusion
       a. Goal: *health teaching* to explain purpose and process to parents:
         (1) Removes anti-Rh antibodies and fetal cells that are coated with antibodies.
         (2) Reduces bilirubin levels—indicated when 20 mg/dL in *term* neonate and 15 mg/dL in *pre-term.*
         (3) Corrects anemia—supplies red blood cells that will not be destroyed by maternal antibodies.
         (4) Rh-negative type O blood elicits no reaction; maximum exchange is 500 mL; duration of exchange: 45–60 min.
       b. Goal: *minimize transfusion hazards*
         (1) Warm blood to room temperature, since cold blood may precipitate cardiac arrest.
         (2) Use only fresh blood—to reduce possibility of hypocalcemia, tetany, convulsions.
         (3) Give calcium gluconate, as ordered, after each 100 mL of transfusion.
       c. Goal: *prepare for transfusion procedure.* Ready necessary equipment—monitor, resuscitation equipment, radiant heater, light.
       d. Goal: *assist with exchange transfusion*
         (1) Continuous monitoring of vital signs; record baseline, and every 15 min during procedure.
         (2) Record: time, amount of blood withdrawn; time and amount injected; medications given.
         (3) *Observe* for: dyspnea, listlessness, bleeding from transfusion site, cyanosis, cardiovascular irregularity or arrest; coolness of lower extremities.
       e. Goal: *posttransfusion care*
         (1) Assessment
           (a) Observe for dyspnea, cyanosis, car-

diac arrest or irregularities, jaundice, hypoglycemia; frequent vital signs.

    (b) Signs of *sepsis*—fever, tachycardia, dyspnea, chills, tremors.

  (2) Nursing care plan/implementation

    (a) Maintain thermal stability—to reduce physiologic stress, possibility of metabolic acidosis.

    (b) Give oxygen—to relieve cyanosis.

    (c) Keep cord moist—to facilitate repeat transfusion, if necessary.

    (d) Maintain nutrition/hydration—feed per schedule.

4. Evaluation/outcome criteria

  a. Infant's hemolytic process ceases; bilirubin level drops.

  b. Infant makes successful transition to extrauterine life.

  c. Infant experiences no complications of therapeutic regimen.

  d. Infant demonstrates evidence of bonding.

B. ABO incompatibility

  1. Pathophysiology—fetal blood carrying antigens A/B enters maternal type O bloodstream → antibody formation → antibodies cross placenta → hemolyze fetal red cells. NOTE: less severe than Rh reaction.

  2. Etiology

    a. Type O mother carries anti-A and anti-B antibodies.

    b. Even first pregnancy is jeopardized if fetal blood enters maternal system.

    c. Reaction possible if fetus is type A, type B, or type AB and mother is type O.

  3. Assessment

    a. Jaundice within first 24 hr.

    b. Rising bilirubin levels.

    c. Enlarged liver and spleen.

  4. Nursing care plan/implementation: goal: *reduce hazard to newborn*

    a. Prepare for exchange transfusion with O-negative blood.

    b. Provide phototherapy (if bilirubin is 10 mg/dL, and anemia is mild or absent.)

    c. Monitor status closely.

    d. Supportive care.

  5. Evaluation/outcome criteria

    a. Infant responds to medical/nursing regimen.

    b. Infant's assessment findings within normal limits.

C. Hyperbilirubinemia

  1. Pathophysiology—bilirubin, a breakdown product of hemolyzed red blood cells, appears at increased levels; exceeds 13–15 mg/dL. Bilirubin is safe when bound with albumin and conjugated by user for body excretion; **danger** is when unconjugated and deposits in CNS.

    a. WARNING: There is no "safe" serum-bilirubin level; kernicterus is a function of the bilirubin level *and* neonatal age and condition; poor fluid-and-caloric balance subjects the infant (especially the premature) to kernicterus at low serum-bilirubin levels.

    b. Kernicterus—high bilirubin levels result in deposition of yellow pigment in basal ganglia of brain → irreversible retardation.

  2. Etiology

    a. Rh or ABO incompatibility, during first 48 hr.

    b. Resolution of an enclosed hemorrhage (e.g., cephalohematoma).

    c. Infection.

    d. Drug-induced—vitamin K injection, maternal ingestion of *sulfisoxazole (Gantrisin)*.

    e. Bile duct blockage.

    f. Albumin-binding capacity is exceeded.

    g. "Breastfeeding jaundice" (e.g., pregnanediol in milk). Breastfeeding is *not* dangerous and not a cause of physiologic jaundice.

    h. Dehydration.

    i. Immature liver (interferes with conjugation).

  3. Assessment

    a. Jaundice noted after *blanching* skin to suppress hemoglobin color; noted in sclera or mucosa in dark-skinned neonates; make sure light is adequate; spreads from head down, with increasing severity.

    b. Pallor.

    c. Concentrated, dark urine.

    d. Blood level determination—hemoglobin or indirect bilirubin (unconjugated, unbound bilirubin deposits in CNS).

    e. *Kernicterus*—similar to intracranial hemorrhage

      (1) Poor feeding and/or sucking.

      (2) Regurgitation, vomiting.

      (3) High-pitched cry.

      (4) Temperature instability.

      (5) Hypertonicity/hypotonicity.

      (6) Progressive lethargy; diminished Moro reflex.

      (7) Respiratory distress.

      (8) Cerebral palsy, mental retardation.

      (9) Death.

  4. Analysis/nursing diagnosis

    a. *Fluid volume (red blood cell) deficit* related to hemolysis secondary to blood incompatibility.

    b. *High risk for injury* (brain damage) related to kernicterus.

    c. *Altered thought processes* (mental retardation) related to brain damage secondary to kernicterus.

    d. *Knowledge deficit (parental)* related to infant condition.

⋈ **5. Nursing care plan/implementation**
   a. *Medical management*
   〰 **(1)** *Prenatal*—amniocentesis.
      (2) *Postnatal*—exchange transfusion, phototherapy.
☞ **b.** Goal: *assist bilirubin conjugation through phototherapy*
   (1) Cover closed eyelids while under light; remove eyepads when not under light (feeding, cuddling, during parental visits)—to protect eyes.
   (2) Expose as much skin as possible—to maximize exposure of circulating blood to light. Remove for only brief time periods.
   (3) *Change position* every hour—to maximize exposure of circulating blood to light.
   (4) NOTE: any loose green stools as bile is cleared through gut; watch for skin breakdown on buttocks.
   (5) Monitor temperature—to identify hyperthermia.
   (6) *Push fluids* (to 25% more than average) between feedings—to counteract dehydration. Breast milk has natural laxative effects that help clear bile.
   c. Goal: *health teaching.* Explain, discuss phototherapy, bilirubin levels, implications.
   d. Goal: *emotional support*
   (1) Encourage verbalization of anxiety, fears, concerns.
   (2) Encourage contact with infant.
   (3) Reassure, as possible.
⋈ **6. Evaluation/outcome criteria**
   a. Infant's hemolytic process ceases; bilirubin level drops.
   b. Infant makes successful transition to extrauterine life.
   c. Infant experiences no complications of therapeutic regimen.
   d. Infant demonstrates evidence of effective bonding.

Emotional Support of the High-Risk Infant

I. *General overview*
  A. The high-risk infant has the same *developmental needs* as the healthy term infant
   1. Social and tactile stimulation.
   2. Comfort and removal of discomfort (hunger, soiling).
   3. Continuous contact with a consistent, parenting person.
  B. Treatment for serious physiologic compromise may result in:
   1. Isolation.
   2. Sensory deprivation or noxious stimuli.
   3. Emotional stress.

⋈ **II. Assessment**—signs of *neonatal emotional stress*
  A. Does not look at person performing care.
  B. Does not cry or protest.
  C. Poor weight gain; failure to thrive.
⋈ **III. Analysis/nursing diagnosis:** *sensory/perceptual alterations* related to isolation in Isolette, oxygen hood.
⋈ **IV. Nursing care plan/implementation**
  A. Goal: *provide consistent parenting contact.* Assign same nurses whenever possible.
  B. Goal: *emotional support*
   1. Comfort when crying.
☞   **2.** Provide positive sensory stimulation. Arrange time to
    a. Stroke skin.
    b. Hold hand.
    c. Hum, sing, talk.
    d. Hold in en-face position (nurse looking into infant's eyes).
    e. Hold when feeding, if possible.
  C. Goal: *encourage parents to participate in care*—to
   1. Reduce their psychological stress, anxiety, fear.
   2. Promote bonding.
   3. Reduce possibility of later child abuse (higher incidence of child abuse against children who have been high-risk infants).
⋈ **V. Evaluation/outcome criteria**
  A. Infant demonstrates successful resolution of physiologic problems.
  B. Parents and infant evidence bonding.
  C. Parents express satisfaction with care and result.

General Aspects: Nursing Care of the High-Risk Infant and Family

I. *General overview:* The birth of a physiologically compromised neonate is psychologically stressful for both infant and family, and physiologically stressful for the neonate. Effective, goal-directed nursing care is directed toward:
  A. Minimizing physiologic and psychological stress.
  B. Facilitating/supporting successful coping and/or adaptation.
  C. Encouraging parental attachment/separation/grieving, as appropriate.
⋈ **II. Assessment**—directed toward determining neonate's present and projected status
  A. Determine neonate's current physical status.
  B. Identify specific status and diagnosis-related problems and needs.
  C. Describe family psychological status, strengths, and coping mechanisms/skills.
  D. Determine medical/surgical/nursing approach to problems—and prognosis.
⋈ **III. Analysis/nursing diagnosis**
  A. Parental *anxiety/fear* related to physiologic compromise of neonate.

B. *Self-esteem disturbance* related to feelings of guilt and/or anger.
C. *Ineffective individual coping* related to severe psychological stress.
D. *Knowledge deficit* related to diagnosis, treatment, prognosis of infant.
E. *Risk for altered parenting* related to concern about infant.

IV. Nursing care plan/implementation
A. Goal: *preoperative and postoperative care*
   1. Maintain/improve physiologic stability
      a. Temperature stabilization—keep warm.
      b. Oxygenation
         (1) Position.
         ☞ (2) Administer oxygen, as ordered and/or necessary.
      c. Nutrition/hydration
         ☞ (1) Administer/monitor intravenous fluids.
         (2) Provide oral fluids, as ordered.
         (3) Feed, as status permits.
   2. Assist with diagnostic testing.
B. Goal: *emotional support of parents*
   1. Encourage exploring and ventilating feelings.
   2. Involve parents in decision-making process.
C. Goal: *health teaching*
   1. Determine knowledge/understanding of problem.
   2. Explain/simplify/clarify, as needed, physician's discussions with parents.
   3. Describe/explain/discuss neonate's present status and any auxiliary equipment; teach CPR to family.
   4. Refer, as needed, to hospital/community resources.
D. Goal: *promote bonding.* encourage parental participation in care of the neonate.

V. Evaluation/outcome criteria
A. Parents verbalize understanding of relevant information; make informed decisions regarding infant care.
B. Parents demonstrate comfort and increasing participation in care of neonate.
C. Infant maintains/increases adequacy of adaptation to extrauterine life.
D. If relevant, parents demonstrate progress in grieving process.

Summary

For some neonates, the transition to extrauterine existence is complicated by **high-risk conditions:** *infections,* maternal disorders such as poorly controlled *diabetes mellitus,* and *maternal drug* and *alcohol dependence.* The life and well-being of other infants are threatened by **preterm** or **postterm** births and/or **congenital** disorders. The nurse must have critical care nursing skills, knowledge of the growth and developmental needs of infants, sensitivity to parental needs, and ability to work with an interdisciplinary team of health care providers.

 Study and Memory Aids

Neonatal Risk Factors: ABC-I

Age, gestational
Birth trauma
Congenital disorders
Infection

Neonatal Infections—Transmission of HBV

Serum to serum
Contact with contaminated urine, feces, saliva, semen
Mother to baby: transplacentally or from infected birth canal

Preterm Infant—Anticipated Problems: TRIES

Temperature regulation
Resistance to infection
Immature liver
Elimination
Sensory-perceptual functions

Respiratory Distress Syndrome: Infant

Avoid placing infant on abdomen.

Prevention of Transmission of Infection (Thrush) and Prevention of Secondary Infections (RDs)

Handwashing—for nurse *and* mother—cannot be overemphasized!

RH Incompatibility

Rh + babies receive Rh −, type O blood in the transfusion.

Questions

1. The nurse would not expect to give tetracycline during pregnancy due to:
   1. Its effect on kidney function in the mother.

2. Its effect on liver function in the mother.
3. The development of Hutchinson's teeth in the child.
4. Its stimulation of bone growth in the fetus/newborn.

2. The plan of care developed by nurses for parents of a drug-dependent baby includes:
   1. Recommendation for minimal contact between parents and infants.
   2. Ways to encourage parent-infant bonding and any positive parental responses to the baby.
   3. Discouraging attachment between the parent and baby.
   4. Acknowledgement that drug-dependent parents are less likely to be interested in their babies.

3. A neonate at 1 min after birth exhibits the following: heart rate, 92; no respiratory effort; muscle tone showing some flexion; grimace in response to slap on sole of foot; pale color. The nurse's first response should be to:
   1. Do nothing because the findings are within normal limits.
   2. Take the neonate to the nursery for further observation.
   3. Administer oxygen by mask until the neonate is pink.
   4. Begin resuscitative actions immediately.

4. Varicella-zoster virus infections are infrequent during pregnancy but can cause serious consequences. Which statement is not relevant to the care of the mother/fetus/newborn?
   1. Transmission occurs through droplet spray (sneeze) or through contact with vesicular fluid and cells from fresh skin lesions.
   2. Infants with varicella embryopathy are highly infectious and should be isolated immediately following birth.
   3. The mother with pneumonia is to be given acyclovir.
   4. Women with chickenpox at the time of birth should not have contact with their newborns until all vesicles have crusted.

5. Health care teaching needs to include information that the most common mode of transmission of herpes simplex virus to an infant is:
   1. Across the placenta.
   2. Vertical infection from a vaginal infection.
   3. During passage through an infected birth canal.
   4. From infected personnel or family.

6. Congenital syphilis is suspected in a newborn infant. For which specific sign should the nurse assess this neonate?
   1. Tremors, sweating.
   2. Seizure activity.
   3. Anemia.
   4. Snuffles.

7. The home health nurse develops a plan of care for a newborn whose mother was diagnosed with a chlamydial infection during pregnancy based on knowledge that *Chlamydia trachomatis* is an intracellular bacterium that causes neonatal conjunctivitis and:
   1. Discolored baby and adult teeth.
   2. Snuffles and rhagades in the newborn.
   3. Pneumonia.
   4. Central and peripheral hearing defects that progress during infancy.

8. Early signs of neonatal infection are nonspecific. The nurse should be aware that the most accurate predictor of neonatal infection is:
   1. Neutropenia.
   2. Neutrophilia.
   3. Leukopenia.
   4. Leukocytosis.

9. A woman's prenatal record reveals a history of alcohol abuse that continued throughout pregnancy. The nurse's plan of care for this woman's newborn includes assessment of fetal alcohol syndrome (FAS) because of which characteristic?
   1. Saddle nose, red rash on chin, and snuffles.
   2. Neonatal conjunctivitis and pneumonia.
   3. Large for gestational age (LGA).
   4. Facial dysmorphia.

10. Birth injury is a concern during a forceps-assisted or breech birth. Erb-Duchenne paralysis is suspected if the nursery nurse observes:
    1. A flaccid arm with the elbow extended.
    2. Absence of Moro reflex on the unaffected side.
    3. Absence of grasp reflex on the affected side.
    4. Torticollis or wry neck.

11. The nurse observes the neonate of the mother whose pregnancy was complicated by the HELLP syndrome for:
    1. High hematocrit.
    2. Hyperglycemia.
    3. Thrombocytopenia.
    4. Cardiomyopathy.

12. What is the most common complication for which the nurse must closely monitor a *preterm* newborn?
    1. Brain damage.
    2. Respiratory distress syndrome.
    3. Meconium aspiration syndrome.
    4. Hemorrhage.

13. The nurse questions the gestational age estimate recorded in the chart if an infant recorded as preterm displays which one of the following?
    1. Absence of lanugo.
    2. Absence of subcutaneous fat.
    3. Parchment-thin skin.
    4. Wrinkled "old-man" appearance.

14. For what complication frequently associated with post-term birth must the nurse closely monitor the *postmature* newborn?
    1. Brain damage.
    2. Respiratory distress syndrome.
    3. Meconium aspiration syndrome.
    4. Hemorrhage.

15. The nurse implements cardiopulmonary resuscitation (CPR) on the newborn by maintaining a compression rate of:
    1. 60/min.
    2. 80/min.
    3. 100/min.
    4. 120/min.

16. An important role of the nurse is in risk management. The nurse reviews all assessment findings to determine which, if any, require further investigation/evaluation. Of the following findings on a full-term newborn, which

one is *not* a normal result of maternal hormone influence, and needs to be reported?
1. "Witch's milk."
2. Vaginal bleeding.
3. Undescended testes.
4. Linea nigra.

17. When forceps are used for the birth of an infant's head, the nurse should assess the newborn for:
1. Torticollis.
2. Facial paralysis.
3. Fractured clavicle.
4. Cephalohematoma.

18. A nurse is evaluating a newborn with hospital-specified criteria for early discharge. The nurse would determine that the newborn who is *not* a candidate for early discharge is one whose:
1. Coombs test is positive, birth weight was 2775 g, and Apgar score was 9, 9.
2. Hematocrit is 52%; respirations, 40/min; feeding is going well.
3. Birth weight was 4000 g, gestational age was 38 wk, and temperature is 98.1°F.
4. Apical heart rate is 122 beats/min, Moro reflex is positive; has passed two meconium stools.

19. The nurse is assessing a newborn on admission to the nursery. In evaluating the findings, the nurse knows that the finding that must be referred for further investigation/evaluation is:
1. Misshapen head.
2. Short neck.
3. Tremors of the extremities.
4. Flat abdomen (scaphoid).

20. The nurse would closely observe a neonate whose:
1. Slight heart murmur, heard at 1 hr, is inaudible at 4 hr.
2. Respiratory rate increased from 30/min to 48/min, then stabilized.
3. Color became cyanotic during the first feeding.
4. Heart rate ranged from 122 to 148 within the same hour.

21. Nursing care for a baby treated for jaundice with phototherapy includes:
1. Discontinuing phototherapy for feedings and parent visits.
2. Monitoring temperature rectally.
3. Replacing fluid loss with an additional 2 mL of formula every 2 hr.
4. Removing eye patches for 5 min every hour.

22. A newborn's record reveals: 42-wk gestation; spontaneous vaginal birth after a 15-hr labor; Apgar scores of 8 and 9; blood glucose of 30 mg/dL. The mother received no sedation, and plans to breastfeed. What is the priority nursing action?
1. Bottle feed with formula, then recheck the blood glucose level.
2. Start an IV of 10% dextrose in water (D/10/W), then recheck the blood glucose level.
3. Let the mother breastfeed for 15 min, then recheck the blood glucose level.
4. Place the baby under a warmer for 15 min, then recheck the blood glucose level.

23. In caring for a preterm infant, the nurse must monitor arterial blood gas readings for oxygen saturation. Following protocol, the nurse discontinues oxygen therapy as soon as possible in order to decrease the possibility of:
1. Necrotizing enterocolitis.
2. Retinopathy of prematurity.
3. Myofibroplasia.
4. Cerebrospinal dysplasia.

24. Which finding would indicate to the nurse that a newborn has thrush (candidiasis)?
1. Bleeding gums.
2. Epstein's pearls on roof of mouth.
3. White patches adherent to mucosa of the mouth.
4. "Milk blisters" on lips.

25. Which laboratory values in suspected Rh incompatibility will be most relevant in planning nursing care for the infant?
1. Oxygen concentration.
2. Direct Coombs test.
3. Glucose level.
4. Hemoglobin A$_{1c}$.

Answers/Rationale

1. **(2)** Tetracycline (used for the treatment of syphilis in penicillin-allergic persons, and for the treatment of chlamydial infection) is contraindicated in pregnancy because of its effects on liver function in the mother. Tetracycline affects liver, *not* kidney **(1)**, function in the mother. It results in tooth *discoloration, not* Hutchinson's teeth **(3)**, fetus. (Hutchinson's teeth is a sequel to congenital syphilis.) Tetracycline also results in *decreased* bone growth in the fetus, *not* increased **(4)**. **EV, 1, PhI**

2. **(2)** Parent-infant bonding and positive parental responses to the baby are encouraged; this may help motivate parents to enter drug rehabilitation. The opposite of the other options is true: Contact **(1)** and attachment **(3)** between parents and baby are *encouraged.* Drug-dependent parents are *not* less likely to be interested in their babies **(4). PL, 7, PsI**

3. **(4)** Begin resuscitative actions immediately; the neonate's Apgar score is only 3. The findings *do* require action **(1)**: immediate resuscitation and further investigation. Resuscitation should *not* wait until the neonate can be taken to the nursery **(2)**. Oxygen **(3)** will not resuscitate the neonate who is not breathing; resuscita-

---

Key to Codes

Nursing process: AS, assessment; **AN,** analysis; **PL,** planning; **IMP,** implementation; **EV,** evaluation. (See Appendix I for explanation of nursing process steps.)

Category of human function: 1, protective; **2,** sensory-perceptual; **3,** comfort, rest, activity, and mobility; **4,** nutrition; **5,** growth and development; **6,** fluid-gas transport; **7,** psychosocial-cultural; **8,** elimination. (See Appendix K for explanation.)

Client need: SECE, safe, effective care environment; **PhI,** physiological integrity; **PsI,** psychosocial integrity; **HPM,** health promotion/maintenance. (See Appendix L for explanation.)

tion, preferably by a trained pediatrician (neonatologist), must be initiated stat. **AN, 6, PhI**

4. **(2)** Infants with varicella embryopathy are *not* considered infectious and do *not* need to be isolated either in the nursery or at home. The other options *are* relevant: Option **1** correctly describes the mode of transmission of chickenpox. Acyclovir **(3)** *is* given to women with marked pulmonary involvement. Women with chickenpox at birth *should not* have contact with their newborns until all vesicles have crusted **(4)**.

   NOTE: There is also a 25% chance that varicella virus will spread vertically from the mother to the fetus or newborn. **PL, 1, SECE**

5. **(3)** The most common mode of transmission of herpes simplex virus to an infant is during passage through an infected birth canal. Transplacental transmission **(1)**, vertical infection from a vaginal infection **(2)**, and transmission by infected personnel or family **(4)** are all possible; however, none of these is *the most common* mode of transmission.

   NOTE: Thorough handwashing should be practiced by health care providers as well as by family members. Gloves should be worn during contact with lesions or secretions. Family members with oral lesions should be discouraged from kissing the newborn. In general, infants born to mothers who are at risk of transmitting the infection should be isolated. **PL, 1, SECE**

6. **(4)** Snuffles (rhinitis), rhagades (cracks, fissures around the mouth), hydrocephaly, and corneal opacity are all sequelae to congenital syphilis. Tremors and sweating **(1)**, seizure activity **(2)**, and anemia **(3)** are *not* sequelae to congenital syphilis. **AS, 1, SECE**

7. **(3)** It causes pneumonia. Newborns exhibit prolonged staccato cough, tachypnea, mild hypoxemia, and eosinophilia. Discolored teeth **(1)** are secondary to treatment of the pregnant woman with *tetracycline*. Snuffles and rhagades **(2)** are sequelae to *congenital syphilis*. *Congenital rubella*, which is not a static disease, results in central and peripheral hearing defects that progress after birth **(4)**.

   NOTE: Snuffles refer to copious, clear, serosanguineous mucous discharge from the obstructed nose. Rhagades refer to circumoral radiating scars that result from rough, cracked mucocutaneous lesions of the lips. **AS, 1, SECE**

8. **(1)** Neutropenia is the most accurate predictor of neonatal infection. This abnormal *decrease* in neutrophils (circulating white blood cells essential for phagocytosis and proteolysis) is associated with a variety of conditions, including infection. Neutropenia is associated with infection, *not* neutrophilia **(2)**, an increase in neutrophils. Leukopenia **(3)** and leukocytosis **(4)** are not accurate predictors of neonatal infection. Leukocytes are of five types; neutrophils are one type of granulocytic leukocytes. **AS, 1, SECE**

9. **(4)** Facial dysmorphia, growth deficits at birth that do not improve with time, and other neurologic dysfunction are characteristically seen in these children. (Additional problems may include anomalies of ocular structure and limbs, and a variety of cardiocirculatory defects, especially ventricular septal defects.) Saddle nose, red rash on chin, and snuffles **(1)** are characteristic of *syphilis* (congenital). Neonatal conjunctivitis and pneumonia **(2)** are characteristic of *chlamydial infection*. FAS newborns may be preterm and *small* for gestational age (SGA), *not* large **(3)**. **AS, 5, HPM**

10. **(1)** The flaccid arm in this paralysis is secondary to damage to spinal nerves C5 and C6. This damage is caused by excessive lateral flexion of the head during birth of the shoulder. The Moro reflex would be absent or lessened on the *affected* side, *not* the unaffected side **(2)**. Injury to C5 and C6 does not affect the grasp reflex **(3)**; Klumpke's paralysis (paralysis of the hand) results from damage to C8. Torticollis, or wry neck **(4)**, is a congenital shortening or spasmodic contraction of the neck (sternocleidomastoid) muscles. **AS, 1, HPM**

11. **(3)** The neonate of the woman whose pregnancy was complicated with the HELLP syndrome must be observed for thrombocytopenia, a common finding with this disorder. A high hematocrit **(1)**, hyperglycemia **(2)**, and cardiomyopathy **(4)** are not associated with HELLP. **AS, 6, HPM**

12. **(2)** Respiratory distress syndrome (RDS) is the most common complication in preterm newborns, secondary to a) insufficient surfactant needed to maintain open alveoli on exhalation; b) small, easily collapsible respiratory passages; c) weak respiratory musculature; and d) immature bony thorax. Brain damage **(1)**, if present, is diagnosed *later*. (If severe hypoxia occurred during birth, brain damage would be of considerable concern.) Meconium aspiration **(3)** is one of the most common complications of the *postterm* newborn. Hemorrhage **(4)** is of concern, but is *not* the *most* common complication seen in the preterm newborn. **AS, 6, HPM**

13. **(1)** Absence of lanugo is characteristic of the *full*-term or *post*term newborn. Absence of subcutaneous fat **(2)**, parchment-thin skin **(3)**, and wrinkled "old-man" appearance **(4)** due to absence of vernix caseosa *are* all characteristic of the preterm newborn. **AS, 1, HPM**

14. **(3)** Meconium aspiration is commonly the cause of respiratory distress in the postterm newborn. It must be suspected if meconium staining is present on the skin, nails, and cord. Brain damage **(1)** if it is present, may be the result of birth trauma, *not* postterm birth. Respiratory distress syndrome **(2)** is seen in *preterm* infants and infants of mothers with poorly controlled diabetes mellitus. Hemorrhage **(4)** is not a frequently associated complication. **AS, 1, HPM**

15. **(3)** A compression rate of a minimum of 100/min is required; assist ventilation on the upstroke of every fifth compression (5 : 1). The rates in the other options are either *too slow* **(1** and **2)** or *too fast* **(4)**. **IMP, 1, SECE**

16. **(3)** Undescended testes are a condition unrelated to maternal hormone influence. Testes begin to descend from the abdominal cavity into the scrotum starting at about 28 wk gestation. Before 36 wk, they should be palpable in the inguinal canal; by 36–38 wk, they should be palpable within the scrotum. "Witch's milk" **(1)** refers to the whitish secretion that comes from the nipples of *some* male or female term newborns. Vaginal bleeding **(2)**, or pseudomenstruation, is seen in *some* full-term female newborns. Linea nigra **(4)** can be seen in *some* full-term male or female newborns. **EV, 5, HPM**

17. (2) Facial paralysis can occur when the forceps blades compress the cranial VII (facial) nerve, anterior to the ears. It is usually mild and temporary, lasting only a few days. Torticollis **(1)**, or wry neck, is caused by a shortened sternocleidomastoid muscle on one side of the fetal neck. Fractured clavicle **(3)** is usually caused during birth of the shoulders, when the infant is large, or the mother's pelvic outlet is small. Cephalohematoma **(4)** is *not* caused by properly placed forceps. This bleeding between the periosteum and one or more of the cranial bones (especially the parietal) is *secondary* to *pressure* from the maternal pelvis. **AN, 2, SECE**

18. (1) If a newborn's Coombs test is positive, further evaluation is needed. If the infant is Coombs positive because of Rh incompatibility, the baby is at risk for anemia and hyperbilirubinemia. (The birth weight of 6 lb 2 oz and the Apgar score of 9, 9 *do* fit the criteria for early discharge.) The hematocrit, respirations, and feeding pattern in option **2** *do* fit the criteria for early discharge. The birth weight, gestational age, and temperature in option **3** *do* fit the criteria for early discharge. The apical heart rate, stooling pattern, and Moro reflex response in option **4** *do* fit the criteria for early discharge. **EV, 6, PhI**

19. (4) A scaphoid abdomen is seen in infants with diaphragmatic hernia, where the abdominal contents have herniated into the thoracic cavity. Within an hour, bowel sounds may be heard in the thoracic cavity and respiratory distress increases markedly. The misshapen head **(1)** is the result of molding (overlapping of cranial bones to accommodate to the dimensions of the maternal pelvis); this is a *normal* finding in infants born vaginally. Normal newborns have very short necks **(2)**, but the neck is flexible and moves easily from side to side. Transient tremors of the extremities **(3)** are *normal* in the newborn. **EV, 8, PhI**

20. (3) Cyanosis during feeding may be a sign of a cardiovascular defect. Some cardiovascular defects become apparent as the newborn experiences cold temperatures, handling, feeding, etc. The findings in options **1**, **2**, and **4** are all *normal* in the newborn infant. **EV, 6, PhI**

21. (1) Phototherapy should be discontinued and eye patches removed during feedings and for parent visits to allow for infant stimulation and to allow for bonding/attachment between parent and child. Option **2** is incorrect; taking the temperature rectally is *not* recommended, since this method can result in injury to the rectum. Option **3** is incorrect because the newborn receiving phototherapy needs to have fluid intake increased by 25% to compensate for insensible water loss;

since the normal intake requirement is 105 mL/kg/24 hr, this newborn would require an increase of *over* 2 mL *per kg* every 2 hr. Option **4** is incorrect because the newborn under phototherapy lights does *not* need this action; the newborn should be *turned* at least every half hour to expose all areas of the skin and to prevent pressure spots. **IMP, 7, HPM**

22. (1) Blood glucose for a newborn should be at least 40 mg/dL; this newborn's level is low and requires immediate replacement of glucose; feeding formula or breast milk, if available, provides longer normal glucose levels. Option **2** is incorrect because an *otherwise healthy* newborn should *not* need the *intrusive* procedure of an IV to obtain an adequate glucose level. Use of D/10/W can result in rebound hypoglycemia (a bolus of glucose stimulates the neonate to produce a large quantity of insulin, which then rapidly uses up the glucose bolus). Options **3** and **4** are incorrect because these do *not* provide for *immediate* glucose replacement: moreover, breast milk **(3)** is *not available* for about 3 days. **IMP, 4, HPM**

23. (2) Retinopathy of prematurity is caused by the effect of high oxygen concentrations; it results in loss of sight in the infant. The conditions in options **1, 3** and **4** are *not* related to the use of high oxygen concentration, but are associated with body damage caused by *other* factors. **IMP, 6, SECE**

24. (3) White patches adherent to mucosa of mouth, gums, and tongue, which tend to bleed when touched, are the lesions of thrush. Bleeding gums **(1)** in the neonate would be an abnormal finding that would necessitate immediate investigation (DIC), but *do not suggest thrush*. Epstein's pearls **(2)**, small white blebs found along the gum margins and at the junction of the soft and hard palates, are a *normal* manifestation commonly seen in the newborn (similar to Bohn's nodules). "Milk blisters" **(4)** are *normally* seen in infants (both breast- and bottle fed); they disappear during weaning. **AS, 1, SECE**

25. (2) Direct Coombs test is used to determine if maternal Rh-positive antibodies are present in fetal cord blood; a positive test result indicates the presence of antibodies (titer). Oxygen concentration **(1)** does *not* give data relevant to the possible presence of anti-Rh positive antibodies. Glucose level **(3)** does *not* provide data relevant to the possible presence of anti-Rh positive antibodies (however, some of these infants may have low glucose levels, which would require intervention). Hgb_{Alc} (glycosylated hemoglobin) **(4)** determines the status of *glucose* metabolism over the previous 120 days. **AN, 6, HPM**

Glossary

Use this list of over 200 terms as an additional way to review content.

ABC   Alternative birthing center. Birthing areas in hospitals located away from the traditional obstetric department.

ABO Incompatibility.   Occurs when the mother's blood type is O and the newborn's is A, B, or AB.

Abortion   The expulsion from the uterus of an embryo or fetus before it is viable and capable of extrauterine existence. See *abortus.*

> **Complete a.**   Abortion in which fetus and all related tissue have been expelled from the uterus.
>
> **Elective a.**   Termination of pregnancy chosen by the woman that is not required for her physical safety.
>
> **Habitual (recurrent) a.**   Loss of three or more successive pregnancies for no known cause.
>
> **Incomplete a.**   Loss of pregnancy in which some but not all the products of conception have been expelled from the uterus.
>
> **Induced a.**   Intentionally produced loss of pregnancy by woman or others.
>
> **Inevitable a.**   Threatened loss of pregnancy that cannot be prevented or stopped and is imminent.
>
> **Missed a.**   Loss of pregnancy in which the products of conception remain in the uterus after the fetus dies.
>
> **Septic a.**   Loss of pregnancy in which there is an infection of the products of conception and the uterine endometrial lining, usually resulting from attempted termination of early pregnancy.
>
> **Spontaneous a.**   Loss of pregnancy that occurs naturally without interference or known cause.
>
> **Therapeutic a.**   Pregnancy that has been intentionally terminated for medical reasons.
>
> **Threatened a.**   Possible loss of a pregnancy; early symptoms are present (e.g., the cervix begins to dilate).

Abortus   An embryo/fetus that is removed or expelled from the uterus at 20 wk gestation or less, or weighing 500 g or less, or measuring 25 cm or less.

Abruptio placentae   Partial or complete premature separation of a normally implanted placenta from the uterine wall, sometimes with massive hemorrhage.

Abstinence   Refraining from sexual intercourse periodically or permanently.

Access to care   Opportunity to receive health care services.

Accreta, placenta   See *placenta accreta.*

Adapted from IM Bobak, M Jensen. *Maternity and Gynecologic Care— the Nurse and the Family* (5th ed). St. Louis: Mosby, 1993; and IM Bobak, DL Lowdermilk, MD Jensen. *Maternity Nursing* (4th ed). St. Louis: Mosby, 1995.

ACHES   Acronym for possible warning signs secondary to use of oral hormone contraceptives. *See text.*

Acini cells   Milk-producing cells in the breast.

Acrocyanosis   Peripheral cyanosis; blue color of hands and feet in most infants at birth that may persist for 7–10 days.

Acromion   Projection of the spine of the scapula (forming the point of the shoulder); used to explain the presentation of the fetus.

Acrosome reaction   Release of proteolytic enzymes from fallopian tubes that enable the sperm to digest the cumulus cells and penetrate the zona pellucida of the ovum.

Adenomyoma   Type of tumor affecting glandular and smooth muscle tissue, such as uterine musculature.

Adnexa   Adjacent or accessory parts of a structure.

> **Uterine a.**   Ovaries and fallopian tubes.

Adult respiratory distress syndrome (ARDS)   Set of symptoms including decreased compliance of lung tissue, pulmonary edema, and acute hypoxemia. The condition is similar to respiratory distress syndrome (RDS) of the newborn.

Afibrinogenemia   Absence or decrease of fibrinogen in the blood such that the blood will not coagulate. In obstetrics, this condition occurs from complications of abruptio placentae or retention of a dead fetus. *See DIC.*

Afterbirth   Lay term for the placenta and membranes expelled after the birth of the child.

Afterpains   Painful uterine cramps that occur intermittently for approximately 2 or 3 days after birth and that result from contractile efforts of the uterus to return to its normal involuted condition; **afterbirth pains.**

AGA   Appropriate (weight) for gestational age.

Agenesis   Failure of an organ to develop.

Agonist-antagonist compounds   An agonist is an agent that activates something; an antagonist is an agent that blocks something.

Alae nasi   Nostrils.

Albuminuria   Presence of readily detectable amounts of albumin in the urine; proteinuria.

Amenorrhea   Absence or suppression of menstruation.

Amniocentesis   Procedure in which a needle is inserted through the abdominal and uterine walls into the amniotic fluid; used for assessment of fetal health and maturity and for elective or therapeutic abortion.

Amnioinfusion   Infusion of normal saline warmed to body temperature, via an intrauterine catheter into the uterine cavity in an attempt to increase the fluid around the umbilical cord and prevent compression during uterine contractions.

Amnion   Inner membrane of two fetal membranes that form the sac and contain the fetus and the fluid that surrounds it in utero.

Amnionitis   Inflammation of the amnion, occurring most frequently after early rupture of membranes.

Amniotic   Pertaining or relating to the amnion.

A. fluid   Fluid surrounding fetus derived primarily from maternal serum and fetal urine.

!A. fluid embolism   Embolism resulting from amniotic fluid entering the maternal bloodstream during labor and birth after rupture of membranes; this is often fatal to the woman if it is a pulmonary embolism.

A. sac   Thin, transparent sac that holds the fetus suspended in amniotic fluid; popularly called the bag of waters.

Amniotomy   Artificial rupture of the fetal membranes (AROM).

Analgesia   Lack of pain without loss of consciousness.

Analgesic   Any drug or agent that will relieve pain.

Android pelvis   Male type of pelvis. See *pelvis.*

Anencephaly   Congenital deformity characterized by the absence of cerebrum, cerebellum, and flat bones of skull.

Anesthesia   Partial or complete absence of sensation with or without loss of consciousness.

Aneuploidy   Having an abnormal number of chromosomes.

Anomaly   Organ or structure that is malformed or in some way abnormal with reference to form, structure, or position.

Anovular menstrual period   Cyclic uterine bleeding not accompanied by the production and discharge of an ovum. Characteristic of early cycles at menarche and after childbirth.

Anovulatory   Failure of the ovaries to produce, mature, or release eggs.

Anoxia   Absence of oxygen.

Antenatal   Occurring before or formed before birth.

Antepartal   Before labor and birth.

Anteroposterior repair   Operation in which the upper and lower walls of the vagina are reconstructed to correct relaxed tissue.

Anthropoid pelvis   Pelvis in which the anteroposterior diameter is equal to or greater than the transverse diameter. See *pelvis.*

Anthropometry   Study of human body measurements.

Antibody   Specific protein substance developed by the body that exerts restrictive or destructive action on specific antigens, such as bacteria, toxins, or Rh factor.

Anticipatory grief   Grief that predates the loss of a beloved person or object, e.g., anticipated loss of a pregnancy or compromised newborn.

Antigen   Protein foreign to the body that causes the body to develop antibodies. Examples: bacteria, dust, Rh factor.

Apgar score   Numeric expression of the condition of a newborn obtained by rapid assessment at 1, 5, and 15 min of age; developed by Dr. Virginia Apgar.

Apnea   Cessation of respirations for more than 10 sec associated with generalized cyanosis.

Apt test   Differentiation of maternal and fetal blood when *vaginal bleeding* is present. It is performed as follows: Add 0.5 mL blood to 4.5 mL distilled water. Shake. Add 1 mL 0.25N sodium hydroxide. Fetal and cord blood remain pink for 1 or 2 min. Maternal blood becomes brown in 30 sec. See *Kleihauer-Betke test.*

Areola   Pigmented ring of tissue surrounding the nipple.

Secondary a.   During the fifth month of pregnancy, a second faint ring of pigmentation seen around the original areola.

Artificial insemination   Introduction of semen by instrument injection into the vagina or uterus for impregnation. Preferred term: *therapeutic insemination.*

Asherman's syndrome   Intrauterine adhesions following inflammation and infection; one cause of impaired fertility.

Asphyxia   Decreased oxygen and/or excess of carbon dioxide in the body.

A. livida   Condition in which the infant's skin is characteristically pale, pulse is weak and slow, and reflexes are depressed or absent; also known as *blue asphyxia.*

A. pallida   Condition in which the infant appears pale and limp and suffers from bradycardia (≤ 80 beats/min) and apnea.

Fetal a.   Condition occurring in utero, with the following biochemical changes: hypoxemia (lowering of PO_2), hypercapnia (increase in PCO_2), and respiratory and metabolic acidosis (reduction of blood pH).

Aspiration pneumonia   Inflammatory condition of the lungs and bronchi caused by the inhalation of vomitus containing acid gastric contents; ARDS may be a sequel.

Aspiration syndrome   See *meconium aspiration syndrome.*

Assault   An unlawful act that places another person, without that person's consent, in fear of immediate bodily harm or battery.

Ataractic   Drug capable of promoting tranquility; a tranquilizer.

Atelectasis   Pulmonary pathosis involving alveolar collapse.

Athetosis   Neuromuscular condition characterized by slow, writhing, continuous, and involuntary movement of the extremities, as seen in some forms of cerebral palsy and in motor disorders resulting from lesions in the basal ganglia.

Atony   Absence of muscle tone.

Atresia   Absence of a normally present passageway.

Choanal a.   Complete obstruction of the posterior nares, which open into the nasopharynx, with membranous or bony tissue.

Esophageal a.   Congenital anomaly in which the esophagus ends in a blind pouch or narrows into a thin cord, thus failing to form a continuous passageway to the stomach.

Attachment   A feeling of affection or loyalty that binds one person to another, which occurs at critical periods, such as birth or adoption; it is unique, specific, and enduring.

Augmentation of labor   Artificial stimulation of uterine contractions after labor has started spontaneously but is not progressing satisfactorily.

Autoimmune disease   Body produces antibodies against itself, causing tissue damage.

Autoimmunization   Development of antibodies against constituents of one's own tissues (e.g., a man may develop antibodies against his own sperm).

Autolysis   "Self-digestive" process by which the uterus returns (involutes) to a nonpregnant state following childbirth. The decrease in estrogen and progesterone levels following childbirth results in this destruction of excess and hypertrophied uterine tissue.

Autosomal inheritance   Characteristics transmitted by genes on the autosomes, not the sex chromosomes.

Autosomes Any of the paired chromosomes other than the sex (X and Y) chromosomes.

Axis, pelvic Imaginary curved line that passes through the centers of all the anteroposterior diameters of the pelvis.

Azoospermia Absence of sperm in the semen.

Baby blues See *postpartum blues.*

Back labor Uncomfortable labor that occurs when fetus, in occiput posterior position, presses on sacral nerves during contractions.

Bacteremic shock Shock that occurs in septicemia when endotoxins are released from certain bacteria in the bloodstream.

Bag of waters Lay term for the sac containing amniotic fluid and fetus.

Ballottement (1) Movability of a floating object (e.g., fetus). (2) Diagnostic technique using palpation: A floating object, when tapped or pushed, moves away and then returns to touch the examiner's hand.

Bandl's ring Abnormally thickened ridge of uterine musculature between the upper and lower segments that follows a mechanically obstructed labor, with the lower segment thinning abnormally.

Barr body (sex chromatin) Chromatin mass located against the inner surface of the nucleus in females, possibly representing the inactive X chromosome.

Bartholin's glands Two small glands situated on either side of the vaginal orifice that secrete small amounts of mucus during coitus and that are homologous to the bulbourethral glands in the male.

Basal body temperature (BBT) Lowest body temperature of a healthy person taken immediately after awakening and before any physical activity.

Battery Repeated beating of or use of force on a person without regard to personal rights; may be physical, sexual, psychological, or social.

Behavioral assessment Assessment of newborn's activity, feeding and sleeping patterns; responsiveness.

Bell's palsy See *palsy, Bell's.*

Bereavement The feelings of loss, pain, desolation, and sadness that occur after the death of a loved one.

Bicornuate uterus Anomalous uterus that may be either a double or single organ with two horns.

Bilirubin Yellow or orange pigment that is a breakdown product of hemoglobin. It is carried by the blood to the liver, where it is chemically changed and excreted in the bile or is conjugated and excreted by the kidneys.

Billings method See *ovulation method.*

Bimanual palpation Examination of a woman's pelvic organs done by placing one hand on the abdomen and one or two fingers of the other hand in the vagina.

Biophysical profile (BPP) Noninvasive assessment of the fetus and its environment using ultrasonography and uterine fetal monitoring; includes fetal breathing movements, gross body movements, fetal muscle tone, reactive fetal heart rate, and qualitative amniotic fluid volume.

Biopsy Removal of a small piece of tissue for microscopic examination and diagnosis.

Biparietal diameter Largest transverse diameter of the fetal head; extends from one parietal bone to the other.

Birth plan A tool by which expectant parents can explore their childbirth options and choose those that are most important to them.

Bishop score Rating system to evaluate inducibility of the cervix; a higher score increases the rate of successful induction of labor.

Blastocyst The stage in development of an embryo following the morula, made of an outer layer of trophoblast and an inner cell mass.

Blastoderm Germinal membrane of the ovum.

B. vesicle Stage in the development of a mammalian embryo that consists of an outer layer, or trophoblast, and a hollow sphere of cells enclosing a cavity.

Blood-brain barrier Obstruction that prevents passage of certain substances from blood into brain tissue.

Bloody show Vaginal discharge that originates in the cervix and consists of blood and mucus; increases as cervix dilates during labor.

Body image Person's subjective concept of his or her physical appearance.

Body mass index (BMI) Method of evaluating the appropriateness of weight for height; formula: BMI = weight/height² (weight in kg/height in m).

Bonding Describes the initial mutual attraction between people, such as between parent and child, at first meeting. Also see *attachment.*

Born out of asepsis (BOA) Pertaining to birth without the use of sterile technique.

Bradley method Preparation for parenthood with active participation of father/coach and mother.

Braxton Hicks sign Mild, intermittent, painless uterine contractions that occur more frequently as pregnancy advances but do not represent true labor.

Braxton Hicks version One of several types of maneuvers designed to turn the fetus from an undesirable position to a more acceptable one to facilitate birth.

Brazelton assessment Criteria for assessing the interactional behavior of a newborn.

Breakthrough bleeding Escape of blood occurring between menstrual periods; may be noted by women using chemical contraception (birth control pill).

Breast milk jaundice See *jaundice, breast milk.*

Breast self-examination (BSE) Self-examination of the breasts.

Breast surgeries for malignant lesions

  Lumpectomy (tylectomy) Excision of tumor and some surrounding normal tissue.

  Quadrectomy (segmental resection) Excision of a quadrant of the mammary gland that includes the tumor.

  Total (simple) mastectomy Removal of all of the mammary gland that includes the tumor.

  Radical mastectomy Removal of mammary gland, pectoralis major, and axillary lymph nodes.

Breech presentation Presentation in which buttocks and/or feet are nearest the cervical opening and are born first; occurs in approximately 3% of all births.

  Complete b.p. Simultaneous presentation of buttocks, legs, and feet.

  Footling (incomplete) b.p. Presentation of one or both feet.

  Frank b.p. Presentation of buttocks, with hips flexed so that thighs are against abdomen.

Bregma Point of junction of the coronal and sagittal sutures of the skull; the area of the anterior fontanel of the fetus.

Brim   Edge of the superior strait of the true pelvis; the inlet.

Bronchopulmonary dysplasia (BPD)   Emphysematous changes caused by oxygen toxicity.

Brown fat   Source of heat unique to neonates that is capable of greater thermogenic activity than ordinary fat. Deposits are found around the adrenals, kidneys, and neck; between the scapulas; and behind the sternum for several weeks after birth.

Bruit, uterine   Sound of passage of blood through uterine blood vessels, synchronous with fetal heart rate.

Calendar method   Method of calculating the fertile days of the *next* menstrual cycle by noting the lengths of the previous 12 cycles; then, subtract 18 from the shortest cycle and 11 from the longest cycle to give the most likely fertile days of the next cycle. *See text.*

Candida **vaginitis**   Vaginal, fungal infection; moniliasis.

Capacitation   Enzymatic process resulting in removal of plasma protein over acrosome of sperm; the process that enables sperm to bind to the egg. (See *Acrosome reaction.*)

Caput   Occiput of fetal head appearing at the vaginal introitus preceding birth of the head.

   C. succedaneum   Swelling of the tissue over the presenting part of the fetal head caused by pressure during labor; swelling *does* cross newborn's suture lines.

Carcinoma   Malignant, often metastatic epithelial neoplasm; cancer.

Cardiac decompensation   Inability of the heart to maintain a sufficient cardiac output.

Cardinal movements of labor   The mechanism of labor in a vertex presentation includes engagement, descent, flexion, internal rotation, extension, external rotation (restitution), and expulsion.

Carpal tunnel syndrome   Pressure on the median nerve at the point at which it goes through the carpal tunnel of the wrist. It causes soreness, tenderness, and weakness of the muscles of the thumb.

Carrier   Individual who carries a gene that does not exhibit itself in physical or chemical characteristics but that can be transmitted to children (e.g., a female carrying the trait for hemophilia, which is expressed in male offspring).

Caul   Hood of fetal membranes covering fetal head during birth.

Cephalhematoma   Extravasation of blood from ruptured vessels between a skull bone and its external covering, the periosteum. Swelling is limited by the margins of the cranial bone affected (usually parietals).

Cephalic   Pertaining to the head.

   C. presentation   Presentation of any part of the fetal head.

Cephalocaudal development   Principle of maturation that development progresses from the head to the feet.

Cephalopelvic disproportion (CPD)   Condition in which the infant's head is of such a shape, size, or position that it cannot pass through the mother's pelvis.

Cerclage   Use of nonabsorbable suture to keep an incompetent cervix closed; released when pregnancy is at term to allow labor to begin.

Cervical cap (custom)   Individually fitted contraceptive covering for the cervix.

Cervical erosion   Alteration of the epithelium of the cervix caused by chronic irritation or infection.

Cervical intraepithelial neoplasm (CIN)   Uncontrolled and progressive abnormal growth of cervical epithelial cells.

Cervical mucus method   See *ovulation method.*

Cervicitis   Cervical infection.

Cervix   Lowest and narrow end of the uterus; the "neck." The cervix is situated between the external os and the body (corpus) of the uterus, and its lower end extends into the vagina.

Cesarean birth   Birth of a fetus by an incision through the abdominal wall and uterus.

Chadwick's sign   Violet color of mucous membrane that is visible from about the fourth week of pregnancy; caused by increased vascularity of the vagina.

Childbed fever   See *puerperal sepsis.*

Chloasma   Increased pigmentation over bridge of nose and cheeks of pregnant women and some women taking oral contraceptives; also known as *mask of pregnancy.*

Choanal atresia   See *atresia, choanal.*

Chorioamnionitis   Stimulated by organisms in the amniotic fluid, which then become infiltrated with polymorphonuclear leukocytes.

Chorion   Fetal membrane closest to the intrauterine wall that gives rise to the placenta and continues as the outer membrane surrounding the amnion.

Chorionic villi   See *villi, chorionic.*

Chorionic villi sampling (CVS)   Removal of fetal tissue from placenta for genetic diagnostic studies; performed after 10 wk gestation.

Chromosome   Element within the cell nucleus carrying genes and composed of DNA and proteins.

Circumcision

   Male   Excision of the prepuce (foreskin) of the penis, exposing the glans.

   Female   Religious or cultural removal of a portion of the clitoris and labia.

Cleavage   Cell division following the fertilization of an ovum.

Cleft lip   Incomplete closure of the lip; *harelip.*

Cleft palate   Incomplete closure of the palate or roof of mouth; a congenital fissure.

Climacterium   The period of a woman's life when she is passing from a reproductive to a nonreproductive state, with regression of ovarian function. The cycle of endocrine, physical, and psychosocial changes that occurs during the termination of the reproductive years.

Clitoris   Female organ analogous to male penis; a small, ovoid body of erectile tissue situated at the anterior junction of the vulva.

   Prepuce of the c.   See *prepuce of the clitoris.*

Clonus (ankle)   Spasmodic alternation of muscular contraction and relaxation; deep tendon reflex (DTR) assessed especially in preeclamptic women.

Coccyx   Small bone at the base of the spinal column.

Coitus   Penile-vaginal intercourse.

   C. interruptus   Intercourse during which penis is withdrawn from vagina before ejaculation.

Cold stress   Excessive loss of heat that results in increased respirations and nonshivering thermogenesis to maintain core body temperature. See *heat loss.*

Colostrum   Yellow secretion from the breast containing mainly serum and white blood corpuscles preceding the onset of true lactation 2 or 3 days after birth.

Conception   Union of the sperm and ovum resulting in fertilization; formation of the one-celled zygote.

Conceptional age   In fetal development, the number of completed weeks since the moment of conception. Because the moment of conception is almost impossible to determine, conceptional age is estimated at 2 wk less than gestational age.

Conceptus   Embryo or fetus, fetal membranes, amniotic fluid, and the fetal portion of the placenta.

Condom   Mechanical barrier worn on the penis for contraception; "rubber"; also provides some protection against transmission of sexually transmitted diseases (STDs).

Condylomata accuminata   Wartlike growth on the skin usually seen near the anus or external genitals caused by human papillomavirus (HPV); genital warts. (Must be differentiated from condyloma latum seen in secondary syphilis.)

Confinement   Period of childbirth and early puerperium.

Congenital   Present or existing before birth as a result of either hereditary or prenatal environmental factors.

Conjoined twins   See *twins, conjoined.*

Conjugate

  Diagonal c.   Radiographic measurement of distance from *inferior border* of symphysis pubis (SP) to sacral promontory; may be obtained by vaginal examination; 12.5 to 13 cm.

  True c. (c. vera)   Radiographic measurement of distance from *upper margin* of SP to sacral promontory; 1.5 to 2 cm less than diagonal conjugate.

Conjunctivitis   Inflammation of the mucous membrane that lines the eyelids and that is reflected onto the eyeball.

Conscious relaxation   Technique used to release the mind and body from tension through conscious effort and practice.

Contraception   Prevention of impregnation or conception.

⊞ **Contraction stress test (CST)**   Test to stimulate uterine contractions for the purpose of assessing fetal response; a healthy fetus does not react to contractions while a compromised fetus demonstrates late decelerations in the fetal heart rate that are indicative of uteroplacental insufficiency.

Contractions

  Duration   The period of time from the beginning of the contraction to the end.

  Frequency   How often the contractions occur—the period of time from the beginning of one contraction to the beginning of the next.

  Intensity   The strength of the contraction at its peak.

  Interval   The period of time between uterine contractions—timed from the end of one contraction to the beginning of the next.

  Resting tone   The tension in the uterine muscle between contractions.

  Increment   An increase, or buildup, as of a contraction.

  Acme   Highest point (e.g., of a contraction).

  Decrement   Decrease or stage of decline, as of a contraction.

⊞ **Coombs test**

  Direct   Determination of maternal Rh-positive antibodies in fetal cord blood. A positive test result indicates the presence of antibodies or titer.

  Indirect   Determination of Rh-positive antibodies in maternal blood.

Copulation   Coitus; sexual intercourse.

Cordocentesis   See *Percutaneous umbilical cord sampling.*

Corpus   Discrete mass of material; body, e.g., body of uterus.

  C. luteum   Yellow body. After rupture of the graafian follicle at ovulation, the follicle develops into a yellow structure that secretes progesterone during the 14 days after ovulation atrophying about 3 days before sloughing of the endometrium in menstrual flow. If impregnation occurs, this structure continues to produce progesterone until the placenta can take over this function.

Cotyledon   One of the 15–28 visible segments of the placenta on the maternal surface, each made up of fetal vessels, chorionic villi, and an intervillous space.

Couplet care   One nurse, educated in both mother and infant care, functions as the primary nurse for both mother and infant (also known as mother-baby care or single-room maternity care).

Couvade   Custom whereby the husband goes through mock labor while his wife is giving birth.

Couvelaire uterus   See *Uterus, Couvelaire.*

CPAP   Continuous positive airway pressure.

Cradle cap   Common seborrheic dermatitis of infants consisting of thick, yellow, greasy scales on the scalp.

Craniotabes   Localized softening of cranial bones.

⊞ **Creatinine**   Substance found in blood and muscle; measurement of levels in maternal urine correlates with amount of fetal muscle mass and therefore fetal size.

Crib death   Unexpected and sudden death of an apparently normal and healthy infant that occurs during sleep and with no physical or autopsic evidence of disease. Also referred to as sudden infant death syndrome (SIDS).

Cri-du-chat **syndrome**   Rare congenital disorder recognized at birth by a kittenlike-cry, which may prevail for weeks, then disappear. Other characteristics include low birth weight, microcephaly, "moon face," wide-set eyes, strabismus, and low-set misshaped ears. Infants are hypotonic; heart defects and mental and physical retardation are common. Also called cat-cry syndrome.

Crisis   Any naturally occurring turning point, such as courtship, marriage, pregnancy, parenthood, or death.

  Developmental crisis   Severe, usually transient, stress that occurs when a person is unable to complete the tasks of a psychosocial stage of development and is therefore unable to move on to the next stage.

  Maturational crisis   Crisis that arises during normal growth and development, e.g., puberty.

  Situational crisis   Crisis that arises suddenly in response to an external event or a conflict concerning a specific circumstance. The symptoms are transient, and the episode is usually brief.

Crisis intervention   Actions taken by the nurse to help an individual deal with an impending, potentially overwhelming crisis, regain his or her equilibrium, grow from the experience, and improve coping skills.

Critical path   The exact timing of all key incidents that must occur to achieve the standard outcomes within the diagnosis-related group (DRG)–specific length of stay.

Crowning   Stage of birth when the top of the fetal head becomes visible at the vaginal opening.

Cryptorchidism   Failure of one or both of the testicles to descend into the scrotum. Also called undescended testis.

Cul-de-sac of Douglas   Pouch formed by a fold of the peritoneum dipping down between the anterior wall of the rectum and the posterior wall of the uterus; also called *Douglas' cul-de-sac,* pouch of Douglas, and rectouterine pouch.

Culdocentesis   Use of needle puncture or incision to remove intraperitoneal fluid (blood, purulent material) by way of the vagina.

Culdotomy   Incision or needle puncture of the cul-de-sac of Douglas by way of the vagina.

!**Cullen's sign**   Faint, irregularly formed, hemorrhagic patches on the skin around the umbilicus. The discolored skin is blue-black and becomes greenish brown or yellow. Cullen's sign may appear 1 to 2 days after the onset of anorexia and the severe, poorly localized abdominal pains characteristic of acute pancreatitis. Cullen's sign is also present in massive upper gastrointestinal hemorrhage, ruptured ectopic pregnancy.

Cultural context   A situation that considers the individual and family's beliefs and practices (culture).

Curettage   Scraping of the endometrium lining of the uterus with a curet to remove the contents of the uterus (as is done after an inevitable or incomplete abortion) or to obtain specimens for diagnostic purposes.

Cutis marmorata   Transient vasomotor phenomenon occurring primarily over extremities when the infant is exposed to chilling. It appears as a pink or faint purple capillary outline on the skin. Occasionally it is seen if the infant is in respiratory distress.

Cycle of violence   Pattern of three phases: period of increasing tension, the abusive episode, and a period of contrition and kindness.

Cystitis   Inflammatory condition or infection of urinary bladder and ureters.

Cystocele   Bladder hernia; injury to the vesicovaginal fascia during labor and birth may allow herniation of the bladder into the vagina.

Daily fetal movement counts (DFMC)   Maternal assessment of fetal activity; the number of fetal movements within a specific time period are counted.

Death   Cessation of life; mortality.

Fetal d.   Intrauterine death. Death of a fetus weighing 500 g or more, of 20 wk gestation or more.

Infant d.   Death during the first year of life.

Maternal d.   Death of a woman during the childbearing cycle.

Neonatal d.   Death of a newborn within the first 28 days after birth.

Perinatal d.   Death of a fetus of 20 wk gestation or older or death of a neonate 28 days old or younger.

Decidua   Mucous membrane, lining of uterus, or endometrium of pregnancy that is shed after giving birth.

D. basalis   Maternal aspect of the placenta made up of uterine blood vessels, endometrial stroma, and glands. It is shed in lochial discharge after birth.

D. capsularis   That part of the decidual membranes surrounding the chorionic sac.

D. vera   Nonplacental decidual lining of the uterus.

Deep tendon reflexes (DTRs)   Reflex caused by stimulation of tendons, such as elbow, wrist, knee, triceps, and ankle jerk reflexes.

Deletion   Loss of a piece of a chromosome that has broken off.

Delivery   Birth of the child with placenta and membranes by the mother or their extraction by the obstetric practitioner.

Abdominal d.   See *cesarean birth.*

D**OD$_{450}$** (read delta OD$_{450}$)   Delta optical density (or absorbance) at 450 nm, obtained by spectral analysis of amniotic fluid. This prenatal test is used to measure the degree of hemolytic activity in the fetus and to evaluate fetal status in women sensitized to Rh(D).

Demand feeding   Infant feeds when hungry, not by schedule.

Deoxyribonucleic acid (DNA)   Intracellular complex protein that carries genetic information, consisting of two purines (adenine and guanine) and two pyrimidines (thymine and cytosine).

Depressive reactions   Depression related to the postpartum period including postpartum blues, postpartum nonpsychotic depression, and postpartum psychosis.

DES   Diethylstilbestrol, used in treating menopausal symptoms. Exposure of female fetus predisposes her to reproductive tract malformations and (later) dysplasia.

Desquamation   Shedding of epithelial cells of the skin and mucous membranes.

Diaphragmatic hernia   Congenital malformation of diaphragm that allows displacement of the abdominal organs into the thoracic cavity.

Diastasis recti abdominis   Separation of the two rectus muscles along the median line of the abdominal wall. This is often seen in women with repeated childbirths or with a multifetal gestation (triplets, etc.). In the newborn it is usually due to incomplete development.

DIC   Disseminated intravascular coagulation.

Dick-Read method   An approach to childbirth based on the premise that fear of pain produces muscular tension, resulting in pain and greater fear. The method includes teaching physiologic processes of labor, exercise to improve muscle tone, and techniques to assist in relaxation and prevent the fear-tension-pain mechanism.

Dilatation and curettage (D and C)   Vaginal operation in which the cervical canal is stretched enough to admit passage of an instrument called a curet. The endometrium of the uterus is scraped with the curet to empty the uterine contents or to obtain tissue for examination.

Dilatation and evacuation (D and E)   A surgical method of pregnancy interruption between weeks 15 and 24; requires extreme cervical dilatation and evacuation of uterine contents using large-bore suction equipment and crushing instruments.

Dilatation of cervix   Stretching of the external os from an opening a few millimeters in size to an opening large enough to allow the passage of the infant.

Diploid number   Having two sets of chromosomes; found normally in somatic (body) cells; 23 pairs or 46 chromosomes.

Discordance   Discrepancy in size (or other indicator) between twins.

Disparate twins   See *twins, disparate.*

Disseminated intravascular coagulation (DIC)   A pathologic form of coagulation in which clotting factors are consumed to such an extent that generalized bleeding can occur; associated with abruptio placentae, eclampsia, intrauterine fetal demise, amniotic fluid embolism, and hemorrhage.

Disseminated lupus erythematosus Chronic inflammatory disease affecting many systems of the body. Also called systemic lupus erythematosus (SLE).

Dizygotic Related to or proceeding from two zygotes (fertilized ova).

Dizygotic twins See *twins, dizygotic*

Döderlein's bacillus Gram-positive bacterium occurring in normal vaginal secretions.

Dominant trait Gene that is expressed whenever it is present in the heterozygous gene state (e.g., brown eyes are dominant over blue).

Doppler blood flow analysis Device for measuring blood flow noninvasively in the fetus and placenta to detect intrauterine growth retardation.

Double set-up A nursing procedure in which an obstetric operating room is prepared for both vaginal birth or cesarean birth; today, ultrasound has made this obsolete in most facilities; used originally to help in diagnosis of vaginal bleeding, to rule out placenta previa.

Douglas' cul-de-sac See *cul-de-sac of Douglas.*

Doula A lay person who provides support during labor.

Down syndrome Abnormality involving the occurrence of a third chromosome (trisomy 21), rather than the normal pair that characteristically results in a typical picture of mental retardation and altered physical appearance. This condition was formerly called *mongolism* or *mongoloid idiocy.*

Dry labor Lay term referring to labor in which amniotic fluid has already escaped. A "dry birth" does not exist.

Dubowitz assessment Estimation of gestational age of a newborn, based on criteria developed for that purpose.

Ductus arteriosus In fetal circulation, an anatomic shunt between the pulmonary artery and arch of the aorta. It is obliterated after birth by a rising PO_2 and change in intravascular pressures in the presence of normal pulmonary function. It normally becomes a ligament after birth but in some instances remains patent.

Ductus venosus In fetal circulation, a blood vessel carrying oxygenated blood between the umbilical vein and the inferior vena cava, bypassing the liver. It is obliterated and becomes a ligament after birth.

Dura (dura mater) Outermost, toughest of the three meninges covering the brain and spinal cord.

Dys- Prefix meaning abnormal, difficult, painful, faulty.

Dysfunctional uterine bleeding Abnormal bleeding from the uterus for reasons that are not readily established.

Dysmaturity See *intrauterine growth retardation (IUGR).*

Dysmenorrhea Difficult or painful menstruation.

Primary dysmenorrhea Painful menstruation beginning 2–6 mo after menarche, related to ovulation.

Secondary dysmenorrhea Painful menstruation related to organic disease such as endometriosis, pelvic inflammatory disease (PID), uterine neoplasm.

Dyspareunia Painful sexual intercourse.

Dystocia Prolonged, painful, or otherwise difficult birth because of mechanical factors produced by the "6 Ps":
Powers—uterine contractions or maternal bearing-down efforts.

Placenta—previa, abruptio.
Passage—pelvic structure; full bladder, rectum.
Position—maternal, during labor, birth.
Passenger—fetal size, abnormal presentation/position, anomalies, number.
Psychological responses—of mother to labor related to past experiences, preparation, culture and heritage, and support system.

Ecchymosis Bruise; bleeding into tissue caused by direct trauma, serious infection, or bleeding diathesis.

Eclampsia Severe complication of pregnancy of unknown cause and occurring more often in the primigravida; characterized by tonic and clonic convulsions, coma, high blood pressure, albuminuria, and oliguria occurring during pregnancy or shortly after birth.

Ectoderm Outer layer of embryonic tissue giving rise to skin, nails, and hair.

Ectopic Occurring in an abnormal location.

E. pregnancy Implantation of the fertilized ovum outside of its normal place in the uterine cavity. Locations include the abdomen, fallopian tubes, and ovaries.

EDB Expected date of birth; "due date."

EDC Expected date of confinement; "due date" (term has been replaced by EDB).

Effacement Thinning and shortening or obliteration of the cervix that occurs during late pregnancy or labor or both.

Effleurage Gentle stroking used in massage.

Ejaculation Sudden expulsion of semen from the male urethra.

ELISA Enzyme-linked *immunosorbent assay* (uses monoclonal antibodies). Laboratory tests: pregnancy, chlamydial infection (Chlamydiazyme), human immunodeficiency virus antibodies.

Embolus Any undissolved matter (solid, liquid, or gaseous) that is carried by the blood to another part of the body and obstructs a blood vessel.

Embryo Conceptus from the second or third wk of development until about the eighth wk after conception, when mineralization (ossification) of the skeleton begins. This period is characterized by cellular differentiation and predominantly hyperplastic growth; embryonic stages are *zygote, morula,* and *blastocyst.*

Emotional lability Rapid mood changes.

Endometriosis Tissue closely resembling endometrial tissue but aberrantly located outside the uterus in the pelvic cavity. Symptomatology may include pelvic pain or pressure, dysmenorrhea, dyspareunia, abnormal bleeding from the uterus or rectum, and sterility.

Endometritis Inflammation of the endometrium.

Endometrium Inner lining of the uterus that undergoes changes caused by hormones during the menstrual cycle and pregnancy; decidua.

Endorphins Endogenous opioids secreted by the pituitary gland that act on the central and peripheral nervous systems to reduce pain.

En face Position in which neonate is held 8 in. (20 cm) away facing the observer to allow for direct eye contact.

Engagement In obstetrics, the entrance of the fetal presenting part into the superior pelvic strait and the beginning of the descent through the pelvic canal.

Engorgement Distention or vascular congestion. In obstetrics, the process of swelling of the breast tissue brought about by an increase in blood and lymph supply to the breast, which precedes true lactation. It lasts about 48 hr and usually reaches a peak between the third and fifth postpartum days.

Engrossment   Sustained involvement of a parent with an infant.

Entoderm   Inner layer of embryonic tissue giving rise to internal organs such as the intestine.

Entrainment   Phenomenon observed in the microanalysis of sound films in which the speaker moves several parts of the body and the listener responds to the sounds by moving in ways that are coordinated with the rhythm of the sounds. Infants have been observed to move in time to the rhythms of adult speech but not to random noises or disconnected words or vowels. Entrainment is thought to be an essential factor in the process of parental infant bonding.

Epicanthus   Fold of skin covering the inner canthus and caruncle that extends from the root of the nose to the median end of the eyebrow; characteristically found in certain races but may occur as a congenital anomaly.

Epidural anesthesia   Injection of anesthetic outside the dura mater (anesthetic does not mix with spinal fluid). See *peridural anesthesia*.

Epidural block   Type of regional anesthesia produced by injection of a local anesthetic into the epidural (peridural) space.

Epidural blood patch   A patch formed by a few milliliters of the mother's blood used to repair a tear or hole in the dura mater around the spinal cord.

Episiotomy   Surgical incision of the perineum at the end of the second stage of labor to facilitate birth and to avoid laceration of the perineum.

Epispadias   Defect in which the urethral canal terminates on dorsum of penis or above the clitoris (rare).

Epstein's pearls   Small, white blebs found along the gum margins and at the junction of the soft and hard palates. They are a normal manifestation and are commonly seen in the newborn. Similar to *Bohn's nodules*.

Epulis   Tumorlike benign lesion of the gingiva seen in pregnant women.

Erb-Duchenne paralysis   Paralysis caused by traumatic injury to the upper brachial plexus, occurring most commonly in childbirth from forcible traction during birth. The signs of Erb's paralysis include loss of sensation in the arm and paralysis and atrophy of the deltoid, the biceps, and the brachialis muscles. Also called *Erb's palsy*.

Ergot   Drug obtained from *Claviceps purpurea*, a fungus, which stimulates the smooth muscles of blood vessels and the uterus, causing vasoconstriction and uterine contractions.

Erythema toxicum   Innocuous pink papular neonatal rash of unknown cause, with superimposed vesicles appearing within 24–48 hr after birth and resolving spontaneously within a few days.

Erythroblastosis fetalis   Hemolytic disease of the newborn usually caused by isoimmunization resulting from Rh incompatibility or ABO incompatibility.

Erythropoiesis   Erythrocyte (RBC) production, which involves the maturation of a nucleated precursor into a hemoglobin-filled, nucleus-free erythrocyte regulated by erythropoietin, a hormone produced by the kidney.

Estimated date of birth   Approximate date of birth. Usually determined by calculation using Nägele's rule, also known as EDC (expected date of confinement).

Estradiol   An estrogen.

Estrangement, psychological   Reaction to the birth of and subsequent separation from a sick and/or preterm infant, whereby the mother is diverted from establishing a normal relationship with her baby.

Estriol   Major metabolite of estrogen that increases during the second half of pregnancy with an intact fetoplacental unit (normal placenta, normal fetal liver and adrenals) and normal maternal renal function.

Estrogen   Female sex hormone produced by the ovaries and placenta.

Estrogen replacement therapy (ERT)   Exogenous estrogen given to women during and after menopause to prevent hot flushes (flashes), mood changes, osteoporosis, and genitourinary symptoms.

Exchange transfusion   Replacement of 75–85% of circulating blood by withdrawing the recipient's blood and injecting a donor's blood in equal amounts, the purposes of which are to prevent an accumulation of bilirubin in the blood above a dangerous level, to prevent the accumulation of other by-products of hemolysis in hemolytic disease, and to correct anemia and acidosis.

Expulsive   Having the tendency to drive out or expel.

  E. contractions   Labor contractions that are characteristic of the second stage of labor.

External cephalic version (ECV)   Turning the fetus to a vertex position by exerting pressure on the fetus externally through the maternal abdomen.

Extrauterine   Occurring outside the uterus.

  E. pregnancy   Ectopic pregnancy in which the fertilized ovum implants itself outside the uterus.

Extrusion reflex   Infant automatically extends tongue when it is stimulated.

Facies   Pertaining to the appearance or expression of the face; certain congenital syndromes typically present with a specific facial appearance.

FAD   Fetal activity determination.

Failure to thrive   Condition in which neonate's or infant's growth and development patterns are below the norms for age.

Fallopian tubes   Two canals or oviducts extending laterally from each side of the uterus through which the ovum travels, after ovulation, to the uterus; uterine tubes.

False labor   Uterine contractions that do not result in cervical dilatation, are irregular, are felt more in front, often do not last more than 20 sec, and do not become longer or stronger.

False pelvis   The part of the pelvis superior to a plane passing through the linea terminalis.

Family dynamics   The process by which family members assume appropriate social roles.

Family functions   Activities carried out within families for the well-being of family members; including biologic, economic, educational, psychological, and socio-cultural.

Family types

  Blended f.   Family form that includes stepparents and stepchildren.

  Communal f.   Groupings vary from highly formalized

structure (Amish) to loosely knit groups; an alternative life-style developed for a variety of ideologic or societal purposes.

Extended f. Family form that includes the nuclear family and other blood-related persons.

Homosexual f. Family form in which parents form a homosexual union. Children may be the offspring of a previous heterosexual union or may be conceived by one member of a lesbian couple through artificial insemination.

Nuclear f. Family form consisting of parents and their dependent children.

Single parent f. Family with only one parent; may result from loss of a spouse/partner (e.g., death), from out-of-wedlock births, or from adoption.

Family violence Interpersonal violence including child, elder, sibling, and spouse/partner.

Fantasy child The imagined dream child; the "ideal" unborn child.

Father—developmental tasks of

Announcement phase The *first* developmental task experienced by expectant fathers as identified by May. During this phase the expectant father accepts the biologic fact of pregnancy.

Moratorium phase The *second* developmental task experienced by expectant fathers as identified by May. During this phase the expectant father adjusts to the reality of pregnancy.

Focusing phase The *third* developmental task experienced by expectant fathers as identified by May. This phase is characterized by the father's active involvement in both the pregnancy and his relationship with his child.

Father—expectant, styles of involvement

Expressive style Expectant father's strong emotional response to partner's pregnancy.

Instrumental style Characteristic style displayed by expectant fathers that emphasizes tasks to be accomplished.

Observer style Characteristic style displayed by expectant fathers who show a detached approach to involvement in their partner's pregnancy.

Ferguson's reflex Reflex contractions of the uterus after stimulation of the cervix, e.g., during sexual intercourse or vaginal examination.

Ferning (arborization) test The appearance of a fernlike pattern in dried smears of uterine cervical mucus, indicating the presence of estrogen.

Ovulation f. t. Test in which cervical mucus, placed on a slide, *dries* in a branching pattern in the presence of high estrogen levels at the time of ovulation.

Pregnancy f. t. Test in which cervical mucus, placed on a slide, does *not* dry in a branching pattern because of high levels of progesterone along with estrogen.

Fertile period The period before and after ovulation during which the human ovum can be fertilized; usually 3 days before ovulation (life span of sperm in woman's reproductive tract) and 24 hr after ovulation (life span of ovum). Since exact moment of ovulation is unknown, fertile period may extend from before to several days after expected ovulation (see *Calendar method*).

Fertility Quality of being able to reproduce.

Fertility rate Number of births per 1000 women aged 15 through 44 yr.

Fertilization Union of an ovum and a sperm.

Fetal Pertaining or relating to the fetus.

F. asphyxia See *asphyxia, fetal.*

F. biophysical profile Noninvasive dynamic assessment, employing ultrasound and external fetal monitoring, of several parameters: breathing movements, movements, tone, amniotic fluid volume, nonstress test, and often placental grading.

F. death See *death, fetal.*

F. distress Evidence such as a change in the fetal heartbeat pattern or activity indicating that the fetus is in jeopardy.

Fetal heart rate (FHR) Beats per minute of the fetal heart. Normal range is 110–160 beats/min.

Acceleration Increase in fetal heart rate, usually seen as a reassuring sign.

Baseline The average fetal heart rate between uterine contractions.

Bradycardia Baseline fetal heart rate below 110 beats/min.

Prolonged deceleration Slowing of fetal heart rate lasting longer than 2 min.

Fetal heart rate deceleration Slowing of fetal heart rate attributed to a parasympathetic response and described in relation to uterine contractions.

Early Onset corresponding to onset of uterine contraction, related to fetal head compression.

Late Onset after peak of contraction, continuing into interval after contraction; caused by uteroplacental insufficiency.

Variable Onset anytime unrelated to contraction; caused by cord compression.

Fetal hemoglobin Hemoglobin of fetal red blood cells has greater affinity for oxygen than adult hemoglobin A; helps to ensure adequate fetal tissue oxygenation.

Fetal membranes

Amnion See *amnion.*

Chorion See *chorion.*

Fetal postures

Attitude Relation of fetal parts to each other in the uterus (all parts flexed, all parts flexed except neck is extended, etc.).

Lie Relation of the fetal spine to the maternal spine; i.e., in *vertical* lie, maternal and fetal spines are parallel and the fetal head or breech presents; in *transverse* lie, fetal spine is perpendicular to the maternal spine and the fetal shoulder presents.

Position Relation of an arbitrarily chosen fetal reference point, such as the occiput, sacrum, chin (mentum), or scapula on the presenting part of the fetus to its location in the front, back, or sides of the maternal pelvis.

Presentation That part of the fetus that first enters the pelvis and lies over the inlet: may be *cephalic* (head): vertex (brow, chin); *breech* (sacrum): complete, frank, or footling; and *shoulder* (scapula).

Fetal syndromes

Fetal alcohol effects (FAE) Set of symptoms that includes prenatal and postnatal growth retardation and CNS malfunctions, including mental retardation; effects may not be evident for several years.

Fetal alcohol syndrome Congenital abnormality or

anomaly resulting from maternal alcohol intake. It is characterized by typical craniofacial and limb defects, cardiovascular defects, intrauterine growth retardation, and developmental delay.

Fetal hydantoin syndrome   Abnormalities such as microcephaly, mental retardation, developmental delay, intrauterine growth retardation, facial clefts, and nail hypoplasia.

Fetofetal transfusion   See *parabiotic syndrome.*

α-Fetoprotein (AFP)   Fetal antigen; elevated levels in amniotic fluid associated with neural tube defects.

Fetotoxic   Poisonous or destructive to the fetus.

Fetus   Child in utero from about the eighth week after conception, until birth.

Fibroid   Fibrous, encapsulated connective tissue tumor, especially of the uterus.

Fimbria   Structure resembling a fringe, particularly the fringelike end of the fallopian tube.

Fissure   Groove or open crack in tissue.

Fistula   Abnormal tubelike passage that forms between two normal cavities, possibly congenital or caused by trauma, abscesses, or inflammatory processes.

Flaccid   Having relaxed, flabby, or absent muscle tone.

! Flaring of nostrils   Widening of nostrils (alae nasi) during inspiration in the presence of air hunger; sign of respiratory distress.

Flexion   In obstetrics, resistance to the descent of the baby down the birth canal causes the head to flex, or bend, so that the chin approaches the chest. Thus the smallest diameter (suboccipitobregmatic) of the vertex presents.

Follicle   Small secretory cavity or sac.

   Graafian f.   Mature, fully developed ovarian cyst containing the ripe ovum and the epithelial cells that surround it. The follicle secretes estrogens, and after ovulation, the corpus luteum develops within the ruptured graafian follicle and secretes estrogen and progesterone.

Follicle stimulating hormone (FSH)   Hormone produced by the anterior pituitary during the first half of the menstrual cycle. Stimulates development of the graafian follicle.

Fomites   Nonliving material on which disease-producing organisms may be conveyed (e.g., bed linen).

Fontanel   Broad area, or soft spot, consisting of a strong band of connective tissue-contiguous with cranial bones and located at the junctions of the bones.

   Anterior f.   Diamond-shaped area between the frontal and two parietal bones just above the baby's forehead at the junction of the coronal and sagittal sutures.

   Mastoid f.   Posterolateral fontanel usually not palpable.

   Posterior f.   Small, triangular area between the occipital and parietal bones at the junction of the lambdoidal and sagittal sutures.

   Sagittal f.   Soft area located in the sagittal suture, halfway between the anterior and posterior fontanels; may be found in normal newborns and in some neonates with Down syndrome.

   Sphenoid f.   Anterolateral fontanel usually not palpable.

Foramen ovale   Septal opening between the atria of the fetal heart. The opening normally closes shortly after birth, but if it remains patent, surgical repair usually is necessary.

Forceps-assisted birth   Birth in which two curved-bladed instruments are used to assist in birth of the fetal head.

Foreskin   Prepuce, or loose fold of skin covering the glans penis.

Fornix   Any structure with an arched or vaultlike shape.

   F. of the vagina   Anterior and posterior spaces, formed by the protrusion of the cervix into the vagina, into which the upper vagina is divided.

Fourth stage of labor   The initial period of recovery from childbirth. It is usually considered to last for the first 1–2 hr after the expulsion of the placenta.

Fourth trimester of pregnancy   Another term for the puerperium, the 6-wk interval between the birth of the newborn and the return of the reproductive organs to their nonpregnant state.

Fowler's position   Posture assumed by patient when head of bed is raised 18 or 20 in. and individual's knees are elevated.

Freestanding birth center   A center that provides prenatal care, labor and birth, and postbirth care outside of a hospital setting.

Frenulum   Thin ridge of tissue in midline of undersurface of tongue extending from its base to varying distances from the tip of the tongue.

Friable   Easily broken. May refer to a fragile condition of the cervix especially during pregnancy that causes the cervix to bleed easily when touched.

Friedman's curve   Labor curve; pattern of descent of presenting part and of dilatation of cervix; partogram.

FSH   See *follicle stimulating hormone.*

Fulguration   Destruction of tissue by means of electricity.

Fundus   Dome-shaped upper portion of the uterus between the points of insertion of the fallopian tubes.

Funic souffle   See *souffle, funic.*

Funis   Cordlike structure, especially the umbilical cord.

Galacto-, galact-   Combining form denoting milk.

Galactorrhea   Excessive flow or secretion of milk.

Galactosemia   Inherited, autosomal recessive disorder of galactose metabolism, characterized by a deficiency of the enzyme galactose-1-phosphate uridyl transferase.

Gamete   Mature male or female germ cell; the mature sperm or ovum.

Gametogenesis   Development of gametes; ova or sperm.

Gastroschisis   Abdominal wall defect at base of umbilical stalk.

Gastrostomy   Surgical creation of an artificial opening into the stomach through the abdominal wall, performed to feed a person when oral feeding is not possible.

Gate control theory   Proposed in 1965 by Melzack and Wall, this theory explains the neurophysical mechanism underlying the perception of pain.

Gavage   Feeding by means of a tube passed to the stomach.

Gender identity   The sense or awareness of knowing to which sex one belongs. The process begins in infancy, continues throughout childhood, and is reinforced during adolescence.

Gene   Factor on a chromosome responsible for hereditary characteristics of offspring.

Genetic   Dependent on the genes. A genetic disorder may or may not be apparent at birth.

Genetic counseling   Process of determining the occurrence or risk of occurrence of a genetic disorder within a family and of providing appropriate information and advice about the courses of action that are available, whether care of a child already affected, prenatal diagnosis, termination of a pregnancy, sterilization, or artificial insemination is involved.

Genitalia   Organs of reproduction.

Genotype   Hereditary combinations in an individual determining physical and chemical characteristics. Some genotypes are not expressed until later in life (e.g., *Huntington's chorea*); some hide recessive genes, which can be expressed in offspring; and others are expressed only under the proper environmental conditions (e.g., diabetes mellitus appearing under the stress of obesity or pregnancy).

Gestation   Period of intrauterine fetal development from conception through birth; the period of pregnancy.

Gestational age   In fetal development, the number of completed weeks counting from the first day of the last normal menstrual cycle.

Gestational diabetes   Glucose intolerance first recognized during pregnancy.

GIFT   Gamete intrafallopian transfer of ova and washed sperm into fallopian tubes.

Gingivitis   Inflammation of the gums characterized by redness, swelling, and tendency to bleed.

Glabella   Bony prominence above the nose and between the eyebrows.

Glans penis   Smooth, round head of the penis, analogous to the female glans clitoris.

Glucose tolerance test   A test of the body's ability to utilize carbohydrates; used as a screening measure for gestational diabetes.

Glycosuria   Presence of glucose (a sugar) in the urine.

Glycosylated hemoglobin   A measurement of glycemic control over time (usually 4–6 wk).

Gonad   Gamete-producing, or sex, gland; the ovary or testis.

Gonadotropic hormone   Hormone that stimulates the gonads.

Goodell's sign   Softening of the cervix, a *probable* sign of pregnancy, occurring during the *second* month.

Graafian follicle (vesicle)   See *follicle, graafian.*

Gravid   Pregnant.

Gravidity   The number of times a woman has been pregnant, regardless of the outcome of the pregnancies.

Grieving process   A complex of somatic and psychological symptoms associated with some extreme sorrow or loss, specifically the death of a loved one.

! Grunt, expiratory   Sign of respiratory distress (*hyaline membrane disease* [respiratory distress syndrome, or RDS] or advanced pneumonia) indicative of the body's attempt to hold air in the alveoli for better gaseous exchange.

Gynecoid pelvis   Pelvis in which the inlet is round instead of oval or blunt. Typical female pelvis.

Gynecology   Study of the diseases of the female, especially of the genital, urinary, and rectal organs.

Habitual (recurrent) abortion   See *abortion, habitual.*

Habituation   An acquired tolerance from repeated exposure to a particular stimulus. Also called negative adaptation; a decline and eventual elimination of a conditioned response by repetition of the conditioned stimulus.

Habitus   Indications in appearance of tendency or disposition to disease or abnormal conditions.

! Haploid number   Having half the normal number of chromosomes found in somatic (body) cells; 23 chromosomes.

Harlequin sign   Rare color change of *no* pathologic significance occurring between the longitudinal halves of the neonate's body. When infant is placed on one side, the dependent half is noticeably pinker than the superior half.

Hawthorne effect   A general *beneficial* effect on a person or group of people as a result of a therapeutic encounter with a health care provider or as a result of a change in the environment (lighting, temperature, or type of room [family-centered versus 4 bed unit]).

hCG   See *human chorionic gonadotropin.*

Heat loss, types   See also *cold stress.*

   Conduction   Heat loss to a cooler surface by direct skin contact.

   Convection   Heat loss from the warm body surface to cooler air currents.

   Evaporation   Heat loss incurred when water on the skin surface is converted to a vapor.

   Radiation   Heat loss incurred when heat transfers to cooler surfaces and objects not in direct contact with the body.

Hegar's sign   Softening of the lower uterine segment that is classified as a *probable* sign of pregnancy and that may be present during the *second* and *third months* of pregnancy and is palpated during bimanual examination.

! HELLP syndrome   Condition characterized by hemolysis, elevated liver enzymes, and low platelet count (it is *not* disseminated intravascular coagulation); it is a form of severe preeclampsia.

Hematocrit   Volume of red blood cells per deciliter (dL) of circulating blood; packed cell volume (PCV).

Hematoma   Collection of blood in a tissue; a bruise or blood tumor.

Hemizygous   Having *only one* of a gene pair that determines a particular genetic trait.

! Hemoconcentration   Increase in the number of red blood cells resulting from either a decrease in plasma volume (as seen in preeclampsia/eclampsia) or increased erythropoiesis.

Hemodilution   An increase in fluid content of blood, resulting in diminution of the proportion of formed elements.

Hemoglobin   Component of red blood cells consisting of globin, a protein, and hematin, an organic iron compound.

H. electrophoresis   Test to diagnose sickle cell disease in newborns. Cord blood is used.

Hemolytic disease of the newborn   Breakdown of fetal red blood cells by maternal antibodies, usually from an Rh-negative mother.

Hemoperitoneum   Blood in the peritoneal cavity.

Hemorrhagic disease of newborn   Bleeding disorder during first few days of life based on a deficiency of vitamin K (intestinal tract needs bacteria to produce vitamin K).

Hemorrhagic shock   A clinical condition in which the peripheral blood flow is inadequate to return sufficient blood to the heart for normal function, particularly oxygen transport to the organs/tissue.

Hereditary   Pertaining to a trait or characteristic transmitted from parent to offspring by way of the genes; used synonymously with *genetic.*

Hermaphrodite   Person having genital and sexual characteristics of both sexes.

Heterozygous   Having two dissimilar genes at the same

site, or locus, on paired chromosomes (e.g., at the sites for eye color, one chromosome carrying the gene for brown, the other for blue).

High risk   An increased possibility of suffering harm, damage, loss, or death. See also *risk factors*.

Hirsutism   Condition characterized by the excessive growth of hair or the growth of hair in unusual places.

Homan's sign   *Early* sign of phlebothrombosis of the deep veins of the calf in which there are complaints of pain when the leg is in extension and the foot is dorsiflexed.

Home birth   Planned birth of the child at home. Usually under the supervision of a midwife.

Homoiothermic   Referring to the ability of warm-blooded animals to maintain internal temperature at a specified level regardless of the environmental temperature. This ability is not fully developed in the human neonate.

Homologous   Similar in structure or origin but not necessarily in function.

Homologous insemination   Insemination in which the semen specimen is provided by the husband. The procedure is used primarily in cases of impotence or when the husband is incapable of sexual intercourse because of some physical disability.

Homozygous   Having two similar genes at the same locus, or site, on paired chromosomes.

Hormone   Chemical substance produced in an organ or gland that is conveyed through the blood to another organ or part of the body, stimulating it to increased functional activity or secretion. See specific hormones.

Hormone replacement therapy (HRT)   Progestin is added to estrogen replacement therapy to prevent endometrial cancer. See *estrogen replacement therapy (ERT)*.

Hot flash (flush)   Transient sensation of warmth experienced by some women during or after menopause, resulting from autonomic vasomotor disturbances that accompany changes in the neurohormonal activity of the ovaries, hypothalamus, and pituitary gland.

Hourglass uterus   Uterus in which a segment of circular muscle fibers contracts during labor. The resultant "constriction ring" *dystocia* is characterized by lack of progress in spite of adequate contractions; by pain experienced before palpation of a uterine contraction and persisting after the observer feels the contraction end; and by recession of the presenting part during a contraction, instead of descent of the presenting part.

Human chorionic gonadotropin (hCG)   Hormone that is produced by chorionic villi; the biologic marker in pregnancy tests. Two main functions are prevention of corpus luteum regression and promotion of testosterone production by the fetal testes.

Hyaline membrane disease (HMD)   Disease characterized by interference with ventilation at the alveolar level, theoretically caused by the presence of fibrinoid deposits lining alveolar ducts. Membrane formation is related to prematurity (especially with fetal asphyxia) and insufficient surfactant production (lecithin-sphingomyelin ratio $\leq 2:1$). Now known as *respiratory distress syndrome (RDS)*.

Hydatidiform mole   Abnormal pregnancy characterized by a degenerative process in the chorionic villi that produces high levels of human chorionic gonadotropin (hCG), multiple cysts, and rapid growth of the uterus with hemorrhage.

Signs and symptoms include vaginal bleeding, the discharge containing grapelike vesicles. Sequela may be chorioadenoma, a highly malignant neoplasm.

Hydramnios (polyhydramnios)   Amniotic fluid in excess of 1.5 liters; often indicative of fetal anomaly and frequently seen in poorly controlled, insulin-dependent, diabetic pregnant women even if no coexisting fetal anomaly is present.

Hydrocele   Collection of fluid in a saclike cavity, especially in the sac that surrounds the testis, causing the scrotum to swell.

Hydrocephalus   Accumulation of fluid in the subdural or subarachnoid spaces.

Hydrops fetalis   Most severe expression of fetal hemolytic disorder, a possible sequela to maternal Rh isoimmunization; infants exhibit gross edema (*anasarca*), cardiac decompensation, and profound pallor from anemia, and seldom survive.

Hymen   Membranous fold that normally partially covers the entrance to the vagina in the virgin.

Hymenal caruncles   Small, irregular bits of tissue that are remnants of the hymen.

Hymenal tag   Normally occurring redundant hymenal tissue protruding from the floor of the vagina that disappears spontaneously in a few weeks after birth.

Hyperbilirubinemia   Elevation of unconjugated serum bilirubin concentrations.

Hyperemesis gravidarum   Abnormal condition of pregnancy characterized by protracted vomiting, weight loss, and fluid and electrolyte imbalance.

Hyperglycemia   Excess glucose in the blood.

Hyperplasia   Increase in number of cells; formation of new tissue.

Hyperreflexia   Increased action of the reflexes.

Hyperthyroidism   Excessive functional activity of the thyroid gland.

Hypertonic uterine dysfunction   Uncoordinated, painful, frequent uterine contractions that do not cause dilatation and effacement; primary dysfunctional labor.

Hypertrophic cardiomyopathy (HCM)   Enlargement of heart walls and septum impacting on the size of the heart chambers.

Hypertrophy   Enlargement, or increase in size, of existing cells.

Hyperventilation   Rapid, shallow (or prolonged, deep) respirations resulting in respiratory alkalosis: a decrease in H^+ concentration and PCO_2 and an increase in the blood pH and the ratio of $NaHCO_3$ to H_2CO_3. Symptoms may include faintness, palpitations, and carpopedal (hands and feet) muscular spasms. Relief may result from rebreathing in a paper bag or into one's cupped hands to replace the carbon dioxide "blown off" during hyperventilation.

Hypofibrinogenemia   Deficient level of a blood-clotting factor, fibrinogen, in the blood; in obstetrics, it occurs following complications of *abruptio placentae* or retention of a dead fetus. See *disseminated intravascular coagulation (DIC)*.

Hypogastric arteries   Branches of the right and left iliac arteries carrying deoxygenated blood from the fetus through the umbilical cord, where they are known as umbilical arteries, to the placenta.

Hypoglycemia   Less-than-normal amount of glucose in the blood, usually caused by administration of too much insulin, excessive secretion of insulin by the islet cells of the pancreas, or by dietary deficiency.

Hypospadias Anomalous positioning of urinary meatus on undersurface of penis or close to or just inside the vagina.

Hypothalamus Portion of the diencephalon of the brain forming the floor and part of the lateral wall of the third ventricle. It activates, controls, and integrates the peripheral autonomic nervous system, endocrine processes, and many somatic functions, as body temperature, sleep, and appetite.

Hypothyroidism Deficiency of thyroid gland activity with underproduction of thyroxine.

! **Hypotonic uterine dysfunction** Weak, ineffective uterine contractions usually occurring in the active phase of labor; often related to cephalopelvic disproportion (CPD) or malposition of the fetus.

! **Hypoxemia** Reduction in arterial PO_2 resulting in metabolic acidosis by forcing anaerobic glycolysis, pulmonary vasoconstriction, and direct cellular damage.

! **Hypoxia** Insufficient availability of oxygen to meet the metabolic needs of body tissue.

Hysterectomy Surgical removal of the uterus.

Panhysterectomy Removal of entire uterus, but ovaries and tubes remain.

Subtotal h. Removal of fundus and body of the uterus, but the cervical stump remains.

TAH-BSO Transabdominal hysterectomy and bilateral salpingo-oophorectomy. Removal of uterus, both tubes, and both ovaries.

Total h. Removal of entire uterus, including the cervix, but the ovaries and tubes remain.

TVH Transvaginal hysterectomy.

Hysterosalpingography X-ray of the uterus and uterine tubes after filling them with radiopaque material.

Hysterotomy Surgical incision into the uterus.

Iatrogenic Caused by a health care provider's words, actions, or treatment.

Icterus neonatorum Jaundice in the newborn.

Idiopathic peripartum cardiomyopathy A primary disease of the maternal heart muscle with no apparent cause, occurring during the peripartum period.

! **Idiopathic respiratory distress syndrome (hyaline membrane disease)** Severe respiratory condition found almost exclusively in preterm infants and in some infants of diabetic mothers regardless of gestational age. See also *hyaline membrane disease (HMD)*.

IDM Infant of a diabetic mother.

IgA Primary immunoglobulin in colostrum.

IgG Transplacentally acquired immunoglobulin that confers passive immunity against the infections to which the mother is immune.

IgM Immunoglobulin that neonate can manufacture soon after birth. Fetus produces it in the presence of amnionitis.

Iliopectineal line Bony ridge on the inner surface of the ilium and pubic bones that divides the true and false pelves; the brim of the true pelvic cavity; the inlet.

Immunity

Acquired i. Protection against microorganisms that develops in response to actual infection or transfer of antibody from an immune donor.

Active natural i. Protection against specific microorganisms that develops in response to actual infection.

Active artificial i. Immunity acquired by Vaccination (e.g., rubella vaccination).

Natural i. Nonspecific protection against microorganisms. Natural immunity is the first line of defense and includes skin and phagocytic cells.

Passive natural i. Protection against specific microorganisms that develops in response to the transfer of antibody or lymphocytes from an immune donor (e.g., maternal antibodies in colostrum).

Passive artificial i. Immunity acquired by infusion of serum/plasma (e.g., Rh.IG).

Immunocompetent The ability of the immune system to respond appropriately to foreign antigens and to develop antigen-specific antibodies.

Immunology The study of the components essential to the recognition and disposal of foreign (nonself or antigenic) material and maintenance of body defenses.

Impaired fertility Inability to conceive or carry to live birth at a time a couple chooses to do so.

Imperforate Without the normal opening.

Implantation Embedding of the fertilized ovum in the uterine mucosa; nidation.

Impotence Archaic term designating a man's inability, partial or complete, to perform sexual intercourse or to achieve orgasm; current term is *erectile dysfunction*.

Inborn error of metabolism Hereditary deficiency of a specific enzyme needed for normal metabolism of specific chemicals (e.g., deficiency of phenylalanine hydroxylase results in *phenylketonuria* [PKU]; a deficiency of hexosaminidase results in *Tay-Sachs disease*).

! **Incompetent cervix** Cervix that is unable to remain closed until a pregnancy reaches term, because of a mechanical defect in the cervix resulting in dilatation and effacement usually during the second or early third trimester of pregnancy.

Induction Artificial stimulation or augmentation of labor.

! **Inertia** Sluggishness or inactivity; in obstetrics, refers to the absence or weakness of uterine contractions during labor.

Infant A child who is under 1 yr of age.

Infective endocarditis Inflammation of the lining membrane of the heart due to invasion of microorganisms.

Infertility Decreased capacity to conceive.

Inlet Passage leading into a cavity.

Pelvic i. Upper brim of the pelvic cavity.

Internal os Inside mouth or opening.

Intertuberous diameter Distance between ischial tuberosities. Measured to determine dimension of pelvic outlet.

Intervillous space Irregular space in the maternal portion of the placenta, filled with maternal blood and serving as the site of maternal-fetal gas, nutrient, and waste exchange.

Intimate partner abuse Violence between intimate adults.

Intrapartum During labor and birth.

Intrathecal Within the subarachnoid space.

IUCD Abbreviation for intrauterine contraceptive device.

Intrauterine device (IUD) Small copper- or progesterone-containing form used for contraception.

Intrauterine growth retardation (IUGR) Fetal undergrowth of any etiology, such as deficient nutrient supply or intrauterine infection, or associated with congenital malformation.

Introitus Entrance into a canal or cavity such as the vagina.

Intromission Insertion of one part or object into another (e.g., introduction of penis into vagina).

Intussusception Prolapse of one segment of bowel into the lumen of the adjacent segment.

In utero Within or inside the uterus.

In vitro fertilization (IVF) Fertilization in a culture dish or test tube.

In vitro fertilization with embryo transplant Fertilization in a culture dish or tube followed by transplant of embryo into uterus (womb).

Inversion Turning end for end, upside down, or inside out.

I. of the uterus Condition in which the uterus is turned inside out so that the fundus intrudes into the cervix or vagina; may be caused by a too-vigorous removal of the placenta before it is detached by the natural process of labor.

Involution Integrated processes (contractions and autolysis) by which uterus returns to nonpregnant size, shape, tone, and consistency.

Isoimmune hemolytic disease Breakdown (hemolysis) of fetal/neonatal Rh-positive red blood cells (RBCs) because of Rh antibodies formed by an Rh-negative mother who had been previously exposed to Rh-positive RBCs.

Isoimmunization Development of antibodies in a species of animal with antigens from the same species (e.g., development of anti-Rh antibodies in an Rh-negative person).

ITP Abbreviation for idiopathic thrombocytopenic purpura.

Jaundice Yellow discoloration of the body tissues caused by the deposit of bile pigments (unconjugated bilirubin); icterus.

Breastfeeding j. Appearing about day three, this jaundice is related to the number of feedings; the greater the number, the lower the bilirubin level (feedings should be ≥ 8 every 24 hr).

Breast milk j. Yellowing of infant's skin from pregnanediol (in mother's milk) inhibition of enzyme (glucuronyl transferase) necessary for conjugation of bilirubin.

! Pathologic j. Jaundice usually first noticeable within 24 hr after birth; caused by some abnormal condition such as an *Rh* or *ABO incompatibility* and resulting in bilirubin toxicity (e.g., *kernicterus*).

Physiologic j. Jaundice usually occurring 48 hr or later after birth, reaching a peak at 5–7 days, gradually disappearing by the seventh to tenth day, and caused by the normal reduction in the number of red blood cells. The infant is otherwise well.

Jet hydrotherapy Use of warm water under pressure to relax muscles and promote comfort.

Kangaroo care Skin-to-skin care. An alternative to technology and maternal-infant separation. Diaper-clad baby is placed under mother's clothing onto her bare chest.

Karyotype Schematic arrangement of the chromosomes within a cell to demonstrate their numbers and morphology.

Kegel's exercises Exercises to strengthen the pubococcygeal muscles.

! Kehr's sign "Referred pain" in the shoulder that indicates intraabdominal bleeding (or rupture of ovarian cyst).

! Kernicterus Bilirubin encephalopathy involving the deposit of unconjugated bilirubin in brain cells, resulting in death or impaired intellectual, perceptive, or motor function, and adaptive behavior.

Kleihauer-Betke test Laboratory test that detects the presence of fetal blood cells in the maternal circulation. See *Apt test.*

Klinefelter's syndrome Sex chromosome abnormality; most common deviation in males; trisomy XXY; poorly developed secondary sex characteristics and small testes; infertile; tall; effeminate. Usually, subnormal intelligence.

Klumpke's palsy Atrophic paralysis of forearm.

Labia Lips or liplike structures.

L. majora Two folds of skin containing fat and covered with hair that lie on either side of the vaginal opening and from each side of the vulva.

L. minora Two thin folds of delicate, hairless skin inside the labia majora.

Labor Series of processes by which the fetus is expelled from the uterus; parturition; childbirth.

Labor-delivery-recovery room (LDR) Unit in which a woman labors, gives birth, and recovers during the fourth stage of labor.

Labor-delivery-recovery-postpartum room (LDRP) An LDR in which a woman continues to stay after recovery until discharge home.

Laceration Irregular tear of wound tissue; in obstetrics, it usually refers to a tear in the perineum, vagina, or cervix caused by childbirth.

Lactation Function of secreting milk, or period during which milk is secreted.

Lactation amenorrhea Amenorrhea caused by the act of suckling and the high levels of prolactin, which has an antigonadotrophic effect.

Lactation suppression Stopping the production of breast milk through the use of medication and/or nonpharmacologic interventions.

Lactogenic Stimulating the production of milk.

L. hormone Gonadotropin produced by anterior pituitary and responsible for promoting growth of breast tissue and lactation; *prolactin;* luteotropin.

Lactose intolerance Inherited absence of the enzyme lactase.

Lactosuria Presence of lactose in the urine during late pregnancy and during lactation. Must be differentiated from glycosuria.

Lamaze method Method of psychophysical preparation for childbirth developed in the 1950s by a French obstetrician, Fernand Lamaze. It requires classes, practice at home, and coaching during labor and birth.

Lambdoid Having the shape of the Greek letter lambda (λ).

L. suture Suture line extending across the posterior third of the skull, separating the occipital bone from the two parietal bones, and forming the base of the triangular posterior fontanel.

Laminaria tent Cone of dried seaweed or synthetic osmotic dilator that swells as it absorbs moisture. Used to dilate the cervix nontraumatically in preparation for an induced abortion or in preparation for induction of labor.

Lanugo Downy, fine hair characteristic of the fetus between 20 wk gestation and birth, that is most noticeable over the shoulder, forehead, and cheeks but is found on nearly all parts of the body except the palms of the hands, soles of the feet, and the scalp.

Laparoscopy Examination of the interior of the abdomen by inserting a small telescope through the anterior abdominal wall.

Large for dates (large for gestational age [LGA]) Exhibiting excessive growth for gestational age.

Last menstrual period (LMP) The date of the first day of the last normal menstrual bleeding.

Learned helplessness Belief that one is powerless and unable to act independently; the result of socialization.

Lecithin A phospholipid that decreases surface tension; surfactant (i.e., surface-active agent).

Lecithin-sphingomyelin ratio Ratio of lecithin to sphingomyelin in the amniotic fluid. This is used to assess maturity of the fetal lung.

Legal terms

Tort A civil offense.

Duty The standard of care, or external code of behavior or expected performance, for a professional nurse. See *standards of care.*

Breach Failure to conform to the standard of care.

Malpractice Professional negligence that is the proximate cause of injury or harm to a patient, resulting from a lack of professional knowledge, experience, or skill that can be expected in others in the profession or from a failure to exercise reasonable care or judgment in the application of professional knowledge, experience, or skill.

Negligence *Commission* of an act that a prudent person would not have done or the *omission* of a duty that prudent person would have fulfilled, resulting in injury or harm to another person. In particular, in a malpractice suit a professional person is negligent if harm to a patient results from such an act or such a failure to act, but it must be proved that other prudent persons of the same profession would ordinarily have acted differently under the same circumstances.

Informed consent Refers to the right of persons to consent to all forms of touching; violation of that right is called **battery.** Includes: information about a procedure, its risks, its anticipated results, and any alternatives to it. The person performing the procedure is usually responsible for obtaining the consent.

Abandonment of care Wrongful cessation of the provision of care to a patient, e.g., leaving a woman in active labor alone. Usually refers to a physician, but can also be the result of a nurse's lack of action.

Reasonably prudent nurse Person who acts with the average degree of skill, care, and diligence as those with similar background, training, and experience. One who acts wisely and judiciously. See *Legal terms, negligence.*

Reasonably prudent person Person who demonstrates the external code of behavior or expected performance (average degree of skill, care, and diligence) exercised by any other person with similar background, training, and experience.

Leopold's maneuver Four maneuvers for diagnosing the fetal position by external palpation of the mother's abdomen. See text.

Let-down reflex Oxytocin-induced flow of milk from the alveoli of the breasts into the milk ducts.

Leukorrhea White or yellowish mucous discharge from the cervical canal or the vagina that may be normal physiologically or caused by pathologic states of the vagina and endocervix (e.g., *Trichomonas vaginalis* infections).

LH See *luteinizing hormone (LH).*

Libido Sexual drive.

Ligation Act of suturing, sewing, or otherwise tying shut.

Tubal l. Abdominal operation in which the fallopian tubes are tied off and a section is removed to interrupt tubal continuity and thus sterilize the woman.

Lightening Sensation of decreased abdominal distention produced by uterine descent into the pelvic cavity as the fetal presenting part settles into the pelvis. It usually occurs 2 wk before the onset of labor in nulliparas.

Linea nigra Line of darker pigmentation seen in some women during the latter part of pregnancy that appears over the midline of the abdomen and extends from the symphysis pubis toward the umbilicus.

Linea terminalis Line dividing the upper (false) pelvis from the lower (true) pelvis.

Lithotomy position Position in which the woman lies on her back with her knees flexed and abducted thighs drawn up toward her chest.

Live birth Birth in which the neonate, regardless of gestational age, manifests any heartbeat, breathes, or displays voluntary movement.

Living ligature In the thick middle myometrial layer of the uterus, the interlaced muscle fibers form a figure-of-eight pattern encircling large blood vessels; contraction of these fibers produces a hemostatic action.

Local infiltration anesthesia Process by which a substance such as a local anesthetic drug is deposited within the tissue to anesthetize a limited region.

Lochia Vaginal discharge during the puerperium, consisting of blood, tissue, and mucus.

L. rubra Red, distinctly blood-tinged vaginal flow that follows birth and lasts 2–4 days.

L. serosa Serous, pinkish brown, watery vaginal discharge that follows lochia rubra until about the tenth postpartum day.

L. alba Thin, yellowish to white, vaginal discharge that follows lochia serosa on about the tenth postpartum day and that may last from the end of the third to the sixth postpartum week.

Low birth weight (LBW) Infant weighing 2500 g or less at birth.

L/S ratio (lecithin-sphingomyelin ratio) Test for fetal lung maturity.

Lunar month Four wk (28 days).

Lutein Yellow pigment derived from the corpus luteum, egg yolk, and fat cells.

L. cells Ovarian cells involved in the formation of the corpus luteum and that contain a yellow pigment.

Luteinizing hormone (LH) Hormone produced by the anterior pituitary that stimulates ovulation and the development of the corpus luteum.

Lymphedema Collection of excessive fluid in tissue when lymph nodes or vessels have been removed.

Lysis of adhesions Operation to free adhesions (bands of scar tissue) that have caused organs to be abnormally drawn or tied to each other. Intraabdominal adhesions, often sequelae to pelvic inflammatory disease, impair fertility.

Lysozyme Enzyme with antiseptic qualities that destroys foreign organisms and that is found in blood cells of the granulocytic and monocytic series and is also normally present in saliva, sweat, tears, and breast milk.

Maceration (1) Process of softening a solid by soaking it in a fluid. (2) Softening and breaking down of fetal skin from prolonged exposure to amniotic fluid as seen in a postterm infant. Also seen in a dead fetus.

Macroglossia Hypertrophy of tongue or tongue large for oral cavity; seen in some preterm neonates and in neonates with Down syndrome.

Macrosomia Large body size as seen in neonates of diabetic or prediabetic mothers; macrosomatia.

Magnetic resonance imaging (MRI) Noninvasive nuclear procedure for imaging tissues with high fat and water content; in obstetrics, uses include evaluation of fetal structures, placenta, amniotic fluid volume.

Mammary gland Compound gland of the female breast that is made up of lobes and lobules that secrete milk for nourishment of the young. Rudimentary mammary glands exist in the male.

Mammography X-ray examination technique used to screen for and evaluate breast lesions.

Manic-depressive psychosis Major affective disorder characterized by episodes of mania and depression. One or the other phase may be predominant at any given time; one phase may appear alternately with the other; or elements of both phases may be present simultaneously. Also called bipolar disorder.

Mask of pregnancy See *chloasma.*

Mastalgia Breast soreness or tenderness.

! **Mastitis** Inflammation of mammary tissue of the breasts.

Maternal role-taking (Reva Rubin)

  Taking-in phase Period after birth characterized by the woman's dependency; maternal needs are dominant, talking about the birth is an important task.

  Taking-hold phase Period after birth characterized by the woman becoming more independent and more interested in learning infant care skills.

  Letting-go phase Interdependent phase after birth in which the mother and family move forward as a system with interacting members.

Maturation (1) Process of attaining maximum development. (2) In biology, a process of cell division during which the number of chromosomes in the germ cells (sperm or ova) is reduced to one-half the number (haploid) characteristic of the species.

McDonald's sign Easy flexion of the fundus on the cervix.

Mean arterial pressure (MAP) Average of systolic and diastolic blood pressures. A MAP of 90 or more in the second trimester is associated with an increase in the incidence of pregnancy-induced hypertension in the third trimester. Example: blood pressure: 108/72; pulse pressure: (108 − 72 = 36), 36 ÷ 3 = 12; MAP (diastolic): 72 + 12 = 84.

Meatus Opening from an internal structure to the outside (e.g., urethral meatus).

Meconium First stools of infant: viscid, sticky; dark greenish brown, almost black; sterile; odorless.

  M. aspiration syndrome Function of fetal hypoxia: with hypoxia, the anal sphincter relaxes and meconium is released; reflex gasping movements draw meconium and other particulate matter in the amniotic fluid into the infant's bronchial tree, obstructing the air flow after birth.

  M. ileus Lower intestinal obstruction by thick, puttylike, inspissated meconium that may be the result of deficiency of trypsin production in the newborn with cystic fibrosis.

  ! **M.-stained fluid** In response to hypoxia, fetal intestinal activity increases and anal sphincter relaxes, resulting in the passage of meconium, which imparts a greenish coloration.

Meiosis Process by which germ cells divide and decrease their chromosomal number by one-half.

Melia Pertaining to a limb or part of a limb or extremity, as in amelia (absence of a limb) or phocomelia (absence of part of arms or legs).

Menarche Onset, or beginning, of menstrual function.

Meningomyelocele Saclike protrusion of the spinal cord through a congenital defect in the vertebral column.

Menopause From the Greek words *men* (month) and *pausis* (to stop), the actual permanent cessation of menstrual cycles.

Menorrhagia Abnormally profuse or excessive menstrual flow.

Menses (menstruation) Periodic vaginal discharge of bloody fluid from the nonpregnant uterus that occurs from the age of puberty to menopause.

Mentum Chin, a fetal reference point in designating position (e.g., "left mentum anterior" [LMA], meaning that the fetal chin is presenting in the left anterior quadrant of the maternal pelvis).

Mesoderm Embryonic middle layer of germ cells giving rise to all types of muscles, connective tissue, bone marrow, blood, lymphoid tissue, and all epithelial tissue.

Metritis Inflammation of the endometrium and myometrium.

Metrorrhagia Abnormal bleeding from the uterus, particularly when it occurs at any time other than the menstrual period.

Microcephaly Congenital anomaly characterized by abnormal smallness of the head in relation to the rest of the body and by underdevelopment of the brain, resulting in some degree of mental retardation.

Micrognathia Abnormal smallness of mandible or chin.

Midwife One who practices the art of helping and aiding a woman to give birth.

Milia Unopened sebaceous glands appearing as tiny, white, pinpoint papules on forehead, nose, cheeks, and chin of a neonate that disappear spontaneously in a few days or weeks.

Milk ejection Milk leaking from the breasts, often before a feeding.

Milk leg See *phlegmasia alba dolens.*

Miscarriage Spontaneous abortion; lay term usually referring specifically to the loss of the fetus between the fourth month and viability.

Misogyny Hatred of women.

Mitleiden Suffering along with, *e.g.,* psychosomatic symptoms sometimes experienced by expectant fathers.

Mitosis Process of somatic cell division in which a single cell divides, but both of the new cells have the same number of chromosomes as the first.

! Mitral valve prolapse (MVP) A disorder in which the cusp(s) of the mitral valve drop into the left atrium during systole characterized by midsystolic click and late systolic murmur.

Mitral valve stenosis Narrowing of the opening of the mitral valve due to stiffening of valve leaflets obstructing free flow from atrium to ventricle.

Mittelschmerz Abdominal pain in the region of an ovary during ovulation, which usually occurs midway through the menstrual cycle. Present in many women, mittelschmerz is useful for identifying ovulation, thus pinpointing the fertile period of the cycle.

Molding Overlapping of cranial bones or shaping of the fetal head to accommodate and conform to the bony and soft parts of the mother's birth canal during labor.

Mongolian spot Bluish-gray or dark, nonelevated pigmented area usually found over the lower back and buttocks present at birth in some infants, primarily nonwhite. The spot fades by school age in African-American or Asian infants and within the first year or two of life in other infants.

Mongolism See *Down syndrome.*

Moniliasis Infection of the skin or mucous membrane by a yeastlike fungus, *Candida albicans; see thrush.*

Monitrice One trained in psychoprophylactic methods and in supporting women during labor.

Monosomy Chromosomal aberration characterized by the absence of one chromosome from the normal diploid complement.

Monozygotic Originating or coming from a single fertilized ovum, such as identical twins.

Mons veneris Pad of fatty tissue and coarse skin that overlies the symphysis pubis in the woman and that, after puberty, is covered with short curly hair.

Montgomery's glands, tubercles Small, nodular prominences (sebaceous glands) on the areolas around the nipples of the breasts that enlarge during pregnancy and lactation.

Mood disorders Depression or depression with manic episodes (bipolar disorders).

Morbidity (1) Condition of being diseased. (2) Number of cases of disease or sick persons in relationship to a specific population; incidence.

Morning sickness Nausea and vomiting that affect some women during the first few months of their pregnancy; may occur at any time of day.

Moro's reflex Normal, generalized reflex in a young infant elicited by a sudden loud noise or by striking the table next to the child, resulting in flexion of the legs, an embracing posture of the arms, and usually a brief cry. Also called *startle reflex.*

Mortality (1) Quality or state of being subject to death. (2) Number of deaths in relation to a specific population; incidence.

    Fetal m. Number of fetal deaths per 1000 births (or per live births).

    Infant m. Number of deaths per 1000 children 1 yr of age or younger.

    Intrauterine m. Death of a fetus weighing 500 g or more, of 20 wk gestation or more.

    Maternal m. Number of maternal deaths per 100,000 births during the childbearing cycle.

    Neonatal m. Statistical rate of infant death during the first 28 days after live birth, expressed as the number of such deaths per 1000 live births in a specific geographic area or institution in a given period of time.

    Perinatal m. Combined fetal and neonatal mortality.

Morula Developmental stage of the fertilized ovum in which there is a solid mass of cells resembling a mulberry.

Mosaicism Condition in which some somatic cells are normal, whereas others show chromosomal aberrations.

Mourning Expressions and behaviors of grief.

Multigravida Woman who has been pregnant two or more times.

Multifetal pregnancy Pregnancy in which there is more than one fetus in the uterus at the same time; multiple pregnancy.

Multipara Woman who has carried two or more pregnancies to viability, whether they ended in live infants or stillbirths and whether the pregnancy yielded one or more babies.

Mutation Change in a gene or chromosome in gametes that may be transmitted to offspring.

Myoepithelial cells Contractile cells that surround the mammary alveoli and contract in response to oxytocin, causing milk let-down.

Nägele's rule Method for calculating the estimated date of confinement (EDC), estimated date of birth (EDB) or "due date."

⬭ Narcotic antagonist A compound such as naloxone (Narcan) that promptly reverses the effects of narcotics such as meperidine (Demerol).

Natal Relating or pertaining to birth.

Navel Depression in the center of the abdomen, where the umbilical cord was attached to the fetus; umbilicus.

! Necrotizing enterocolitis (NEC) Acute inflammatory bowel disorder that occurs primarily in preterm, low-birthweight, or cocaine-exposed neonates. It is characterized by ischemic necrosis (death) of the gastrointestinal mucosa that may lead to perforation and peritonitis.

! Neonatal hypovolemic shock Cardiovascular collapse resulting from a diminished volume of circulating fluid in the cardiovascular system.

Neoplasia Growth of new tissue; tumor that serves no physiologic function; may be benign or malignant.

Neural tube Tube formed from fusion of the neural folds from which develops the brain and spinal cord.

    N. t. defect Improper development of tube resulting in malformation of brain and/or spinal cord; see (α) *fetoprotein (AFP).*

Neutral temperature range That grouping of environmental conditions in which the neonate's oxygen consumption is at a minimum and temperature is within normal limits.

Nevus Natural blemish or mark; a congenital circumscribed deposit of pigmentation in the skin; mole.

    N. flammeus Port-wine stain; reddish, usually flat, discoloration of the face or neck. Because of its large size and color, it is considered a serious deformity.

    N. vasculosus (strawberry hemangioma) Elevated lesion of immature capillaries and endothelial cells that regresses over a period of years.

Nidation Implantation of the fertilized ovum in the endometrium, or lining, of the uterus.

Nondisjunction   Failure of homologous pairs of chromosomes to separate during the first meiotic division or of the two chromatids of a chromosome to split during anaphase of mitosis or the second meiotic division. The result is an abnormal number of chromosomes in the daughter cells.

Nonreassuring fetal heart rate pattern   Fetal heart rate pattern that indicates the fetus is not well oxygenated and requires intervention.

Nonshivering thermogenesis   Infant's method of producing heat by increasing metabolic rate.

Nonstress test (NST)   Evaluation of fetal response (fetal heart rate) to natural contractile uterine activity or to an increase in fetal activity.

Nosocomial   Pertaining to a hospital.

Nuchal cord   Encircling of fetal neck by one or more loops of umbilical cord.

Nulligravida   Woman who has never been pregnant.

Nullipara   Woman who has not yet carried a pregnancy to viability.

Nurse practitioner   Registered nurse who has additional education to practice nursing in an expanded role.

Obstetrix   Midwife; from *obstare*, to stand by.

Occipitobregmatic   Pertaining to the occiput (the back part of the skull) and the bregma (junction of the coronal and sagittal sutures) or anterior fontanel; the smallest diameter of the fetal head.

Occiput   Back part of the head or skull.

Oligohydramnios   Abnormally small amount or absence of amniotic fluid; often indicative of fetal urinary tract defect.

Oliguria   Diminished secretion of urine by the kidneys.

Omphalic   Concerning or pertaining to the umbilicus.

Omphalitis   Inflammation of the umbilical stump characterized by redness, edema, and purulent exudate in severe infections.

Omphalocele   Congenital defect resulting from failure of closure of the abdominal wall or muscles and leading to hernia of abdominal contents through the navel.

Oogenesis   Formation and development of the ovum.

Oophorectomy   Excision or removal of an ovary.

Operculum   Plug of mucus that fills the cervical canal during pregnancy.

Ophthalmia neonatorum   Infection in the neonate's eyes, usually resulting from gonorrheal or other infection contracted when the fetus passes through the birth canal (vagina).

Oral GTT   Test for blood sugar following oral ingestion of a concentrated sugar solution.

Orchitis   Inflammation of one or both of the testes, characterized by swelling and pain, often caused by mumps, syphilis, or tuberculosis; may result in infertility in males.

Organogenesis period   Period of embryonic development (between weeks 3–4 and 8) during which all major organ systems are formed. Period of extreme vulnerability to teratogens (e.g., environmental hazards and toxic substances).

Orifice   Normal mouth, entrance, or opening, to any aperture.

Os   Mouth, or opening.

External o.   External opening of the cervical canal.

Internal o.   Internal opening of the cervical canal.

O. uteri   Mouth, or opening, of the uterus.

Ossification   Mineralization of fetal bones.

Osteoporosis   Deossification of bone tissue resulting in structural weakness.

-Otomy   Combining form meaning cutting, incision, section.

Outlet   Opening by which something can exit.

pelvic o.   Inferior aperture, or opening, of the true pelvis.

Ovary   One of two glands in the female situated on either side of the pelvic cavity that produce the female reproductive cell, the ovum, and two known hormones, estrogen and progesterone.

Ovulation   Periodic ripening (maturation) and discharge of the unimpregnated ovum from the ovary, usually 14 days before the onset of menstrual flow.

O. method   Evaluation of cervical mucus throughout the menstrual cycle; ovulation occurs just after the appearance of the peak mucus sign; Billings method.

Ovum   Female germ, or reproductive cell, produced by the ovary; egg.

Oxygen toxicity   Oxygen overdosage that results in pathologic tissue changes (e.g., retinopathy of prematurity, bronchopulmonary dysplasia in the neonate).

Oxytocics   Drugs that stimulate uterine contractions, thus accelerating childbirth and preventing postbirth hemorrhage. They may be used to increase the let-down reflex during lactation.

Oxytocin   Hormone produced by the posterior pituitary gland that stimulates uterine contractions and the release of milk in the mammary gland (let-down reflex).

O. challenge test (OCT)   Evaluation of fetal response (fetal heart rate) to contractile activity of the uterus stimulated by exogenous oxytocin (Pitocin).

Palmar erythema   Redness on the surface of the palms sometimes seen in pregnancy, caused by estrogen.

Palsy   Permanent or temporary loss of sensation or ability to move and control movement; paralysis.

Bell's p.   Peripheral facial paralysis of the facial nerve (cranial nerve VII), causing the muscles of the unaffected side of the face to pull the face into a distorted position.

Erb's p.   See *Erb-Duchenne paralysis.*

Papanicolaou (Pap) test   Microscopic examination using scrapings from the cervix, endocervix, or other mucous membranes that will reveal, with a high degree of accuracy, the presence of premalignant or malignant cells.

Para   Term used to refer to past pregnancies that reached viability regardless of whether the infant(s) was dead or alive at birth.

Parabiotic syndrome   Fetofetal blood transfer caused by placental vascular anastomoses occurring in a small plethoric twin (polycythemia) and one pale twin (anemia).

Paracervical block   Type of regional anesthesia produced by injection of a local anesthetic into the lower uterine segment just beneath the mucosa adjacent to the outer rim of the cervix (9 and 3 o'clock positions) after the cervix is more than 5 cm dilated. Used primarily for gynecologic surgery.

Parity   Number of pregnancies that reached viability, 20–22 wk gestation.

Parturient   Woman giving birth.

Parturition   Process or act of giving birth.

Patent   Open.

Pathologic hyperbilirubinemia   High (toxic) levels of serum bilirubin resulting from a disease process causing hemolysis (e.g., *Rh incompatibility*); jaundice apparent within first 24 hr. See *jaundice, pathologic.*

Patulous   Open or spread apart.

Peak mucus sign   Lubricative, cloudy-to-clear egg white cervical mucus occurring under high estrogen levels close to time of ovulation; ferns; good spinnbarkheit.

Peau d'orange   "Orange-peel"-like skin secondary to cancerous lesions and seen over edematous breasts.

Pelvic inflammatory disease (PID)   Infection of internal reproductive structures and adjacent tissues usually secondary to sexually transmitted disease infection.

Pelvic relaxation   Refers to the lengthening and weakening of the fascial supports of pelvic structures.

Pelvic tilt (rock)   An exercise used to help relieve low-back discomfort during pregnancy.

Pelvis   Bony structure formed by the sacrum, coccyx, innominate bones, and symphysis pubis, and the ligaments that unite them. Types:

Android   Male, heart-shaped.

Anthropoid   Oval.

False   Pelvis above the linea terminalis and symphysis pubis.

Gynecoid   Female, round.

Platypelloid   Flat.

True   Pelvis below the linea terminalis.

Penis   Male organ used for urination and copulation.

Percutaneous umbilical blood sampling (PUBS)   Procedure during the second or third trimester which the fetal umbilical vessel is accessed under ultrasound for blood sampling or for transfusions of severely anemic fetuses. Indications: prenatal diagnosis of inherited organic disorders; fetal infection; assessment of acid-base status of intrauterine growth–retarded (IUGR) fetuses; assessment and treatment of isoimmunization and thrombocytopenia in women.

Peridural anesthesia   Injection of anesthetic outside the dura mater (anesthetic does not mix with spinal fluid); epidural anesthesia.

Perinatal   Of or pertaining to the time and process of giving birth or being born.

Perinatal period   Period extending from the twentieth or twenty-eighth week of gestation through the end of the twenty-eighth day after birth.

Perinatologist   Physician who specializes in fetal and neonatal care.

Perineum   Area between the vagina and rectum in the female and between the scrotum and rectum in the male.

Periodic breathing   Sporadic episodes of cessation of respirations for periods of 10 sec or less not associated with cyanosis; commonly noted in preterm infants.

Periods of reactivity (newborn infant)   *First period* (within 30 min after birth): brief cyanosis, flushing with crying; crackles (rales), nasal flaring, grunting, retractions; heart sounds loud, forceful, irregular; alert; mucus; no bowel sounds; followed by period of sleep. *Second period* (4–8 hr after birth): swift color changes; irregular respiratory and heart rates; mucus with gagging; meconium passage; and temperature stabilizing.

Pessary   Device placed inside the vagina to function as a supportive structure for the uterus or a contraceptive device.

Petechiae   Pinpoint hemorrhagic areas caused by numerous disease states involving infection and thrombocytopenia and occasionally found over the face and trunk of the newborn because of increased intravascular pressure in the capillaries during birth.

pH   Hydrogen ion concentration.

Phenotype   Expression of certain physical or chemical characteristics in an individual, resulting from interaction between genotype and environmental factors.

Phenylketonuria (PKU)   Recessive hereditary disease that results in a defect in the metabolism of the amino acid phenylalanine caused by the lack of an enzyme, phenylalanine hydroxylase, that is necessary for the conversion of the amino acid phenylalanine into tyrosine. If PKU is not treated, brain damage may occur, causing severe mental retardation.

Phimosis   Tightness of the prepuce, or foreskin, of the penis.

Phlebitis   Inflammation of a vein with symptoms of pain and tenderness along the course of the vein, inflammatory swelling and acute edema below the obstruction, and discoloration of the skin because of injury or bruise to the vein, possibly occurring in acute or chronic infections or after operations or childbirth.

Phlebothrombosis   Formation of a clot or thrombus in the vein; inflammation of the vein with secondary clotting.

Phlegmasia alba dolens   Phlebitis of the femoral vein with thrombosis leading to a venous obstruction, causing acute edema of the leg, and occurring occasionally after birth; also called *milk leg*.

Phocomelia   Developmental anomaly characterized by the absence of the upper portion of one or more limbs so that the feet or hands or both are attached to the trunk of the body by short, irregularly shaped stumps, resembling the fins of a seal.

Phosphatidylglycerol   A phospholipid, a component of pulmonary surfactant; its presence in amniotic fluid is considered a sign of fetal lung maturity when the pregnancy is complicated by maternal diabetes.

Phototherapy   Utilization of lights to reduce serum bilirubin levels by oxidation of bilirubin into water-soluble compounds that are then processed in the liver and excreted in bile and urine.

Physiologic hyperbilirubinemia   Hemolysis of excessive fetal red blood cells in the early neonatal period; jaundice not apparent during first 24 hr. Levels are nontoxic to the individual. See *jaundice, physiologic*.

Pica   Unusual craving during pregnancy (e.g., for laundry starch, dirt, or red clay).

PID   Abbreviation for pelvic inflammatory disease.

Pinch test   Determines if nipples are erectile or retractile.

Pinna   Ear cartilage.

Placenta   Latin, flat cake; afterbirth; specialized vascular disk-shaped organ for maternal-fetal gas and nutrient exchange.

Abruptio p.   See *abruptio placentae*.

Battledore p.   Umbilical cord insertion into the margin of the placenta.

Circumvallate p.   Placenta having a raised white ring at its edge.

P. accreta   Invasion of the uterine muscle by the placenta, thus making separation from the muscle difficult if not impossible.

P. previa   Placenta that is abnormally implanted in the thin, lower uterine segment and that is typed according to proximity to cervical os: *total*—completely occludes os; *partial*—does not occlude os completely; and *marginal*—placenta encroaches on margin of internal cervical os.

P. succenturiata   Accessory placenta.

Placental   Pertaining or relating to the placenta.

⚡ **P. dysfunction**   Failure of placenta to meet fetal needs and requirements; placental insufficiency.

P. dystocia   See *dystocia, placental.*

P. infarct   Localized, ischemic, hard area on the fetal or maternal side of the placenta.

P. souffle   See *souffle, placental.*

Platypelloid pelvis   Broad pelvis with a shortened antero-posterior diameter and a flattened, oval, transverse shape.

Plethora   Deep beefy-red coloration ("boiled lobster" hue) of a newborn caused by an increased number of red blood cells (polycythemia) per volume of blood.

Podalic   Concerning or pertaining to the feet.

P. version   Shifting of the position of the fetus so as to bring the feet to the outlet during labor.

Polycythemia   Increased number of erythrocytes per volume of blood, which may be caused by large placental transfusion, fetofetal transfusion (in twin pregnancy), or maternal-fetal transfusion, or it may be due to hypovolemia resulting from movement of fluid out of vascular into interstitial compartment.

Polydactyly   Excessive number of digits (fingers or toes).

Polygenic   Pertaining to the combined action of several different genes.

Polyhydramnios   See *hydramnios.*

Polyuria   Excessive secretion and discharge of urine by the kidneys.

Position   Relationship of an arbitrarily chosen fetal reference point, such as the occiput, sacrum, chin, or scapula, on the presenting part of the fetus to its location in the front, back, or sides of the maternal pelvis.

Positive sign of pregnancy   Definite indication of pregnancy (e.g., hearing the fetal heartbeat, visualization and palpation of fetal movement by the examiner, sonographic examination).

! **Postmature infant**   Infant born at or after the beginning of week 43 of gestation or later and exhibiting signs of dysmaturity.

Postnatal   Happening or occurring after birth (newborn).

Postpartum   Happening or occurring after birth (mother).

Postpartum blues   A letdown feeling, accompanied by irritability and anxiety, which usually begins 2–3 days after giving birth and disappears within a week or two. Sometimes called the "baby blues."

Postpartum depression   Depression occurring within 6 mo of childbirth; lasts longer than postpartum blues and is characterized by a variety of symptoms.

Postpartum psychosis   Symptoms begin as postpartum blues or depression but are characterized by a break with reality. Delusions, hallucinations, confusion, delirium, and panic can occur.

Postterm birth   Birth of an infant after 42 wk gestation.

Precipitous labor   Rapid or sudden labor of less than 3 hr duration beginning from onset of cervical changes to completed birth of neonate.

Preconception care   Care designed for health maintenance before pregnancy.

⚡ **Preeclampsia**   Disease encountered after 20 wk gestation or early in the puerperium; a vasospastic disease process characterized by increasing hypertension, proteinuria, and hemoconcentration with or without generalized edema; pregnancy-induced hypertension (PIH); toxemia.

Pregnancy   Period between conception through complete delivery of the products of conception. The usual duration of pregnancy in the human is 280 days, 9 calendar mo, or 10 lunar mo.

⚡ **Pregnancy-induced hypertension (PIH)**   Hypertensive disorders of pregnancy including preeclampsia, eclampsia, and transient hypertension.

! **Premature infant**   Infant born before completing week 37 of gestation, irrespective of birth weight; preterm infant.

Premenstrual syndrome (PMS)   Syndrome of nervous tension, irritability, weight gain, edema, headache, mastalgia, dysphoria, and lack of coordination occurring during the last few days of the menstrual cycle preceding the onset of menstruation.

Premonitory   Serving as an early symptom or warning.

Prenatal   Occurring or happening before birth.

Prepartum   Before birth; before giving birth.

Prepuce   Fold of skin, or foreskin, covering the glans penis of the male.

P. of the clitoris   Fold of the labia minora that covers the aroused glans clitoris.

Presenting part   That part of the fetus that lies closest to the internal os of the cervix.

Pressure edema   Edema of the lower extremities caused by pressure of the heavy pregnant uterus against the large veins; edema of fetal scalp after cephalic presentation (caput succedaneum).

Presumptive signs   Manifestations that suggest pregnancy but that are not absolutely positive. These include the cessation of menses, Chadwick's sign, morning sickness, and quickening.

Preterm birth   Birth occurring before completion of week 37 of gestation; premature birth.

Preterm infant   See *premature infant.*

Primigravida   Woman who is pregnant for the first time.

Primipara   Woman who has carried a pregnancy to viability without regard to the child's being dead or alive at the time of birth.

Primordial   Existing first or existing in the simplest or most primitive form.

Probable signs   Manifestations or evidence indicating that there is a definite likelihood of pregnancy. Among the probable signs are enlargement of abdomen, Goodell's sign, Hegar's sign, Braxton Hicks' sign, and positive hormonal tests for pregnancy.

Prodromal   Serving as an early symptom or warning of the approach of a disease or condition (e.g., prodromal labor).

Progesterone   Hormone produced by the corpus luteum, adrenal cortex, and placenta whose function is to prepare the endometrium of the uterus for implantation of the fertilized ovum, develop the mammary glands, and maintain the pregnancy.

Prolactin   See *lactogenic hormone.*

! **Prolapsed cord**   Protrusion of the umbilical cord in advance of the presenting part of the fetus.

Proliferative phase of menstrual cycle   Preovulatory, follicular, or estrogen phase of the menstrual cycle.

! **PROM**   Premature (before 38 wk gestation) rupture of membranes.

Promontory of the sacrum   Superior projecting portion of the sacrum at the junction of the sacrum and the L5 vertebra.

Prophylactic Pertaining to prevention or warding off of disease or certain conditions; condom, or "rubber."

Proscription Establish taboos. See *taboo.*

Prostaglandin (PG) Substance present in many body tissues; has a role in many reproductive tract functions.

Proteinuria Excretion of protein into urine.

Pruritus Itching.

Pruritus gravidarum Itching of the skin caused by pregnancy.

Pseudocyesis (pseudopregnancy) Condition in which the woman has all the usual signs of pregnancy, such as enlargement of the abdomen, cessation of menses, weight gain, and morning sickness, but is not pregnant; phantom or false pregnancy.

Pseudomenstruation Blood-tinged mucus from the vagina in the newborn female infant; caused by withdrawal of maternal hormones that were present during pregnancy.

Psychoprophylaxis Mental and physical education of the parents in preparation for childbirth, with the goal of minimizing the fear and perception of pain and promoting positive family relationships.

Ptyalism Excessive salivation.

Puberty Period in life in which the reproductive organs mature and one becomes functionally capable of reproduction.

Pubic Pertaining to the pubis.

Pubis Pubic bone forming the front of the pelvis.

PUBS See *percutaneous umbilical blood sampling.*

Pudendal block Injection of a local anesthetizing drug at the pudendal nerve root in order to produce numbness of the genital and perianal region.

Pudendum External genitalia of either sex; Latin, "that of which one should be ashamed."

Puerperal sepsis Infection of the pelvic organs during the postbirth period; childbed fever.

Puerperium Time following the third stage of labor and lasting until involution of the uterus takes place, usually about 3–6 wk.

Pulse oximetry Noninvasive method of monitoring oxygen levels by detecting the amount of light absorbed by oxygen-carrying hemoglobin.

Pyrosis A burning sensation in the epigastric and sternal region from stomach acid; **heartburn.**

Quickening Maternal perception of fetal movement; usually occurs between weeks 16 and 20 of gestation.

Radioimmunoassay Pregnancy test that tests for the beta subunit of hCG using radioactive labeled markers.

Rape Sexual intercourse that is inflicted forcibly on another person, against that person's will; sexual assault.

Rape trauma syndrome Characteristic symptoms seen in victims of rape, consisting of several phases; similar to post-traumatic stress syndrome.

RDS See *respiratory distress syndrome.*

Recessive trait Genetically determined characteristic that is expressed only when present in the homozygotic state (e.g., blue eyes, blond hair).

Rectocele Herniation or protrusion of the rectum into the posterior vaginal wall.

Referred pain Discomfort originating in a local area such as cervix, vagina, or perineal tissues; the discomfort is felt in the back, flanks, or thighs.

Reflex Automatic response built into the nervous system that does not need the intervention of conscious thought (e.g., in the newborn, rooting, gagging, grasp).

Regional block anesthesia Anesthesia of an area of the body by injecting a local anesthetic to block a group of sensory nerve fibers.

Regurgitation Vomiting or spitting up of solids or fluids.

Relaxin A water-soluble protein secreted by the corpus luteum that causes relaxation of the symphysis and cervical dilatation.

Respiratory distress syndrome (RDS) Condition resulting from decreased pulmonary gas exchange, leading to retention of carbon dioxide (increase in arterial PCO_2). Most common neonatal causes are prematurity, perinatal asphyxia, and maternal diabetes mellitus; hyaline membrane disease (HMD).

Restitution In obstetrics, the turning of the fetal head to the left or right after it has completely emerged from the introitus (vaginal opening) as it assumes a normal alignment with the infant's shoulders.

Retained placenta Retention of all or part of the placenta in the uterus after birth.

Retinopathy of prematurity Associated with hyperoxemia, resulting in eye injury and blindness.

Retraction (1) Drawing in or sucking in of soft tissues of chest, indicative of an obstruction at any level of the respiratory tract from the oropharynx to the alveoli. (2) Retraction of uterine muscle fiber. After contracting, the muscle fiber does not return to its original length but remains slightly shortened, a unique attribute of uterine muscle that aids in preventing postbirth hemorrhage and results in involution.

Retroflexion Bending backward.

R. of the uterus Condition in which the body of the womb is bent backward at an angle with the cervix.

Retrolental fibroplasia (RLF) *Retinopathy of prematurity* associated with hyperoxemia, resulting in eye injury and blindness.

Retroversion Turning or a state of being turned back.

R. of the uterus Displacement of the uterus; the body of the uterus is tipped backward with the cervix pointing forward toward the symphysis pubis.

Retrovirus A single piece of ribonucleic acid (RNA) surrounded by a protein coat, or envelope. A unique enzyme, reverse transcriptase, allows this RNA retrovirus to go backward, *against the "flow of life."* The RNA becomes a piece of deoxyribonucleic acid (DNA) which infects the cell's DNA nucleus and remains in the cell until its death (e.g., human immunodeficiency virus). (The normal flow of genetic information in life is from DNA to RNA to protein.)

Rh factor Inherited antigen present on erythrocytes. The individual with the factor is known as *positive* for the factor.

Rh immune globulin Solution of gamma globulin that contains Rh antibodies produced by another person; an example of passive artificial immunity giving a short-term immune response. Intramuscular (IM) administration of Rh immune globulin (trade name Rh_oGAM) prevents sensitization in Rh-negative women who have been exposed to Rh-positive red blood cells.

Rheumatic heart disease Permanent damage of heart valves secondary to an autoimmune reaction in the heart tissue precipitated by rheumatic heart disease.

Rhythm method   Contraceptive method in which a woman abstains from sexual intercourse during the ovulatory phase of her menstrual cycle and at least 3 days before and 1 day after the ovulation date.

Ribonucleic acid (RNA)   Element responsible for transferring genetic information within a cell; a template, or pattern.

Ring of fire   Burning sensation as vagina stretches and fetal head crowns.

Risk factors   Factors that cause a person or a group of people to be particularly vulnerable to an unwanted, unpleasant, or unhealthful event.

Risk management   Actions taken to eliminate or minimize either the chance of injury to a patient or the harm that occurs. Requires nurse to be skilled in all steps of the nursing process.

Risk-taking   Intentional behaviors with uncertain outcomes. Characteristic of adolescence.

Rite of passage   Significant life event indicating movement from one maturational level to another.

Ritgen maneuver   Procedure used to control the birth of the head.

Role playing   Psychotherapeutic technique in which a person acts out a real or simulated situation as a means of understanding intrapsychic conflicts.

Roll-over test   Sometimes used in the second trimester as a predictor of a potential hypertensive problem in the *third trimester*. An increase of 20 mm Hg in diastolic blood pressure (BP) from the side position to the supine position indicates a *positive roll-over test* reaction; even if BP is within normal limits, pregnancy-induced hypertension or preeclampsia will develop at least 60% of the time. Institute home self-care measures.

Rooming-in unit   Maternity unit designed so that the newborn's crib is at the mother's bedside or in a nursery adjacent to the mother's room.

Rooting reflex   Normal response in newborns when the cheek is touched or stroked along the side of the mouth to turn the head toward the stimulated side, to open the mouth, and to begin to suck. The reflex disappears by 3–4 mo of age but in some infants may persist until 12 mo.

Rotation   In obstetrics, the turning of the fetal head as it follows the curves of the birth canal downward.

Round ligaments   Ligaments that arise from the side of the uterus near the fallopian tube insertion to help the broad ligament keep the uterus in place.

Rubella vaccine   Live attenuated rubella virus given to women who have not had rubella or who are serologically negative (i.e., titer <1 : 3). Exposure to the rubella virus through vaccination causes the woman to form antibodies, producing active artificial immunity. (The person who contracts the infection will develop active *natural* immunity.) Notes:

1. Lactating mothers can receive the live attenuated virus.
2. A transient arthralgia or rash may develop, but is benign.
3. Women should not become pregnant for 2–3 mo after vaccination.
4. Women allergic to duck eggs may develop a hypersensitivity reaction.
5. If woman also receives Rh$_o$GAM at or around the time of rubella vaccination, the vaccination may not "take"; her titer needs to be retested 3 mo later.

Rubin, Reva   See *maternal role-taking*.

Rubin's test   Transuterine insufflation of the fallopian tubes with carbon dioxide to test their patency.

Rugae   Folds of vaginal mucosa; creases in scrotum.

Sacroiliac   Of or pertaining to the sacrum and ilium.

Sacrum   Triangular bone composed of five united vertebrae and situated between L5 and the coccyx; forms the posterior boundary of the true pelvis.

Saddle block anesthesia   Type of regional anesthesia produced by injection of a local anesthetic solution into the cerebrospinal fluid intrathecal (subarachnoid) space in the spinal canal; "low spinal" anesthesia.

Safe passage   Normal, uneventful birth process for mother and child.

Safe period   The days in the menstrual cycle that are not designated as fertile days, i.e., before and after ovulation.

Sagittal suture   Band of connective tissue separating the parietal bones, extending from the anterior to the posterior fontanel.

Salpingo-oophorectomy   Removal of a fallopian tube and an ovary.

! Scaphoid abdomen   Abdomen with a sunken interior wall. In newborn, usually indicates a diaphragmatic hernia that allowed abdominal contents to enter the chest cavity during fetal development, thereby compromising development of heart and lungs; a surgical emergency.

Sclerema   Hardening of skin and subcutaneous tissue that develops in association with such life-threatening disorders as severe cold stress, septicemia, and shock.

Scrotum   Pouch of skin containing the testes and parts of the spermatic cords.

Sebaceous glands   Oil-secreting glands found in the skin.

Secretory phase of menstrual cycle   Postovulatory, luteal, progestational, premenstrual phase of menstrual cycle; 14 days in length.

Secundines   Fetal membranes and placenta expelled after childbirth; afterbirth.

Self-care   Patient provides care for self as part of plan of care.

Self-quieting activity   Infant's ability to use personal resources to quiet and console him or herself.

Semen   Thick, white, viscid secretion discharged from the urethra of the male at orgasm; the transporting medium of the sperm.

Semen analysis   Examination of semen specimen to determine liquefaction, volume, pH, sperm density, and normal morphology.

Sensitization   Development of antibodies to a specific antigen.

Sensory behavior   Responses of the five senses; indicate a readiness for social interaction.

! Sepsis   Bacterial infections of the bloodstream in infants during the first 4 wk of life.

Sex chromosome   Chromosome associated with determination of gender: the X (female) and Y (male) chromosomes. The normal female has two X chromosomes and the normal male has one X and one Y chromosome.

Sexual assault   Penetration of any orifice by the penis, other male appendage, or object without the victim's consent; achieved through use of actual or implied threats, force, intimidation, or deception.

Sexual decision making   Selection of choices concerned with intimate and sexual behavior.

Sexual history   Past and present health conditions, life-style behaviors, knowledge, and attitudes related to sex and sexuality.

Sexual response cycle   The phases of physical changes that occur in response to sexual stimulation and sexual tension release.

Sexuality   The part of life that has to do with being male or female.

Sexually transmitted diseases (STDs)   Disease acquired as a result of sexual activity with an infected individual.

⊞ **Shake test**   "Foam" test for lung maturity of fetus; more rapid than determination of lecithin-sphingomyelin ratio.

Sibling rivalry   Competition that occurs between brothers and sisters.

! **Sickle cell hemoglobinopathy**   Abnormal crescent shape red blood corpuscles in the blood.

! **Simian line**   A single palmar crease frequently found in children with Down syndrome.

Sims' position   Position in which the person lies on the left side with the right knee and thigh drawn upward toward the chest.

Single-parent family   Family form characterized by one parent in the household. This may result from loss of spouse by death, divorce, separation, desertion, out-of-wedlock birth of a child, or adoption.

Singleton   Pregnancy with a single fetus.

Sitz bath   Application of moist heat to the perineum by sitting in a tub or basin filled with warm water.

Sleep-wake cycles   Variations in states of newborn consciousness.

Small for dates (small for gestational age [SGA])   Refers to inadequate growth for gestational age.

Smegma   Whitish secretion around labia minora.

Somatic   Pertaining to the body, not reproductive, cells.

Souffle   Soft, blowing sound or murmur heard by auscultation.

   Funic s.   Soft, muffled, blowing sound produced by blood rushing through the umbilical vessels and synchronous with the fetal heart sounds.

   Placental s.   Soft, blowing murmur caused by the blood current in the placenta and synchronous with the maternal pulse.

   Uterine s.   Soft, blowing sound made by the blood in the arteries of the pregnant uterus and synchronous with the maternal pulse.

Sperm   Male sex cell. Also called spermatozoon.

Spermatogenesis   Process by which mature spermatozoa are formed, during which the diploid chromosome number (46) is reduced by half (haploid, 23).

⊙ **Spermicide**   Chemical substance (usually nonoxynol-9) that kills sperm by reducing their surface tension, causing the cell wall to break down by a bactericidal effect or by creating a highly acidic environment.

! **Spina bifida occulta**   Congenital malformation of the spine in which the posterior portion of laminas of the vertebrae fails to close but there is no herniation or protrusion of the spinal cord or meninges through the defect. The newborn may have a dimple in the skin or growth of hair over the malformed vertebrae.

⊙ **Spinal block anesthesia**   See *saddle block anesthesia.*

Spinnbarkheit   Formation of a stretchable thread of cervical mucus under estrogen influence at time of ovulation.

Splanchnic engorgement   Excessive filling or pooling of blood within the visceral vasculature that occurs following the removal of pressure from the abdomen, e.g., birth of a child, removal of an excess of urine from bladder ($\geq$1000 mL), removal of large tumor.

⊞ **Square window**   Angle of wrist between hypothenar prominence and forearm; one criterion for estimating gestational age of neonate.

Standard body weight   An appropriate weight for height, a body mass index (BMI) within the normal range.

Standards of care   Actions that a reasonably prudent person would have performed or omitted under specific conditions; conduct against which the defendant's actions are judged in a malpractice/negligence case.

State-related behavior   Behavioral responses dependent on current state of infant.

Station   Relationship of the presenting fetal part to an imaginary line drawn between the ischial spines of the pelvis.

Sterility   (1) State of being free from living microorganisms. (2) Complete inability to reproduce offspring.

Sterilization   Process or act that renders a person unable to produce children, e.g., fallopian tube occlusion or ligation; vasectomy or occlusion of vas deferens.

Stillbirth   The birth of a baby after 20 wk gestation and 1 day and/or 350 g (depending on the state code) who does not show any signs of life.

Stork bites   See *telangiectatic nevi.*

Striae gravidarum ("stretch marks")   Shining reddish lines caused by stretching of the skin, often found on the abdomen, thighs, and breasts during pregnancy. These streaks turn to a fine pinkish white or silver tone in time in fair-skinned women and brownish in darker-skinned women.

! **Subinvolution**   Failure of a part (e.g., the uterus) to reduce to its nonpregnant size and condition after enlargement from functional activity (i.e., pregnancy).

Suboccipitobregmatic diameter   Smallest diameter of the fetal head—follows a line drawn from the middle of the anterior fontanel to the under surface of the occipital bone.

Succedaneum   See *caput succedaneum.*

! **Supine hypotension**   Shock; fall in blood pressure caused by impaired venous return when gravid uterus presses on ascending vena cava, when woman is lying flat on her back; vena caval syndrome.

Support systems   Network from which people receive help in times of crisis.

Surfactant   Phosphoprotein necessary for normal respiratory function that prevents the alveolar collapse (*atelectasis*). See also *lecithin* and *lecithin-sphingomyelin ratio.*

Suture   (1) Junction of the adjoining bones of the skull. (2) Operation uniting parts by sewing them together.

Symphysis pubis   Fibrocartilaginous union of the bodies of the pubic bones in the midline.

Syndactyly   Malformation of digits, commonly seen as a fusion of two or more toes to form one structure.

Synostosis   Articulation by osseous tissue of adjacent bones; union of separate bones by osseous tissue.

Systemic analgesia Analgesics, either intramuscular (IM) or intravenous (IV), that cross the blood-brain barrier and provide central analgesic effects.

Systemic lupus erythematosus A connective tissue disease affecting the mucous membranes, skin, kidneys, and nervous system. It is inflammatory and chronic in nature.

Taboo Proscribed (forbidden) by society as improper and unacceptable.

Tachypnea Excessively rapid respiratory rate (e.g., in neonates, respiratory rate of 60 breaths/min or more).

Talipes equinovarus Deformity in which the foot is extended and the person walks on the toes.

Telangiectasia Permanent dilatation of groups of superficial capillaries and venules.

Telangiectatic nevi ("stork bites") Clusters of small, red, localized areas of capillary dilatation commonly seen in neonates at the nape of the neck or lower occiput, upper eyelids, and nasal bridge that can be blanched with pressure of a finger.

Teratogenic agent Any drug, virus, or irradiation, the exposure to which can cause malformation of the fetus.

Teratogens Nongenetic factors that cause embryonic/fetal malformations and disease syndromes in utero; examples: rubella, thalidomide, X-ray.

Teratoma Tumor composed of different kinds of tissue, none of which normally occur together or at the site of the tumor.

Term infant Infant born between weeks 38 and 42 of completed gestation.

Testis One of the two glands contained in the male scrotum that produce the male reproductive cell, or sperm, and the male hormone testosterone; testicle.

! Tetany, uterine Extremely prolonged uterine contractions.

Tetralogy of Fallot Congenital cardiac malformation consisting of pulmonary stenosis, intraventricular septal defect, dextroposed aorta that receives blood from both ventricles, and hypertrophy of the right ventricle.

Thalassemia anemia Affecting Mediterranean and Southeast Asian populations in which there is an insufficient amount of globin produced to fill the red blood cells.

Therapeutic intrauterine insemination See *artificial insemination.*

Therapeutic rest Administration of analgesics to decrease pain and induce rest for management of hypertonic uterine dysfunction.

Thermoneutral environment Environment that enables the neonate to maintain a body temperature of 36.5°C (97.7°F) with minimum use of oxygen and energy.

! Thrombocytopenia Abnormal hematologic condition in which the number of platelets is reduced, usually by destruction of erythroid tissue in bone marrow owing to certain neoplastic diseases or to an immune response to a drug.

Thrombocytopenic purpura Hematologic disorder characterized by prolonged bleeding time, decreased number of platelets, increased cell fragility, and purpura, which result in hemorrhages into the skin, mucous membranes, organs, and other tissue.

Thromboembolism Obstruction of a blood vessel by a clot that has become detached from its site of formation.

Thrombophlebitis Inflammation of a vein with secondary clot formation.

Thrombus Blood clot obstructing a blood vessel that remains at the place it was formed.

Thrush Fungal infection of the mouth or throat characterized by the formation of white patches on a red, moist, inflamed mucous membrane and caused by *Candida albicans.*

Toco- (toko-) Combining form that means childbirth or labor.

Tocolytic drug Drug used to suppress preterm labor, e.g., ritodrine (Yutopar), terbutaline (Brethine), magnesium sulfate.

Tocotransducer Electronic device for measuring uterine contractions.

Tongue-tie Congenital shortening of the frenulum, which, if severe, may interfere with sucking and articulation; a rare condition.

TORCH organisms Organisms that damage the embryo or fetus; acronym for *t*oxoplasmosis, *o*ther (e.g., syphilis), *r*ubella, *c*ytomegalovirus, and *h*erpes simplex.

Torticollis Congenital or acquired stiff neck caused by shortening or spasmodic contraction of the neck (sternocleidomastoid) muscles that draws the head to one side with the chin pointing in the other direction; wryneck.

Toxemia Term previously used for hypertensive states of pregnancy.

Tracheoesophageal fistula Congenital malformation in which there is an abnormal tubelike passage between the trachea and esophagus.

Trait A distinguishing feature or characteristic.

Transition—labor Last phase of first stage of labor; 8–10 cm cervical dilatation.

Transition period—newborn Period from birth to 4–6 hr later; infant passes through period of reactivity, sleep, and second period of reactivity.

Translocation Condition in which a chromosome breaks and all or part of that chromosome is transferred to a different part of the same chromosome or to another chromosome.

Trauma Physical or psychic injury.

Trial of labor (TOL) Period of observation to determine if a laboring woman is likely to be successful in progressing to a vaginal birth.

Trichomonas vaginitis Inflammation of the vagina caused by *Trichomonas vaginalis,* a parasitic protozoan and characterized by persistent burning and itching of the vulvar tissue and a profuse, frothy, white discharge.

Trimester Period of 3 mo.

Trisomy Condition in which any given chromosome exists in triplicate instead of the normal duplicate pattern.

Trophoblast Outer layer of cells of the developing blastodermic vesicle that develops the trophoderm or feeding layer which will establish the nutrient relationships with the uterine endometrium.

! Trophoblastic disease, gestational (GTD) A condition in which trophoblastic cells covering the chorionic villi proliferate and undergo cystic changes that may be malignant. See *hydatidiform mole.*

TSS Toxic shock syndrome.

Tubercles of Montgomery Small papillae on surface of nipples and areolae that secrete a fatty substance that lubricates the nipples.

Turner's syndrome Most common sex chromosome abnormality; monosomy X; juvenile external genitalia with undeveloped ovaries; short stature; webbed neck.

Twins Two neonates from the same impregnation developed within the same uterus at the same time.

    Conjoined t. Twins who are physically united; Siamese twins.

    Disparate t. Twins who are different (e.g., in weight) and distinct from one another.

    Fraternal twins Nonidentical twins who come from two separate fertilized ova. Dizygotic.

    Identical twins Come from one fertilized ovum that then divides; same sex; same genotype. Monozygotic.

    Dizygotic t. Twins developed from two separate ova fertilized by two separate sperm at the same time; fraternal twins.

    Monozygotic twins Twins developed from a single fertilized ovum; identical twins.

Ultrasonography High-frequency sound waves to discern fetal heart rate or placental location or body parts.

Ultrasound transducer External signal source for monitoring fetal heart rate electronically.

Umbilical cord (funis) Structure connecting the placenta and fetus and containing two arteries and one vein encased in a tissue called *Wharton's jelly*. The cord is ligated at birth and severed; the stump falls off in 4–10 days.

Umbilicus Navel, or depressed point in the middle of the abdomen that marks the attachment of the umbilical cord during fetal life.

Universal precautions Universal blood and body-fluid precautions, recommended by the Centers for Disease Control (CDC); infection control measures to protect care providers and to prevent nosocomial infection of patients.

Urachus Epithelial tube connecting the apex of the urinary bladder with the allantois. Its connective tissue forms the median umbilical ligament.

    ! **U. persistent** Urachus does not close; urine can be seen oozing from the umbilical cord.

Urethra Small tubular structure that drains urine from the bladder.

Urinary frequency Need to void often or at close intervals.

Urinary meatus Opening, or mouth, of the urethra.

Uterine Referring or pertaining to the uterus.

    U. adnexa See *adnexa, uterine.*

    U. bruit Abnormal sound or murmur heard while auscultating the uterus.

    ! **U. ischemia** Decreased blood supply to the uterus.

    ! **U. prolapse** Falling, sinking, or sliding of the uterus from its normal location in the body.

    U. souffle See *souffle, uterine.*

Uteroplacental insufficiency Decline in placental function—exchange of gases, nutrients, and wastes—leading to fetal hypoxia and acidosis; evidenced by late fetal heart rate decelerations in response to uterine contractions.

Uterus Hollow muscular organ in the female designed for the implantation, containment, and nourishment of the fetus during its development until birth.

    Couvelaire u. Interstitial myometrial hemorrhage following premature separation (abruptio) of placenta. A purplish-bluish discoloration of the uterus and boardlike rigidity of the uterus are noted.

Vaccination Intentional injection of antigenic material given to stimulate antibody production in the recipient.

Vacuum curettage Uterine aspiration method of early abortion.

Vacuum extraction Birth involving attachment of vacuum cup to fetal head and using negative pressure to assist in birth of the fetus.

Vagina Normally collapsed musculomembranous tube that forms the passageway between the uterus and the entrance to the vagina.

Vaginal birth after cesarean (VBAC) Giving birth vaginally after having had a previous cesarean birth.

Valsalva maneuver The process of making a forceful attempt at expulsion while holding one's breath and tightening the abdominal muscles (as in pushing during the second stage of labor).

Variability Normal irregularity of fetal cardiac rhythm; short term—beat-to-beat changes; long term—rhythmic changes (waves) from the baseline, usually 3–5 beats/min.

Varices (varicose veins) Swollen, distended, and twisted veins that may develop in almost any part of the body but are most commonly seen in the legs, caused by pregnancy, obesity, congenitally defective venous valves, and occupations that require much standing.

Varicocele Enlargement of veins of the spermatic cord.

Varicosity See *Varices (varicose veins).*

Vascular spiders See *telangiectasia.*

Vasectomy Ligation or removal of a segment of the vas deferens, usually done bilaterally to produce sterility in the male.

VBAC Vaginal birth after cesarean.

VDRL test Abbreviation for Venereal Disease Research Laboratory test, a serologic flocculation test for syphilis.

Velocimetry See *Doppler blood flow analysis.*

Vernix caseosa Protective gray-white fatty substance of cheesy consistency covering the fetal skin.

Version Act of turning the fetus in the uterus to change the presenting part and facilitate birth.

    Podalic v. Shifting of the fetus' position so as to bring the feet to the outlet during birth.

Vertex Crown or top of the head.

    V. presentation Presentation in which the fetal skull is nearest the cervical opening and born first.

Very low birth weight (VLBW) Infant weighing 1500 g or less at birth.

Viable Capable of living, such as a fetus that has reached a stage of development, usually 22 menstrual (20 wk gestation), which will permit it to live outside the uterus.

Villi Short, vascular processes or protrusions growing on certain membranous surfaces.

    Chorionic v. Tiny vascular protrusions on the chorionic surface that project into the maternal blood sinuses of the uterus and that help to form the placenta and secrete hCG.

Visceral pain Discomfort from cervical changes and uterine ischemia located over the lower portion of the abdomen; radiates to the lumbar area of the back and down the thighs.

Voluntary abortion See *abortion, elective.*

Vulva External genitalia of the female that consist of the labia majora, labia minora, clitoris, urinary meatus, and vaginal introitus.

Vulvar self-examination (VSE)   Systematic examination of the vulva by the woman herself.

Weaning   Process of changing from breastfeeding or bottle feeding to drinking from a cup.

Wharton's jelly   White, gelatinous material surrounding the umbilical vessels within the cord.

Witch's milk   Secretion of a whitish fluid for about a week after birth from enlarged mammary tissue in the neonate, presumably resulting from maternal hormonal influences.

Womb   See *uterus*.

X chromosomes   Sex chromosome in humans existing in duplicate in the normal female and singly in the normal male.

X linkage   Genes located on the X chromosome.

X-linked inheritance   Characteristics transmitted by genes on the X chromosome.

Y chromosome   Sex chromosome in the human male necessary for the development of the male gonads.

Zona pellucida   A thin layer of proteins and polysaccharides that surrounds the oocyte and provides protection during transport in the female genital tract.

Zona reaction   After one sperm has entered an egg, other sperm cannot; this process causes destruction of sperm receptors and hardening of the zona pellucida.

Zygote   Cell formed by the union of two reproductive cells or gametes; the fertilized ovum resulting from the union of a sperm and an ovum.

Common Acronyms and Abbreviations

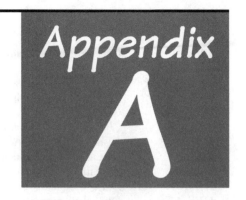

This list provides a review of over 350 *need-to-know* acronyms and abbreviations used in charting, verbal communication, directives, and study guides.

a	Before (*ante*)
Ab	Antibody/Abortion
ABC	Alternative birthing center
Abd	Abdomen/Abdominal
ABG	Arterial blood gas
ABO	Blood typing system
ac	Before meals (*ante cibum*)
ACHES	Acronym for possible warning signs secondary to use of oral hormone contraceptives (see text)
ADH	Antidiuretic hormone
ad lib	As much as desired (*ad libitum*)
ADLs	Activities of daily living
AFB	Acid-fast bacillus
Afib	Atrial fibrillation
Aflutter	Atrial flutter
AFP	Alpha-fetoprotein
AG	Antigen
AGA	Average (weight) for gestational age
AIDS	Acquired immunodeficiency syndrome
A-K (or AKA)	Above-the-knee (amputation)
ALL	Acute lymphocytic (lymphoblastic) leukemia
ALT	Alanine aminotransferase (formerly SGPT)
AMA	Against medical advice
A&O × 3	Alert, oriented to person, place, time
AP	Anteroposterior/Alkaline phosphatase
ARC	AIDS-related complex
ARDS	Adult respiratory distress syndrome
ARF	Acute renal failure
aPPT	Activated partial thromboplastin time
ASA	Acetylsalicylic acid (aspirin)
ASAP	As soon as possible
ASD	Atrial septal defect
AST	Aspartate aminotransferase (formerly SGOT)
AV	Atrioventricular/Arteriovenous/Aortic valve
AVB	Atrioventricular block
AVM	Arteriovenous malformation

BBT	Basal body temperature
bid	Twice daily (*bis in die*)
BKA	Below-the-knee (amputation)
BM	Bowel movement/Bone marrow
BMI	Body mass index
BMR	Basal metabolic rate
BOA	Born out of asepsis
BP	Blood pressure
BPH	Benign prostatic hyperplasia
BPD	Biparietal diameter/Bronchopulmonary dysplasia
BPM	Beats per minute
BPP	Biophysical profile
BSE	Breast self-examination
BUN	Blood urea nitrogen
Bx	Biopsy
c̄	With (*cum*)
CA	Carcinoma/Cancer
CABG	Coronary artery bypass graft operation (× 1,2,3,4 = number of grafts)
CAD	Coronary artery disease
CBC	Complete blood count
CC	Chief complaint
CCU	Cardiac (intensive) care unit
CDC	Centers for Disease Control
CF	Cystic fibrosis
CHD	Congenital heart disease
CIN	Cervical intraepithelial neoplasm
CK	Creatine kinase
CMV	Cytomegalovirus
CNS	Central nervous system/Coagulase-negative staphylococcus
C/O	Complains of
CO_2	Carbon dioxide
COPD	Chronic obstructive pulmonary disease
CPAP	Continuous positive airway pressure
CPD	Cephalopelvic disproportion
CPK	Creatine phosphokinase (now creatine kinase [CK])
CPR	Cardiopulmonary resuscitation
CRF	Chronic renal failure/Cardiac risk factors
CRP	C-reactive protein
CSF	Cerebrospinal fluid
CSM	Circulation motion checks
CST	Contraction stress test
CT	Computed tomography

Adapted from P. Fine. *The Wards: An Introduction to Clinical Clerkships.* Boston: Little, Brown, 1994.

CVA	Cerebrovascular accident/Costovertebral angle	**GI**	Gastrointestinal
CVP	Central venous pressure	**GIFT**	Gamete intrafallopian transfer
CVS	Chorionic villi sampling	**GT**	Gastric tube
Cx	Cervix	**GTD**	Gestational trophoblastic disease
D	Change (Greek letter delta)	**GTT**	Glucose tolerance test
D/C	Discharge/Discontinue	**gtt(s)**	Drop(s) (*guttae*)
D&C	Dilatation and curettage	**GU**	Genitourinary
D&E	Dilatation and evacuation	**GYN**	Gynecologic
DBM	Diabetes mellitus	**Hb, Ag**	Hepatitis B antigen
DES	Diethylstilbestrol	**HBV**	Hepatitis B virus
DFMC	Daily fetal movement counts	**hCG**	Human chorionic gonadotropin
DI	Diabetes insipidus	**Hct**	Hematocrit
DIC	Disseminated intravascular coagulation	**HDL**	High-density lipoprotein
Dig	Digitalis	**HEENT**	Head, eyes, ears, nose, and throat
DM	Diabetes mellitus (also called DBM)	**HELLP**	Hemolysis, elevated liver enzymes, low platelets
DNA	Deoxyribonucleic acid	**HF**	Heart failure
DNR	Do not resuscitate	**Hgb**	Hemoglobin
DOA	Dead on arrival	**Hgb$_{Alc}$**	Glycosylated hemoglobin
DOB	Date of birth	**HIV**	Human immunodeficiency virus
DOE	Dyspnea on exertion	**HMO**	Health maintenance organization
DPT	Diphtheria, pertussis, and tetanus	**HOB**	Head of bed
DRG	Diagnosis-related group	**HR**	Heart rate
DTs	Delirium tremens	**HRT**	Hormone replacement therapy
DTR	Deep tendon reflex	**hs**	Bedtime (*hora somni*)
DVT	Deep-venous thrombosis	**HSV**	Herpes simplex virus
D$_5$W	5% dextrose in water	**HTN**	Hypertension
Dx	Diagnosis	**Hx**	History
ECG	Electrocardiogram (purist's version)	**ICN**	Intensive care nursery
Echo	Echocardiogram	**ICP**	Intracranial pressure
ECT	Electroconvulsive therapy	**ICU**	Intensive care unit
EDB	Estimated date of birth	**I&D**	Incision and drainage
EDC	Estimated date of "confinement" (old term)	**IDDM**	Insulin-dependent diabetes mellitus
EEG	Electroencephalogram	**IDM**	Infant of a diabetic mother
EKG	Electrocardiogram (common version)	**Ig**	Immunoglobulin
ELISA	Enzyme-linked immunosorbent assay	**IM**	Intramuscular
EMG	Electromyogram	**INH**	Isoniazid
EMT	Emergency medical technician	**I&O**	Intake and output
ENT	Ear, nose, and throat	**IPPB**	Intermittent positive-pressure breathing
ER	Emergency room	**ITP**	Idiopathic thrombocytopenic purpura
ERT	Estrogen replacement therapy	**IUD**	Intrauterine device
ESR	Erythrocyte sedimentation rate	**IUGR**	Intrauterine growth retardation
ETOH	Alcohol (ethanol)	**IV**	Intravenous
FAD	Fetal activity determination	**IVC**	Inferior vena cava
FAS	Fetal alcohol syndrome	**IVF**	In vitro fertilization
FBS	Fasting blood sugar	**IVP**	Intravenous pyelogram/Intravenous push
FEV$_1$	Forced expiratory volume in 1 sec	**IZ**	Immunization
FHR	Fetal heart rate	**JRA**	Juvenile rheumatoid arthritis
FRC	Functional residual capacity	**JVD**	Jugular venous distention
FSH	Follicle stimulating hormone	**KUB**	Kidneys, ureters, and bladder (flat/upright abdominal X-ray)
FTT	Failure to thrive		
FUO	Fever of unknown origin	**KVO**	Keep vein open
FVC	Forced vital capacity	**LDR**	Labor-delivery-recovery room
Fx	Fracture	**LDRP**	Labor-delivery-recovery-postpartum room
g	Gram		
G	Gravida	**LGA**	Large for gestational age
GB	Gallbladder	**LH**	Luteinizing hormone
GC	Gonococcus/Gonorrhea	**LLL**	Left lower (lung) lobe
GFR	Glomerular filtration rate	**LLQ**	Left lower quadrant
G-6-P-D	Glucose-6-phosphate dehydrogenase		

LMP	Last menstrual period
LNMP	Last normal menstrual period
LOC	Loss of consciousness/Level of consciousness
LPN	Licensed practical nurse
L/S	Lecithin-sphingomyelin ratio
LUL	Left upper (lung) lobe
LUQ	Left upper quadrant
LVN	Licensed vocational nurse
MAP	Mean arterial pressure
MCL	Midclavicular line
Med	Medication
MI	Myocardial infarction
MMR	Measles, mumps, and rubella
MODS	Multiple organ dysfunction syndrome
MOM	Milk of magnesia
Mono	Mononucleosis
MR	Mitral regurgitation/Mental retardation
MRI	Magnetic resonance imaging
MRSA	Methicillin- resistant *Staphylococcus aureus*
MS	Mental status/Mitral stenosis/Multiple sclerosis/Morphine sulfate
MVP	Mitral valve prolapse
MVR	Mitral valve replacement
NA	Not applicable
NEC	Necrotizing enterocolitis
NG	Nasogastric
NIDDM	Non–insulin-dependent diabetes mellitus
NL	Normal
NOC	Night (nocturnal)
NPH	Neutral-protamine-Hagedorn (intermediate-acting insulin)
NPO	Nothing by mouth (*nil per os*)
NS	Normal saline
NSAID	Nonsteroidal anti-inflammatory drug
NSR	Normal sinus rhythm
NST	Nonstress test
NTG	Nitroglycerin
N/V	Nausea, vomiting
NVD	Nausea, vomiting, and diarrhea
O_2	Oxygen
OB	Obstetrics
OCT	Oxytocin stress test (oxytocin challenge test)
OD	Right eye (*oculus dexter*)/Overdose
OOB	Out of bed/Out of breath
O&P	Ova and parasites
OR	Operating room
OS	Left eye (*oculus sinister*)/Opening snap
OT	Occupational therapy
OU	Both eyes (*oculo utro*)
P	Para/Pulse
p̄	Post (after)
PA	Posteronterior/Physician's assistant/Pulmonary artery
PAINS	Acronym for possible warning signs of problems related to use of the intrauterine device (see text)
PAO_2	Alveolar oxygen pressure
PaO_2	Arterial partial pressure of oxygen
Pap	Papanicolaou test
PAS	Para-aminosalicylic acid
PAT	Paroxysmal atrial tachycardia
pc	After meals (*post cibum*)
PCA	Patient-controlled analgesia (pump)
PCP	*Pneumocystis carinii* pneumonia/Phencyclidine
PDA	Patent ductus arteriosus
PEEP	Positive end-expiratory pressure
PERRL(A)	Pupils equally round and reactive to light (and accommodation)
PG	Prostaglandin
pH	Hydrogen ion concentration
PID	Pelvic inflammatory disease
PIH	Pregnancy-induced hypertension
PKU	Phenylketonuria
PMI	Point of maximum impulse
PMS	Premenstrual syndrome
PND	Paroxysmal nocturnal dyspnea
PO	By mouth (*per os*)
PPD	Purified protein derivative (tuberculosis skin test)
PPO	Preferred provider organization
prn	When necessary (*pro re nata*)
PROM	Premature (prolonged) rupture of membranes
PSA	Prostate-specific antigen
Pt	Patient
PT	Prothrombin time/Physical therapy
PTA	Prior to admission
PTCA	Percutaneous transluminal coronary angioplasty
PTT	Partial thromboplastin time
PUBS	Percutaneous umbilical blood sampling
PUD	Peptic ulcer disease
PVC	Premature ventricular contraction
q	Each, every (*quaque*)
qd	Each day (*quaque die*)
qhs	Every night before sleep (*quaque hora somni*)
qid	Four times a day (*quarter in die*)
qod	Every other day
R	Respirations
RA	Rheumatoid arthritis/Right atrium
RBC	Red blood cell
RDS	Respiratory distress syndrome
REEDA	Acronym for warning signs of problems related to episiotomy (see text)
RHD	Rheumatic heart disease
RLL	Right lower (lung) lobe
RLQ	Right lower quadrant
RML	Right middle (lung) lobe
RNA	Ribonucleic acid
R/O	Rule out
ROM	Range of motion/Rupture of membranes
ROP	Retinopathy of prematurity
ROS	Review of systems
RUL	Right upper (lung) lobe
RUQ	Right upper quadrant

Rx	Prescription/Therapy/Treatment		tid	Three times a day (*ter in die*)
s̄	Without (*sine*)		TKO	To keep open
S_1	First heart sound		TLC	Total lung capacity/Tender loving care
S_2	Second heart sound		Toco-(Toko-)	Combining form meaning childbirth or labor
S_3	Third heart sound			
S_4	Fourth heart sound		TOL	Trial of labor
SBE	Subacute bacterial endocarditis		TPN	Total parenteral nutrition
SC	Subcutaneously		TPR	Temperature, pulse, and respirations
SGA	Small for gestational age		TSH	Thyroid-stimulating hormone
SIADH	Syndrome of inappropriate antidiuretic hormone		TSS	Toxic shock syndrome
			TURP	Transurethral resection of prostate
SICU	Surgical intensive care unit		TV	Total volume/Tidal volume
SIDS	Sudden infant death syndrome		TVH	Transvaginal hysterectomy
SIRS	Sudden inflammatory response syndrome		Tx	Treatment
			UA	Urinalysis
SL	Sublingually		UGI	Upper gastrointestinal
SLE	Systemic lupus erythematosus		UOQ	Upper outer quadrant
SOB	Short(ness) of breath		UQ	Upper quadrant
SQ	Subcutaneously		URI	Upper respiratory infection
SR	Sinus rhythm		UTI	Urinary tract infection
S/S	Signs, symptoms		UV	Ultraviolet
Stat	Immediately (*statim*)		VBAC	Vaginal birth after cesarean
STD	Sexually transmitted disease		VC	Vital capacity
SVD	Spontaneous vaginal delivery		VDRL	Venereal Disease Research Laboratory test
SVT	Supraventricular tachycardia			
Sx	Symptoms		Vfib (VF)	Ventricular fibrillation
T	Temperature		VLBW	Very low birth weight
T&A	Tonsillectomy and adenoidectomy		VS	Vital signs
TAH-BSO	Transabdominal hysterectomy and bilateral salpingo-oophorectomy		VSD	Ventricular septal defect
			VTx	Vertex
TB	Tuberculosis		WBC	White blood count/White blood cells
TIA	Transient ischemic attack		WNL	Within normal limits
			w/o	Without

Quick Guide to Common Clinical Signs

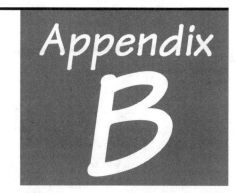

Appendix B

Many clinical signs have been named for the physicians who first described them, or the phenomena they resemble. Following is a list of 28 of the most common clinical signs, for use as a quick reference as you review.

Babinski reflex Dorsiflexion of the big toe after stimulation of the lateral sole; normal response in newborn, but associated with *corticospinal tract lesions in the adult*

Blumberg's sign Transient pain in the abdomen after approximated fingers pressed gently into abdominal wall are suddenly withdrawn—rebound tenderness; associated with *peritoneal inflammation*

Braxton Hicks sign Mild, intermittent, painless uterine contractions that occur more frequently as pregnancy advances, but do *not* represent *true* labor

Brudzinski's sign Flexion of the hip and knee induced by flexion of the neck; associated with *meningeal irritation*

Chadwick's sign Cyanosis of vaginal and cervical mucosa; associated with *pregnancy*

Cheyne-Stokes respiration Rhythmic cycles of deep and shallow respiration, often with apneic periods; associated with *central nervous system respiratory center dysfunction*

Chvostek's sign Facial muscle spasm induced by tapping on the facial nerve branches; associated with *hypocalcemia*

Coppernail's sign Ecchymoses on the perineum, scrotum, or labia; associated with *fracture* of the *pelvis*

Cullen's sign Bluish discoloration of the umbilicus; associated with acute *pancreatitis* or *hemoperitoneum*, especially *rupture of fallopian tube* in ectopic pregnancy

Doll's eye sign Dissociation between the movements of the head and eyes: as the head is raised the eyes are lowered, and as the head is lowered the eyes are raised; associated with global-diffuse disorders of the *cerebrum*

Fluid wave Transmission across the abdomen of a wave induced by snapping the abdomen, associated with *ascites*

Goldstein's sign Wide distance between the great toe and the adjoining toe; associated with *cretinism* and *trisomy 21*

Goodell's sign Softening of the cervix, a *probable* sign of pregnancy, occurring during the second month

Harlequin sign In the newborn infant, reddening of the lower half of the laterally recumbent body and blanching of the upper half, due to a *temporary vasomotor disturbance*

Hegar's sign Softening of the isthmus of the uterus; associated with the *first trimester of pregnancy*

Homans' sign Pain behind the knee, induced by dorsiflexion of the foot; associated with peripheral vascular disease, especially *venous thrombosis* in the calf

Kehr's sign Severe pain in the left upper quadrant, radiating to the top of the shoulder; associated with *splenic rupture*

Kernig's sign Inability to extend leg when sitting or lying with the thigh flexed on the abdomen; associated with *meningeal irritation*

Knie's sign Unequal dilatation of the pupils; associated with *Graves'* disease

Kussmaul's respiration Paroxysmal air hunger; associated with acidosis, especially *diabetic ketoacidosis*

McBurney's sign Tenderness at McBurney's point (located two-thirds of the distance from the umbilicus to the anterosuperior iliac spine); associated with *appendicitis*

Ortolani's (click) sign "Click" sound sometimes heard if hip *dysplasia* is present; on assessment, head of femur can be felt (or heard as a click) to slip forward in acetabulum and slip back when pressure is released and legs are returned to their original position

Osler's sign Small painful erythematous swellings in the skin of the hands and feet; associated with *bacterial endocarditis*

Psoas sign Pain induced by hyperextension of the right thigh while lying on the left side; associated with *appendicitis*

Setting-sun sign Downward deviation of the eyes so that each iris appears to "set" beneath the lower lid, with white sclera exposed between it and the upper lid; associated with *increased intracranial pressure* or irritation of the *brain stem*

Tinel's sign Tingling sensation felt from light percussion on the radial side of the palmaris longus tendon; associated with *carpal tunnel syndrome*

Trousseau's sign Carpopedal spasm that develops when BP cuff is inflated above systolic pressure for 3 minutes; associated with *hypocalcemia*

Williamson's sign Markedly diminished blood pressure in the leg as compared with that in the arm on the same side; associated with *pneumothorax* and *pleural effusions*

Adapted from RM Macklis, et al. *Introduction to Clinical Medicine* (3rd ed). Boston: Little, Brown, 1994.

Common Diagnostic Tests and Procedures

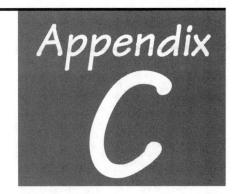

For a quick review, use this index to locate over 60 diagnostic tests and procedures covered in this book as they relate to specific conditions.

Electronic fetal monitoring (EFM), 55, 62, 91, 112, 122–124, 128
  Contraction stress test (CST): oxytocin stress test (OST)/ oxytocin challenge test (OCT); 55, 80, 187
  Nonstress test (NST) or fetal activity determination (FAD), 55, 70, 75, 80, 110, 122, 187

Hemodynamic status tests: symptoms of shock
  Central venous pressure (CVP), 68
  Pulmonary arterial wedge pressure (PAWP) with Swan-Ganz catheter, 68, 154
  Pulmonary flow test, 65
  Pulse oximetry, 217

Laboratory tests (selected)
  Alpha-fetoprotein (AFP or α-FP): amnionic fluid or maternal serum, 37, 81
  Antibody titers, 14, 188
    Anti-Rh, 37, 71, 99, 108
    Coombs (direct, with fetal cord blood; indirect, with maternal blood), 53, 71, 77, 108, 143, 173, 188
    Rubella, 35
  Blood values—comparison between prepregnant, pregnant, and postpartum, 30, 73
  CBC, 173
    Creatinine clearance, 32
    Hgb, Hct, 152
    Platelets, 165
  Enzyme-linked immunosorbent assay (ELISA) tests, 58, 62
  Fasting blood sugar (FBS), 54
  Fibrinogen levels, 152–154
  Glucose tolerance test (GTT), 54, 55
  Glycosylated hemoglobin, 54
  Huhner test, 12
  Inborn errors of metabolism (amnionic fluid or newborn blood), 66, 80, 170, 173
  Papanicolaou (Pap) smear, 8, 35, 58, 60, 63
  Pregnancy tests, 14, 35, 73
  Semen analysis, 14
  Sexually transmitted disease (STD) tests, 8, 35–37, 59–63, 99
  Tuberculin tests, 37

Magnetic resonance imaging (MRI), 212

Radiography (roentgenography)
  Amniography, 72
  Hysterosalpingography, 12
  Mammography/mammogram, 6, 8
  Rubin test, 12
  X-ray pelvimetry, 55, 126, 127
  X-ray (other), 67, 72, 186–188

Surgical tests
  Amniocentesis: chromosome analysis of cultured amniotic fluid cells (e.g., for Down syndrome); biochemical (e.g., for *AFP, fetal hemolytic* disease, *fetal lung maturity* [lecithin-sphingomyelin ratio, phosphatidylglycerol]), 53, 55, 64, 79–81, 104, 110, 114, 128, 188, 190
  Biopsy, 6
  Chorionic villous sampling (CVS), 81
  Dilatation and curettage (D&C), 17, 71
  Fetal blood sampling, 114, 122, 129
  Laparoscopy, 12
  Needle aspiration/needle localization, 6
  Percutaneous umbilical blood sampling (PUBS), or cordocentesis, 215

Ultrasound (abdominal, transvaginal sonography), 6, 36, 37, 55, 72, 78–80, 122, 126, 127, 187

Urinalysis
  Culture and sensitivity, 156, 157, 180, 183, 189
  Ketones, 126
  Protein, sugar, 99, 137, 140

Miscellaneous tests
  APGAR, 107, 143, 173
  Biophysical profile, 80, 114
  Body mass index (BMI), 199
  Cardiac catheterization, 187, 188
  Echocardiogram (ECG or EKG), 188
  Mean arterial pressure, 212
  Measurement of fundal height, 28, 37
  Roll-over test, 218
  Tests for rupture of membranes (ROM): pH, color, character, amount, 71

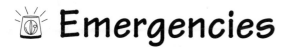 # Emergencies

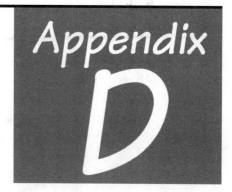 **Appendix D**

For a quick review, use this index to locate content on over 30 maternal–newborn emergencies covered in this book.

● Index to Diets

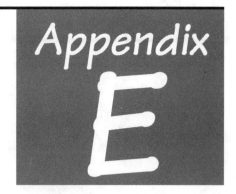

For a quick review, use this index to locate over 30 special dietary considerations covered in this book as they relate to specific conditions situations.

Index to Positioning the Patient

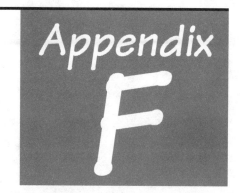

For a quick reference as you study or review, use this index to locate 20 positions of choice (or contraindicated) for various conditions.

Index to Nursing Treatments

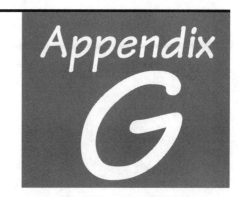

Appendix G

(Essential "Hands-On" Skills, Nursing Procedures)

Use this index as a quick checklist of over 58 skills and procedures mentioned in this book that nurses need to know about or be able to perform in giving patient care.

NANDA-Approved Nursing Diagnoses

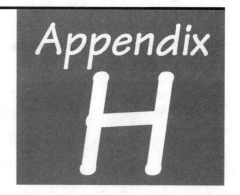

Appendix H

This list represents the North American Nursing Diagnosis Association (NANDA) approved nursing diagnoses for clinical use and testing (1994).

Pattern 1: Exchanging

Altered Nutrition: More than Body Requirements
Altered Nutrition: Less than Body Requirements
Altered Nutrition: Potential for More Than Body Requirements
Risk for Infection
Risk for Altered Body Temperature
Hypothermia
Hyperthermia
Ineffective Thermoregulation
Dysreflexia
Constipation
Perceived Constipation
Colonic Constipation
Diarrhea
Bowel Incontinence
Altered Urinary Elimination
Stress Incontinence
Reflex Incontinence
Urge Incontinence
Functional Incontinence
Total Incontinence
Urinary Retention
Altered (Specify Type) Tissue Perfusion (Renal, cerebral, cardiopulmonary, gastrointestinal, peripheral)
Fluid Volume Excess
Fluid Volume Deficit
Risk for Fluid Volume Deficit
Decreased Cardiac Output
Impaired Gas Exchange
Ineffective Airway Clearance
Ineffective Breathing Pattern
Inability to Sustain Spontaneous Ventilation
Dysfunctional Ventilatory Weaning Response (DVWR)
Risk for Injury
Risk for Suffocation
Risk for Poisoning
Risk for Trauma
Risk for Aspiration

Risk for Disuse Syndrome
Altered Protection
Impaired Tissue Integrity
Altered Oral Mucous Membrane
Impaired Skin Integrity
Risk for Impaired Skin Integrity
Decreased Adaptive Capacity: Intracranial
Energy Field Disturbance

Pattern 2: Communicating

Impaired Verbal Communication

Pattern 3: Relating

Impaired Social Interaction
Social Isolation
Risk for Loneliness
Altered Role Performance
Altered Parenting
Risk for Altered Parenting
Risk for Altered Parent/Infant/Child Attachment
Sexual Dysfunction
Altered Family Processes
Caregiver Role Strain
Risk for Caregiver Role Strain
Altered Family Process: Alcoholism
Parental Role Conflict
Altered Sexuality Patterns

Pattern 4: Valuing

Spiritual Distress (Distress of the Human Spirit)
Potential for Enhanced Spiritual Well-Being

Pattern 5: Choosing

Ineffective Individual Coping
Impaired Adjustment
Defensive Coping
Ineffective Denial
Ineffective Family Coping: Disabling
Ineffective Family Coping: Compromised
Family Coping: Potential for Growth
Potential for Enhanced Community Coping
Ineffective Community Coping

From NANDA. *Nursing Diagnoses: Definitions and Classification, 1995–1996.* Philadelphia: North American Nursing Diagnosis Association, 1994.

Ineffective Management of Therapeutic Regimen
   (Individuals)
Noncompliance (Specify)
Ineffective Management of Therapeutic Regimen: Families
Ineffective Management of Therapeutic Regimen:
   Community
Ineffective Management of Therapeutic Regimen:
   Individual
Decisional Conflict (Specify)
Health-Seeking Behaviors (Specify)

Pattern 6: Moving

Impaired Physical Mobility
Risk for Peripheral Neurovascular Dysfunction
Risk for Perioperative Positioning Injury
Activity Intolerance
Fatigue
Risk for Activity Intolerance
Sleep Pattern Disturbance
Diversional Activity Deficit
Impaired Home Maintenance Management
Altered Health Maintenance
Feeding Self-Care Deficit
Impaired Swallowing
Ineffective Breastfeeding
Interrupted Breastfeeding
Effective Breastfeeding
Ineffective Infant Feeding Pattern
Bathing/Hygiene Self-Care Deficit
Dressing/Grooming Self-Care Deficit
Toileting Self-Care Deficit
Altered Growth and Development
Relocation Stress Syndrome
Risk for Disorganized Infant Behavior
Disorganized Infant Behavior
Potential for Enhanced Organized Infant Behavior

Pattern 7: Perceiving

Body Image Disturbance
Self-Esteem Disturbance
Chronic Low Self-Esteem
Situational Low Self-Esteem
Personal Identity Disturbance
Sensory/Perceptual Alterations (Specify) (Visual, Auditory,
   Kinesthetic, Gustatory, Tactile, Olfactory)
Unilateral Neglect
Hopelessness
Powerlessness

Pattern 8: Knowing

Knowledge Deficit (Specify)
Impaired Environmental Interpretation Syndrome
Acute Confusion
Chronic Confusion
Altered Thought Processes
Impaired Memory

Pattern 9: Feeling

Pain
Chronic Pain
Dysfunctional Grieving
Anticipatory Grieving
Risk for Violence: Self-Directed or Directed at Others
Risk for Self-Mutilation
Post-Trauma Response
Rape-Trauma Syndrome
Rape-Trauma Syndrome: Compound Reaction
Rape-Trauma Syndrome: Silent Reaction
Anxiety
Fear

NCLEX-RN Test Plan: Nursing Process Definitions/Descriptions

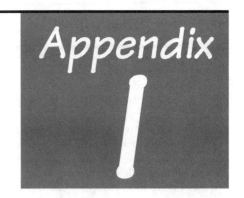

The phases of the nursing process include the following:

I. Assessment: establishing a database
  A. *Gather objective and subjective information relative to the client*
    1. Collect information from the client, significant others, and/or health care team members; current and prior health records; and other pertinent resources
    2. Utilize assessment skills appropriate to client's condition
    3. Recognize *symptoms* and significant findings
    4. Determine client's ability to assume care of daily health needs (self-care)
    5. Determine health team member's ability to provide care
    6. Assess *environment* of client
    7. Identify own or staff reactions to client, significant others, and/or health care team members
  B. *Confirm data*
    1. *Verify* observation or perception by obtaining additional information
    2. *Question* prescriptions and decisions by other health care team members when indicated
    3. *Observe* condition of client directly when indicated
    4. *Validate* that an appropriate client assessment has been made
  C. *Communicate information gained in assessment*
    1. Document assessment findings thoroughly and accurately
    2. Report assessment findings to relevant members of the health care team

II. Analysis: identifying actual or potential health care needs and/or problems based on assessment
  A. *Interpret data*
    1. Validate data
    2. Organize related data
    3. Determine need for additional data
    4. Determine client's unique needs and/or problems
  B. *Formulate client's nursing diagnoses*
    1. Determine significant relationship between data and client needs and/or problems

  2. Utilize *standard taxonomy* for formulating nursing diagnoses
  C. *Communicate results of analysis*
    1. Document client's *nursing diagnoses*
    2. Report results of analysis to relevant members of the health care team

III. Planning: setting goals for meeting client's needs and designing strategies to achieve these goals
  A. *Prioritize nursing diagnoses*
    1. Involve client, significant others, and/or health care team members when establishing nursing diagnoses
    2. Establish *priorities* among nursing diagnoses
    3. Anticipate needs and/or problems on the basis of established priorities
  B. *Determine goals of care*
    1. Involve client, significant others, and/or health care team members in setting goals
    2. Establish *priorities among goals*
    3. Anticipate needs and/or problems on the basis of established priorities
  C. *Formulate outcome criteria for goals of care*
    1. Involve client, significant others, and/or health care team members in formulating outcome criteria for goals of care
    2. Establish *priorities* among outcome *criteria* for goals of care
    3. Anticipate needs and/or problems on the basis of established priorities
  D. *Develop plan of care and modify as necessary*
    1. Involve the client, significant others, and/or health care team members in designing strategies
    2. Individualize the plan of care based on such information as *age, gender, culture, ethnicity, and religion*
    3. Plan for client's safety, comfort, and maintenance of optimal functioning
    4. Select nursing interventions for delivery of client's care
    5. Select *appropriate* teaching approaches
  E. *Collaborate with other health care team members when planning delivery of client's care*
    1. Identify health or social resources available to the client and/or significant others
    2. *Select appropriate health care team members* when planning assignments

Source: National Council of State Boards of Nursing, Inc., *NCLEX-RN Test Plan*, 1994.

3. Coordinate care provided by health care team members
  F. *Communicate plan of care*
     1. Document plan of care thoroughly and accurately
     2. Report plan of care to relevant members of the health care team
     3. Review plan of care with client
IV. **Implementation: initiating and completing actions necessary to accomplish the defined goals**
  A. *Organize and manage client's care*
     1. Implement a plan of care
     2. Arrange for a client care conference
  B. *Counsel and teach client, significant others, and/or health care team members*
     1. Assist client, significant others, and/or health care team members to recognize and manage stress
     2. Facilitate client relationships with significant others and health care team members
     3. *Teach* correct principles, procedures, and techniques for maintenance and promotion of health
     4. Provide client with health status information
     5. Refer client, significant others, and/or health care team members to appropriate *resources*
  C. *Provide care to achieve established goals of care*
     1. Use *safe* and appropriate techniques when administering client care
     2. Use precautionary and *preventive* interventions in providing care to client
     3. *Prepare client for surgery, delivery,* or other *procedures*
     4. Institute interventions to compensate for adverse responses
     5. *Initiate life-saving interventions* for emergency situations
     6. Provide an *environment* conducive to attainment of goals of care
     7. Adjust care in accord with client's expressed or implied needs, problems, and/or preferences
     8. Stimulate and motivate client to achieve *self-care* and independence
     9. Encourage client to follow a treatment regime
     10. Assist client to maintain optimal functioning
  D. *Supervise and coordinate the delivery of client's care provided by nursing personnel*
     1. *Delegate* nursing interventions to appropriate nursing personnel
     2. *Monitor* and follow up on delegated interventions
     3. Manage health care team members' *reactions* to factors influencing therapeutic relationships with clients

  E. *Communicate nursing interventions*
     1. Record actual client responses, nursing interventions, and other information relevant to implementation of care
     2. Provide complete, accurate reports on assigned client(s) to relevant members of the health care team
V. **Evaluation: determining the extent to which goals have been achieved and interventions have been successful**
  A. *Compare actual outcomes with expected outcomes of care*
     1. Evaluate responses (*expected and unexpected*) in order to determine the degree of success of nursing interventions
     2. Determine impact of therapeutic interventions on the client and significant others
     3. Determine need for modifying the plan of care
     4. Identify factors that may interfere with the client's ability to implement the plan of care
  B. *Evaluate the client's ability to implement self-care*
     1. Verify that *tests or measurements are performed correctly* by the client and/or other caregivers
     2. Ascertain client's, and/or others' *understanding* of information given
  C. *Evaluate health care team members' ability to implement client care*
     1. Determine impact of teaching on health care team members
     2. Identify factors that might alter health care team members' response to teaching
  D. *Communicate evaluation findings*
     1. Document client's response to therapy, care, and/or teaching
     2. Report client's response to therapy, care, and/or teaching to relevant members of the health care team
     3. Report and document others' responses to teaching
     4. Document other caregivers' responses to teaching

The practice questions in this book are coded as to the phase of the nursing process being tested; the codes are found following the answer/rationale for each question. *Key to Nursing Process Codes:*

AS	Assessment
AN	Analysis
PL	Planning
IMP	Implementation
EV	Evaluation

For an index to questions relating to each phase of the nursing process, see Appendix J.

◤ Index: Questions Related to Nursing Process

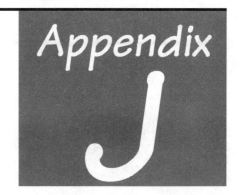

Use this index to locate *practice questions* throughout the book, in each of the five *phases of the nursing process.*

Chapter	Assessment (AS) Question No.	Analysis (AN) Question No.	Planning (PL) Question No.	Implementation (IMP) Question No.	Evaluation (EV) Question No.
1—Growth and Development	14, 19	5, 6, 20, 24, 27	11	1, 3, 4, 7, 8, 9, 12, 13, 15, 16, 18, 23, 25, 26	2, 10, 17, 21, 22
2—Normal Pregnancy	1	6, 9, 16, 21, 27	2, 7, 15, 29	4, 8, 10, 12, 13, 14, 18, 20, 23, 24, 25, 26, 28, 32	3, 5, 11, 17, 19, 22, 30, 31
3—High-Risk Conditions and Complications During Pregnancy	11, 20, 29, 39, 41, 45, 53	1, 10, 14, 27, 43, 44, 49, 52	5, 8, 16, 17, 18, 19, 21, 25, 34, 37, 38	2, 3, 6, 12, 15, 23, 28, 33, 35, 36, 40, 42, 46, 47, 48, 51, 54	4, 7, 9, 13, 22, 24, 26, 30, 31, 32, 50
4—The Intrapartal Experience	21, 24, 26	2, 8, 9, 11, 28	4, 16, 22, 25	1, 3, 5, 12, 14, 15, 17, 18, 20, 23, 27	6, 7, 10, 13, 19, 29, 30, 31
5—Complications During the Intrapartal Period	17	4, 5	16	2, 3, 7, 8, 9, 12, 14, 18, 19	1, 6, 10, 11, 13, 15
6—The Postpartal Period	13, 15, 23	9, 16, 20, 21	4, 6, 18, 19	1, 2, 5, 8, 10, 11, 12, 14, 22, 25, 26	3, 7, 17, 24, 27
7—Complications During the Postpartal Period		6, 8, 13, 14	2, 9	3, 4, 5, 10, 11, 12, 15	1, 7, 16
8—The Newborn Infant	11	5, 14		1, 3, 4, 6, 7, 10, 13, 15, 16, 17, 18	2, 8, 9, 12
9—Complications During the Neonatal Period: The High-Risk Newborn	6, 7, 8, 9, 10, 11, 12, 13, 23, 25	3, 16, 24	2, 4, 5	14, 20, 21, 22	1, 15, 17, 18, 19

Index: Questions Related to Categories of Human Functions

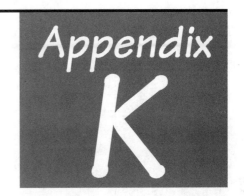

Appendix K

This index lists *practice questions* for you to use in reviewing *categories of human functions* (which are *detailed* examples of what subtopics are covered by the four *broad* client needs categories).

The eight categories of human functions include:

Protective Functions   client's ability to maintain defenses and prevent physical and chemical trauma, injury, and threats to health status (e.g., communicable diseases, abuse, safety hazards, poisoning, skin disorders, and pre- and post-operative complications).

Sensory-Perceptual Functions   client's ability to perceive, interpret, and respond to sensory and cognitive stimuli (e.g., auditory, visual, verbal impairments, brain tumors, aphasia, sensory deprivation or overload, body image, reality orientation, learning disabilities).

Comfort, Rest, Activity, and Mobility Functions   client's ability to maintain mobility, desirable level of activity, adequate sleep, rest, and comfort (e.g., pain, sleep disturbances, joint impairment).

Nutrition   client's ability to maintain the intake and processing of essential nutrients (e.g., obesity, gastric and metabolic disorders that primarily affect the nutritional status).

Growth and Development   client's ability to maintain maturational processes throughout the life span (e.g., child bearing, child rearing, maturational crisis, changes in aging, psychosocial development).

Fluid-Gas Transport Functions   client's ability to maintain fluid-gas transport (e.g., fluid volume deficit/overload, acid-base balance, CPR, anemias, cardiopulmonary diseases).

Psychosocial-Cultural Functions   client's ability to function (intrapersonal/interpersonal relationships; e.g., grieving, death/dying, psychotic behaviors, self concept, therapeutic communication, ethical-legal aspects, community resources, situational crises, substance abuse).

Elimination Functions   client's ability to maintain functions related to relieving the body of waste products (e.g., conditions of GI and/or GU systems).

Chapter	Protective Functions (1) Question No.	Sensory-Perceptual Functions (2) Question No.	Comfort, Rest, Activity, and Mobility Functions (3) Question No.	Nutrition (4) Questions No.	Growth and Development (5) Question No.	Fluid-Gas Transport Functions (6) Question No.	Psychosocial-Cultural Functions (7) Question No.	Eliminations Functions (8) Question No.
1—Growth and Development	3, 4, 16, 17, 18, 19, 21, 25		1, 22	2	5, 6, 7, 8, 9, 10, 12, 13, 14, 15, 23, 24, 26, 27	11, 20		
2—Normal Pregnancy	12	19	13, 22, 23	1, 2, 3, 4, 18, 24, 25, 26, 31, 32	5, 6, 9, 10, 15, 16, 17, 20, 21, 27	7, 8, 11, 29, 30	14, 28	
3—High-Risk Conditions and Complications During Pregnancy	2, 3, 12, 20, 22, 30, 33, 34, 39, 43, 44, 47, 50, 51, 52, 53	9, 25, 27, 28, 49	24, 37,	8, 17, 18	15, 21, 31, 38, 42, 54	4, 5, 6, 7, 10, 11, 13, 14, 16, 19, 23, 26, 32, 35, 36, 40, 41, 44, 45, 46, 48	1	29
4—The Intrapartal Experience	10, 25		6, 8, 9, 14, 20		1, 2, 3, 5, 7, 11, 15, 17, 19, 22, 23, 24, 26, 27, 28, 29, 30, 31	4, 12, 13, 21	16, 18	
5—Complications during the Intrapartal Period	7, 13, 14, 15, 18		3, 12		2, 4, 5, 10	1, 6, 8, 9, 11, 16, 17, 19		
6—The Postpartal Period	4, 5, 14, 16, 24		8, 11	9, 25, 27	2, 3, 10, 12, 13, 26	1, 18, 19, 20, 21, 22, 23,	6, 7	15, 17
7—Complications During the Postpartal Period	1, 2, 7, 12, 13			4, 5		3, 6, 8, 9, 10, 11, 14, 15, 16		
8—The Newborn Infant	7, 8, 10, 15, 16, 17		5, 14		1, 2, 4, 6, 9, 11, 12, 13, 18	3		
9—Complications During the Neonatal Period: The High-Risk Newborn	1, 4, 5, 6, 7, 8, 10, 13, 14, 23, 25	16		21	9, 15	17, 19, 22, 24	20	18

Index: Questions Related to Client Needs

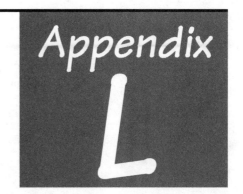

To *practice questions* in each of the four categories of *client needs* that are tested on NCLEX-RN, refer to the questions listed.

The four broad categories of client needs include:

Safe, Effective Care Environment *coordinated care, environmental safety, safe* and *effective treatment* and procedures (e.g., client rights, confidentiality, principles of teaching/learning, control of infectious agents).

Physiologic Integrity *physiologic adaptation, reduction of risk potential, provision of basic care* (e.g., drug administration, emergencies, nutritional therapies).

Psychosocial Integrity *psychosocial adaptation; coping* (e.g., behavioral norms, chemical dependency, communication skills, family systems, mental health concepts, psychodynamics of behavior, psychopathology, treatment modalities).

Health Promotion and Maintenance *normal growth and development* from birth to death, *self-care* and *support systems, prevention* and *early treatment of disease* (e.g., newborn care, normal perinatal care, family planning, human sexuality, parenting, death/dying, life-style choices, immunity).

Chapter	Safe, Effective Care Environment (SECE) Question No.	Physiologic Integrity (PhI) Question No.	Psychosocial Integrity (PsI) Question No.	Health Promotion and Maintenance (HPM) Question No.
1—Growth and Development	1, 3, 16, 25	11, 20	17	2, 4, 5, 6, 7, 8, 9, 10, 12, 13, 14, 15, 18, 19, 21, 22, 23, 24, 26, 27
2—Normal Pregnancy		1, 2, 30	28, 29	3, 4, 5, 6, 7, 8, 9, 10, 11, 12, 13, 14, 15, 16, 17, 18, 19, 20, 21, 22, 23, 24, 25, 26, 27, 31, 32
3—High Risk Conditions and Complications During Pregnancy	2, 3, 8, 12, 15, 20, 22, 23, 27, 33, 34, 39, 44, 50, 53	7, 9, 11, 14, 16, 18, 19, 24, 25, 26, 28, 29, 35, 36, 37, 38, 40, 41, 45, 46, 47, 48, 49	1	4, 5, 6, 10, 13, 17, 21, 30, 31, 32, 42, 43, 51, 52, 54
4—The Intrapartal Experience	25	10, 12, 13, 20, 21, 27, 30	18	1, 2, 3, 4, 5, 6, 7, 8, 9, 11, 14, 15, 16, 17, 19, 22, 23, 24, 26, 28, 29, 31
5—Complications During the Intrapartal Period	12, 13, 14, 19	1, 2, 3, 7, 8, 9, 11, 15, 16, 17, 18		4, 5, 6, 10
6—The Postpartal Period	4, 16, 24	19, 20, 22, 23	6, 7	1, 2, 3, 5, 8, 9, 10, 11, 12, 13, 14, 15, 17, 18, 21, 25, 26, 27
7—Complications During the Postpartal Period	2, 5, 7, 12, 13	10, 11, 14, 15, 16		1, 3, 4, 6, 8, 9
8—The Newborn Infant	7, 8, 15			1, 2, 3, 4, 5, 6, 9, 10, 11, 12, 13, 14, 16, 17, 18
9—Complications During the Neonatal Period: The High-Risk Newborn	4, 5, 6, 7, 8, 14, 16, 22, 23	1, 3, 17, 18, 19	2	9, 10, 11, 12, 13, 15, 20, 21, 24, 25

Resources

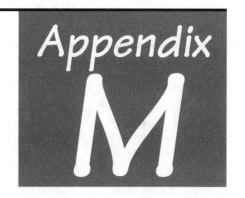

Appendix M

Selected sources of information and services. (Every effort has been made to provide current names and addresses; however, addresses do change frequently.)

Health and Welfare Agencies/Associations

American Cancer Society
1599 Clifton Rd. NE
Atlanta, GA 30329
404-320-3333

American Diabetes Association
National Center
1660 Duke St.
Alexandria, VA 22314
800-232-3472

Centers for Disease Control
Department of Health and Human Services
U.S. Public Health Service
Atlanta, GA 30333
404-639-3534

Endometriosis Association
238 West Wisconsin Ave.
PO Box 92187
Milwaukee, WI 53202
414-962-8972

HELP (Herpes Resource Center)
PO Box 100
Palo Alto, CA 94302
919-361-2120

La Leche League International
9616 Minneapolis Ave.
Franklin Park, IL 60131
800-LA-LECHE

Maternity Center Association, Inc.
48 East 92nd St.
New York, NY 10028
212-269-7300

National Coalition Against Domestic Violence
2401 Virginia Ave., NW, Suite 305
Washington, DC 20037
1-800-333-SAFE (24-hr line)

National Coalition Against Sexual Assault
c/o Fern Ferguson, President
Volunteers of America of Illinois
8787 State St., Suite 202
East St. Louis, IL 62203

National Safety Council
444 N. Michigan Ave.
Chicago, IL 60611
800-621-7619

Parenthood After Thirty
451 Vermont
Berkeley, CA 94707
415-524-6635

AIDS Information and Hotlines

American Foundation for AIDS Research	212-719-0033
American Red Cross AIDS Education Office	202-737-8300
Centers for Disease Control—Statistics:	
AIDS cases and deaths	404-330-3020
Distribution-categories	404-330-3021
Demographics	404-330-3022
Hearing Impaired AIDS Hotline	800-243-7889
National AIDS Hotline	800-342-AIDS
National AIDS Information Clearing House	800-458-5231
National AIDS Network	202-293-2437
National Gay/Lesbian Crisis Line	800-767-4297
Pediatric and Pregnancy AIDS Hotline	212-340-3333
Project Inform (Drug Information)	800-822-7422
National Sexually Transmitted	
Diseases Hotline	800-227-8022
Spanish AIDS Hotline	800-344-7432

Professional Organizations/ Associations

American Academy of Ambulatory Nursing Administration
N. Woodbury Rd., Box 56
Pitman, NJ 08071

American Academy of Nurse Practitioners
45 Foster St., Suite A
Lowell, MA 01851

The American Assembly for Men in Nursing
PO Box 31753
Independence, OH 44131

American College of Nurse Midwives
1522 K St., NW, Suite 1120
Washington, DC 20005
202-347-5445

American Holistic Nurses' Association
4101 Lake Boon Tr., Suite 201
Raleigh, NC 27607

American Nurses Association
1101 14th St., NW, Suite 200
Washington, DC 20005
202-789-1800;
Head office
600 Maryland Ave., SW
Washington, DC

Association of Nurses in AIDS Care
704 Stonyhill Rd., Suite 106
Yardley, PA 19067

Association of Rehabilitation Nurses
5700 Old Orchard Rd., 1st floor
Skokie, IL 60077

The Association of Women's Health, Obstetric, and Neonatal Nurses (AWHONN—formerly NAACOG)
700 14th St., NW, Suite 600
Washington, DC 20005-2019
202-662-1600

Canadian Nurses Association
50 The Driveway
Ottawa, Ont., Canada K2P 1E2

Midwives Alliance of North America
United States and Canada
c/o Concord Midwifery Service
30 South Main St.
Concord, NH 03301
603-225-9586

NAACOG: The Organization for Obstetric, Gynecologic, and Neonatal Nurses
409 12th St., SW
Washington, DC 20024-2191

National Association of Hispanic Nurses
6905 Alamo Downs Pkwy.
San Antonio, TX 78238

National Association of Neonatal Nurses
191 Lynch Creek Way, Suite 101
Petaluma, CA 94954

National Association of Nurse Practitioners in Reproductive Health (NANPRH)
325 Pennsylvania Ave., SE
Washington, DC 20002

National Black Nurses Association, Inc.
1912 10th St., NW
Washington, DC 20001

National League for Nursing (NLN)
Ten Columbus Circle
New York, NY 10019
212-582-1022

Transcultural Nursing Society
Department of Nursing
Madonna College
36600 Schoolcraft Rd.
Livonia, MI 48150

Patient Education Materials

Abbott Laboratories
Professional Services—D383
Abbott Park
N. Chicago, IL 60064

Childbirth Graphics
PO Box 21207
Waco, TX 76702
1-800-229-3366

Ed-U-Press
760 Ostrum Ave.
Syracuse, NY 13210

Eli Lilly and Company
Educational Resources Program
PO Box 100B
Indianapolis, IN 46206

Healthy Mothers, Healthy Babies Coalition
600 Maryland Ave., SE, Suite 300E
Washington, DC 20024-2588

Maternity Center Association
42 E. 92nd St.
New York, NY 10128

National Woman's Health Network
1325 G St., NW
Washington, DC 20005

Nutrition Education Association
PO Box 20301
Houston, TX 77225

Planned Parenthood Federation of America, Inc.
810 Seventh Ave.
New York, NY 10019
1-800-829-7732

Ross Laboratories
Creative Services and Information Department
625 Cleveland Ave.
Columbus, OH 43216

Schering Corporation
Professional Film Library
Galloping Hill Rd.
Kenilworth, NJ 07033

Videotapes for Parents

All are available from Childbirth Graphics Ltd, Rochester, NY.

Baby Basics (VHS, 110 min)
Excellent and entertaining resource on infant care in the first few months. Topics include the newborn at birth, parents caring for themselves postpartum, the first few days at home, daily care, feeding, health and safety, crying and sleeping, growth and development.
Baby Talk (VHS, 60 min)
Excellent new video on early parenting concerns and baby care. Topics include newborn appearance, sleep and awake patterns, crying and colic, illness and doctor visits, bottle feeding, and the importance of parents taking care of themselves.
Hey, What About Me? (VHS, 25 min)
Video on sibling adjustment. Contains songs about feelings, games and lullabies, bouncing rhymes to do with the new baby, and suggestions on what the siblings can do when they feel angry or lonely.

Nursing Journals

"Bereavement" Magazine
305 Gradle Dr.
Carmel, IN 46032
317-846-9429

Birth: Issues in Prenatal Care and Education
(formerly *Birth and Family Journal*)
110 El Camino Real
Berkeley, CA 94705
415-658-5099

Bookmarks
ICEA Supplies Center
PO Box 20048
Minneapolis, MN 55420
 Complimentary annotated catalogue of book reviews.

Canadian Nurse
The Canadian Nurses Association
50 The Driveway
Ottawa, Ont., Canada K2P 1E2

The Female Patient
Division Excerpta Medica
301 Gibraltar Dr.
PO Box 528
Morris Plains, NJ 07950

Journal of Nurse-Midwifery
Editor
82 Willow Ln.
Tenafly, NJ 07670

Journal of Obstetric, Gynecologic and Neonatal Nursing (JOGNN)
J.B. Lippincott Co.
12107 Insurance Way
Hagerstown, MD 21740

Journal of Perinatal and Neonatal Nursing
Aspen Publishers, Inc.
7201 McKinney Circle
Frederick, MD 21701

Maternal/Newborn Advocate
The National Foundation/March of Dimes
PO Box 2000
White Plains, NY 10602

MCN The American Journal of Maternal Child Nursing
555 W. 57th St.
New York, NY 10019

Newsletter
(a multiple birth loss support network)
PO 1064
Palmer, AK 99645
907-745-2706

Nurse Practitioner: A Journal of Primary Nursing Care
3845 42nd Ave, NE
Seattle, WA 98105

Nursing Network on Violence Against Women Newsletter
Trauma Program, UHN-66
Oregon Health Sciences University
3181 SW Sam Jackson Pk. Rd.
Portland, OR 97201-3098
Fax: 503-494-4357

Nursing Research
555 W. 57th St.
New York, NY 10019

Perinatal Press
Perinatal Press Subscriptions
The Perinatal Center
Sutter Memorial Hospital
52nd and F Sts.
Sacramento, CA 95819

Women's Health Nursing Scan
J.B. Lippincott Co.
Downsville Pike, Rte. 3, Box 20-B
Hagerstown, MD 21740

Index to Memory Aids (Mnemonics and Acronyms)

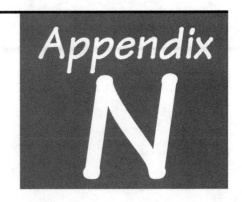

Appendix
N

Condition	Memory Aid	Page
Blood vessels in cord	AVA	116
Dystocia: etiology	Six P's	130
Episiotomy: assessment	REEDA	116
Gestational diabetes: assessment	3 P's	81
Infections during pregnancy	TORCH	81
IUDs: signs of potential problems	PAINS	19
Neonatal risk factors	ABC.I	191
Newborn assessment components	APGAR	116
Oral contraceptives: signs of potential problems	ACHES	19
Preterm infant: anticipated problems	TRIES	191
Recording gravidity/parity	GT PAL	43
Severs pre-eclampsia	HELLP	82

Cervical Dilatation and Gestation Wheel

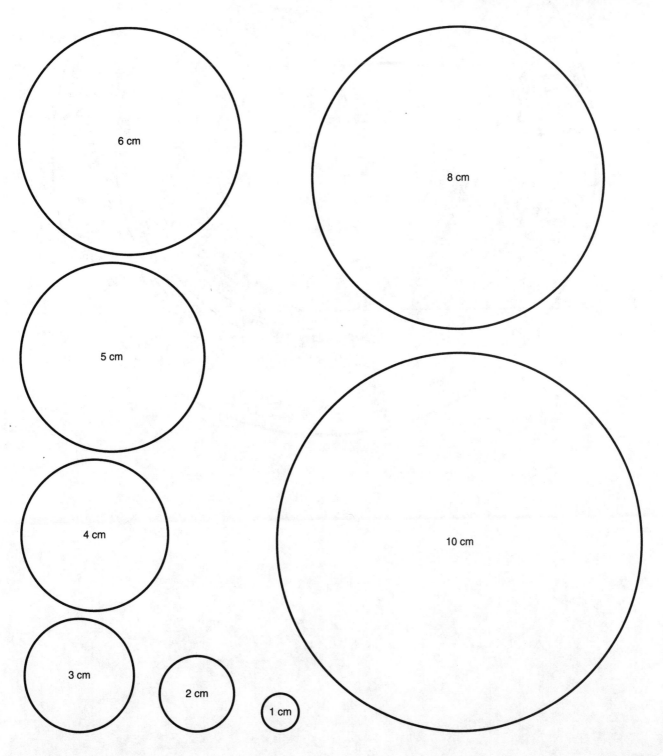

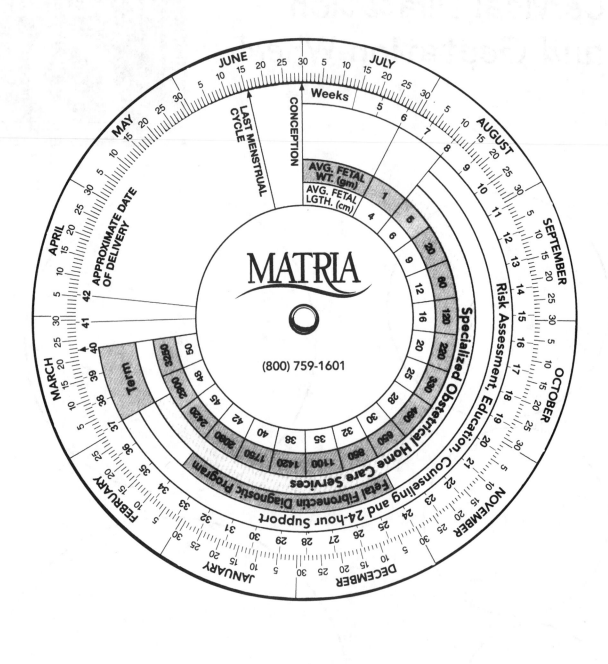

Bibliography

Texts

Bobak IM, Jensen MD. *Maternity and Gynecologic Care: The Nurse and the Family* (5th ed). St. Louis: Mosby, 1993.

Bobak IM, Lowdermilk DL, Jensen MD. *Maternity Nursing* (4th ed). St. Louis: Mosby, 1995.

Caroline NL. *Emergency Care in the Streets* (5th ed). Boston: Little, Brown, 1995.

Craig CR, Stitzel RE. *Modern Pharmacology* (4th ed). Boston: Little, Brown, 1994.

Cunningham FG, MacDonald PC, Gant NF. *Williams Obstetrics* (19th ed). Norwalk, CT: Appleton & Lange, 1993.

DiSaia PF, Creasman WT. *Clinical Gynecologic Oncology* (4th ed). St. Louis, Mosby–Year Book, 1992.

Ebadi M. *Pharmacology: A Review with Questions and Explanations* (2nd ed). Boston: Little, Brown, 1995.

Fanaroff AA, Martin RJ. *Neonatal-Perinatal Medicine: Diseases of the Fetus and Infant* (5th ed). St. Louis: Mosby, 1992.

Geissler E. *Pocket Guide to Cultural Assessment.* St. Louis: Mosby, 1994.

Guyton A. *Textbook of Medical Physiology.* Philadelphia: Saunders; 1991.

Hatcher RA, et al. *Contraceptive Technology: 1994–1996,* (16th ed). New York Irvington Publishers, 1994.

Judge RD, Zuidema GD, Fitzgerald FT. *Clinical Diagnosis: A Physiologic Approach:* (5th ed). Boston/Toronto, Little, Brown, 1989.

Lawrence RA. *Breastfeeding: A Guide for the Medical Profession* (4th ed). St. Louis: Mosby, 1994.

Rhoades RA, Tanner GA. *Medical Physiology.* Boston: Little, Brown, 1995.

Rogers P. *The Medical Student's Guide to Top Board Scores.* Boston: Little, Brown, 1996.

Scott JR, et al. *Danforth's Obstetrics and Gynecology,* (7th ed). Philadelphia, Lippincott, 1994.

Varney H. *Nurse-Midwifery* (3rd ed). Boston: Blackwell Scientific, 1991.

Whaley LF, Wong DL. *Nursing Care of Infants and Children* (5th ed). St. Louis: Mosby, 1995.

Willson JR, Carrington ER. *Obstetrics and Gynecology* (9th ed). St. Louis: Mosby, 1991.

Zimmerman J, Jacobson S. *Anatomy.* Boston/Toronto: Little, Brown, 1989.

Journals

Aderhold KJ, Roberts JE. Phases of second stage labor: Four descriptive care studies. *J Nurse Midwife* 36:267, 1991.

Ament LA: Maternal tasks of the puerperium reidentified. *JOGNN* 19:330, 1990.

American College of Obstetricians and Gynecologists. More women now deliver in alternative birth sites. *ACOG Newsletter* 37:8, 1993.

Andrews CM, Chrzanowski M. Maternal position, labor, and comfort. *Appl Nurs Res* 3:7, 1990.

Beck CT, Reynolds MA, Rutowski P. Maternity blues and postpartum depression. *JOGNN* 21:287, 1992.

Chapman LL. Expectant fathers' roles during labor and birth. *JOGNN* 21:114, 1992.

Coffman S. Parent and infant attachment: Review of nursing research 1981–1990. *Pediatric Nursing* 18:421, 1992.

Contraception choices for women over age 35: Focus on benefits and risks. *The Contraception Report* 3:4, 1992.

Davis MS. Natural family planning. *NAACOG Clin Issues Perinat Women Health Nurs* 3:280, 1992.

Denehy JA. Interventions related to parent-infant attachment. *Nurs Clin North Am* 27:425, 1992.

Gillerman H, Beckham MH. The postpartum early discharge dilemma: An innovative solution. *J Perinat Neonat Nurs* 5:9, 1991.

Harrison LL. Patient education in early postpartum discharge programs. *MCN* 15:39, 1990.

Hinkle LT. Counseling for the Norplant user. *JOGNN* 23:387, 1994.

Horn B. Cultural concepts and postpartal care. *J Transcultural Nurs* 2:48, 1990.

Lantican S, Corona D. Comparison of the social support networks of Filipinos and Mexican American primigravidas. *Health Care Women Int.* 13:329, 1992.

Luegenbiehl DL. Postpartum bleeding. *NAACOG Clin Issues. Perinat Women Health Nurs* 2:402, 1991.

Luegenbiehl DL, et al. Standardized assessment of blood loss. *MCN* 15:241, 1990.

Lukacs A: Issues surrounding early postpartum discharge: effects on the caregiver. *J Perinat Neonatal Nurs* 5:33, 1991.

Malestic SL. Fathers need help during labor, too. *RN* 53:23, 1990.

McKay S, Roberts J. Obstetrics by ear. Maternal and caregiver perceptions of the meaning of maternal sounds during second stage labor. *J Nurse Midwife* 35:266, 1990.

Metzer BL, Therrien B. Effect of position on cardiovascular response during the Valsalva maneuver. *Nurs Res* 39:198, 1990.

NAACOG. Physical assessment of the neonate. *OGN Nursing Practice Resource,* Washington, DC: NAACOG, 1991.

NAACOG. Postpartum nursing care. Vaginal delivery. *OGN Nursing Practice Resource,* Washington, DC: NAACOG, 1991.

NAACOG. Neonatal skin care. *OGN Nursing Practice Resource,* Washington, DC: NAACOG, 1992.

Queenan JT. Partners in the delivery room: A natural evolution. *Contemp OB/GYN* 35:8, 1990.

Thomson AM. Pushing techniques in the second stage of labour. *J Adv Nurs* 18:171, 1993.

Wheeler DG. Intrapartum bleeding. *NAACOG Clin Issues Perinat Women Health Nurs* 2:381, 1991.

Index

The Lippincott's NurseNotes Series Disk Instructions

System Requirements

- A PC compatible computer with an Intel 386 or better processor. Windows 3.1 or later.
- 4 Megabytes RAM (minimum); but recommend 8 MB RAM on Windows 3.1.
- 8 Megabytes RAM (minimum); but recommend 12 MB RAM minimum on Windows 95.
- 3 Megabytes of available hard disk space.

Installation

Installing *NurseNotes: Maternal–Newborn* for Windows

1. Start up Windows.
2. Insert the *Maternal–Newborn* disk into the floppy disk drive.
3. From the Program Manager's File Menu, choose the Run command.
4. When the Run dialog box appears, type a:\setup (or b:\setup if you're using the B drive) in the Command Line box. Click OK or press the Enter button.
5. The installation process will begin. A dialog proposing the directory "nnpm" on the drive containing Windows will appear. If the name and location are correct, click OK. If you want to change this information, type over the existing data, then click OK.
6. When the *Maternal–Newborn* setup routine is complete, a new group called "Nurse Notes" will appear on your desktop.
7. Start the *Maternal–Newborn* program by double-clicking on its icon.

NurseNotes: Maternal–Newborn disk program

Lippincott's *NurseNotes* Series consists of two modes: Test Mode and Study Mode.

TEST MODE

To begin a test, click the Start Over button with your mouse cursor. As a result, the first question will appear on the screen. If you decide to stop the test before you complete it, your answers will be saved. You can resume the test by selecting the Resume button from the Main Menu screen. You may clear your answers for a test at any time by clicking on the Start Over button.

NurseNotes: Maternal–Newborn—Toolbar

The Toolbar contains a series of buttons that provide direct access to all test program functions. When you move the cursor over a button, an explanation of its function displays in the Status Bar which is immediately above the ToolBar.

From left to right, the Toolbar buttons are:
- Program Help
- Pause
- Mark Question
- Table of Contents
- First Question Arrow
  (go to the first question in the section)
- Prior Question Arrow
  (go to the previous question in the test)
- Next Question Arrow
  (go to the next question in the test)
- Last Question Arrow
  (go to the last question in the section)
- Stop

To get help at any time during the test, choose the Program Help button. Program Help reviews basic functions of the program. To close the Program Help window, click on the Program Help button again. Answer each question by clicking on the oval to the left of an answer selection or by selecting the appropriate letter on the keyboard (A, B, C, or D). When an answer is selected, its oval will darken. If you change your mind about an answer, simply select that choice, by mouse or keyboard, again.

To register your answer selection and proceed to the next question, click on the Next Question Arrow button or press the Enter key.

If you are unsure about an answer to a particular question, the program allows you to mark it for later review. Flag the question by clicking on the Mark Question button. To review all marked questions for a test, click on the Table of Contents button, which is immediately to the right of the Mark button. This will open the Table of Contents window.

The Table of Contents window lists every question included on the test and summarizes whether it has been answered, left unanswered, or marked for later review. Click on an item in the Table of Contents window and the program will move to that test question, or use the Arrow buttons to move to the first, previous, next, or last question. To close the Table of Contents window, click on the Table of Contents button again.

At any time during the test or when you are finished taking the test, click on the Stop button. If you wish, you may return to the session at a later time without erasing your existing answers by selecting the Resume button.

After taking the test, you may receive your score by clicking the Results Button on the Main Menu Screen. There are four different ways to review your results: Test Results, Nursing Process, Category of Human Function, and Client Need.

STUDY MODE

After taking the test and receiving your score, you may wish to enter the Study Mode. This mode supplies you with the test questions, the answers that you chose, and the rationale for correct and incorrect answers. To enter the Study Mode, click the Study Mode button with your mouse cursor. You will not be able to modify the answers you have given; however, you can select any of the answer choices for an explanation of that answer. You may also wish to use the Table of Contents button to show you which questions you marked for review. Each of these windows may be closed by clicking again on their respective buttons.

To exit the *Maternal–Newborn* program, click the Exit button on the Main Menu.